Food and Nutrition: A Health Perspective

Food and Nutrition: A Health Perspective

Editor: Dave Stewart

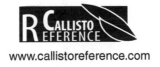

www.callistoreference.com

Callisto Reference,
118-35 Queens Blvd., Suite 400,
Forest Hills, NY 11375, USA

Visit us on the World Wide Web at:
www.callistoreference.com

ISBN: 978-1-63239-898-7 (Hardback)

Cataloging-in-Publication Data

Food and nutrition : a health perspective / edited by Dave Stewart.
    p. cm.
Includes bibliographical references and index.
ISBN 978-1-63239-898-7
1. Health. 2. Nutrition. 3. Food. 4. Public health. 5. Medical policy. 6. Diet. I. Stewart, Dave.
RA776.5.F66 2017
613--dc23

Table of Contents

Preface...IX

Chapter 1   Association between intimate partner violence and child morbidity in
             South Asia..1
             Elma Z. Ferdousy and Mohammad A. Matin

Chapter 2   Water use practices, water quality, and household's diarrheal encounters
             in communities along the Boro-Thamalakane- Boteti river system,
             Northern Botswana..8
             G. Tubatsi, M. C. Bonyongo and M. Gondwe

Chapter 3   From home deliveries to health care facilities: establishing a traditional
             birth attendant referral program in Kenya.......................................20
             Angelo Tomedi, Sophia R. Stroud, Tania Ruiz Maya,
             Christopher R. Plaman and Mutuku A. Mwanthi

Chapter 4   The validity of birth and pregnancy histories in rural Bangladesh............27
             Donna Espeut and Stan Becker

Chapter 5   Groundwater arsenic and education attainment in Bangladesh...................38
             Michael P. Murray and Raisa Sharmin

Chapter 6   White rice consumption and risk of esophageal cancer in Xinjiang
             Uyghur Autonomous Region, northwest China....................................48
             Li Tang, Fenglian Xu, Taotao Zhang, Jun Lei, Colin W. Binns and
             Andy H. Lee

Chapter 7   The opioid effects of gluten exorphins: asymptomatic celiac disease.........53
             Leo Pruimboom and Karin de Punder

Chapter 8   "Girl Power!": The Relationship between Women's Autonomy and
             Children's Immunization Coverage in Ethiopia................................61
             Jane O. Ebot

Chapter 9   Perception and attitudes towards preventives of malaria infection
             during pregnancy in Enugu State, Nigeria.......................................70
             Nkechi G. Onyeneho, Ngozi Idemili-Aronu, Ijeoma Igwe and
             Felicia U. Iremeka

Chapter 10   Predictors of maternal health services utilization by poor, rural
             women: a comparative study in Indian States of Gujarat and
             Tamil Nadu...80
             Kranti Suresh Vora, Sally A. Koblinsky and Marge A. Koblinsky

Chapter 11   **Magnitude of undernutrition in children aged 2 to 4 years using CIAF and conventional indices in the slums of Mumbai city**................................89
Mitravinda S. Savanur and Padmini S. Ghugre

Chapter 12   **Is there a value for probiotic supplements in gestational diabetes mellitus?**................................96
Neda Dolatkhah, Majid Hajifaraji, Fatemeh Abbasalizadeh, Naser Aghamohammadzadeh, Yadollah Mehrabi and Mehran Mesgari Abbasi

Chapter 13   **Antiretroviral therapy adherence strategies used by patients of a large HIV clinic in Lesotho**................................104
Johanna Maria Axelsson, Sofie Hallager and Toke S. Barfod

Chapter 14   **Caesarean delivery and its correlates in Northern Region of Bangladesh: application of logistic regression and cox proportional hazard model**................................113
Mostafizur Rahman, Asma Ahmad Shariff, Aziz Shafie, Rahmah Saaid and Rohayatimah Md. Tahir

Chapter 15   **High risk of malnutrition associated with depressive symptoms in older South Africans living in KwaZulu-Natal, South Africa**................................124
I. Naidoo, Karen E. Charlton, TM Esterhuizen and B. Cassim

Chapter 16   **Socio-economic determinants of household food security and women's dietary diversity in rural Bangladesh**................................132
Helen Harris-Fry, Kishwar Azad, Abdul Kuddus, Sanjit Shaha, Badrun Nahar, Munir Hossen, Leila Younes, Anthony Costello and Edward Fottrell

Chapter 17   **High prevalence of typhoidal *Salmonella enterica* serovars excreting food handlers in Karachi-Pakistan: a probable factor for regional typhoid endemicity**................................144
Taranum Ruba Siddiqui, Safia Bibi, Muhammad Ayaz Mustufa, Sobiya Mohiuddin Ayaz and Adnan Khan

Chapter 18   **Women's participation in household decision-making and higher dietary diversity: findings from nationally representative data from Ghana**................................153
Dickson A. Amugsi, Anna Lartey, Elizabeth Kimani and Blessing U. Mberu

Chapter 19   **Water Quality Index for measuring drinking water quality in rural Bangladesh**................................161
Tahera Akter, Fatema Tuz Jhohura, Fahmida Akter, Tridib Roy Chowdhury, Sabuj Kanti Mistry, Digbijoy Dey, Milan Kanti Barua, Md Akramul Islam and Mahfuzar Rahman

Chapter 20   **What does quality of care mean for maternal health providers from two vulnerable states of India?**..173
Shilpa Karvande, Devendra Sonawane, Sandeep Chavan and
Nerges Mistry

Chapter 21   **Out-of-pocket expenditure on prenatal and natal care post Janani Suraksha Yojana**..183
Dipti Govil, Neetu Purohit, Shiv Dutt Gupta and Sanjay Kumar Mohanty

Chapter 22   **Are there changes in the nutritional status of children of *Oportunidades* families in rural Chiapas, Mexico?**..194
Esmeralda García-Parra, Héctor Ochoa-Díaz-López,
Rosario García-Miranda, Laura Moreno-Altamirano,
Roberto Solís-Hernández and Raúl Molina-Salazar

Chapter 23   **Bacteriological quality of bottled drinking water versus municipal tap water in Dharan municipality, Nepal**...202
Narayan Dutt Pant, Nimesh Poudyal and Shyamal Kumar Bhattacharya

Permissions

List of Contributors

Index

Preface

Every book is a source of knowledge and this one is no exception. The idea that led to the conceptualization of this book was the fact that the world is advancing rapidly; which makes it crucial to document the progress in every field. I am aware that a lot of data is already available, yet, there is a lot more to learn. Hence, I accepted the responsibility of editing this book and contributing my knowledge to the community.

This book on food and nutrition deals with the right practices that maintain human health, growth and well-being. Nutrition and dietetics provide dietary patterns that can alleviate problems such as obesity as well as malnutrition. This book is appropriate for students seeking detailed information in this area as well as for experts. It strives to provide a fair idea about this discipline and to help develop a better understanding of the latest advances within this field. Different approaches, evaluations, methodologies and advanced studies on food and nutrition have been included herein. It will provide comprehensive knowledge to the readers.

While editing this book, I had multiple visions for it. Then I finally narrowed down to make every chapter a sole standing text explaining a particular topic, so that they can be used independently. However, the umbrella subject sinews them into a common theme. This makes the book a unique platform of knowledge.

I would like to give the major credit of this book to the experts from every corner of the world, who took the time to share their expertise with us. Also, I owe the completion of this book to the never-ending support of my family, who supported me throughout the project.

Editor

Association between intimate partner violence and child morbidity in South Asia

Elma Z. Ferdousy[*] and Mohammad A. Matin

Abstract

Background: This study investigates the association between intimate partner violence (IPV) against women and its impact on child morbidity in the south Asian region.

Methods: The analysis uses logistic regression models with cross sectional nationally representative data from three countries - Bangladesh, India and Nepal. The data have been pooled from 'Demographic and Health Surveys' (DHS) of Bangladesh, Nepal and 'National Family and Health Survey' (NFHS) of India.

Results: The study revealed that after controlling for potential confounders, children of mothers experiencing physical violence, sexual violence or both were more likely to have Acute Respiratory Infection (ARI) (OR_{adj} 1.57; 95 % CI 1.48–1.67), fever (OR_{adj} 1.44; 95 % CI 1.35–1.54) and diarrhea (OR_{adj} 1.56; 95 % CI 1.44–1.69).

Conclusions: The results highlight that IPV can influence childhood morbidity and support the need to address IPV with a greater focus within current child nutrition and health programs and policies.

Keywords: Intimate partner violence, Childhood morbidity, South Asian Region, Bangladesh DHS, India DHS, Nepal DHS

Background

During the last decade several studies investigated the impact of intimate partner violence (IPV) on children's health. A recent study by World Health Organization (WHO) shows that the global prevalence of physical and/or sexual intimate partner violence among all ever-partnered women was 30.0 % [39]. The estimates of physical and sexual violence are substantially higher in the developing countries in general [12, 14, 25]. South Asia reports some of the highest rates of violence [17, 20, 30].

Evidence is available on negative consequences of IPV for women's health and well-being [6]. Several studies reported the link between IPV and women's mental health and depression [8, 28]. Some of the studies also highlighted an association between such violence and reproductive health outcomes like non-use of contraception, gynecological problems, unintended pregnancy and sexually transmitted infections including HIV/AIDS. These results suggest there may be direct or indirect impact of IPV on children as well.

Significant attention has also been dedicated to the potential negative role of IPV on the health and survival of infants. Some population based studies have reported considerable adverse effects of IPV upon gestational and birth outcomes [3]. This also contributes in part to the association between IPV and prematurity or low birth weight [31, 38].

Studies on the association between IPV and childhood mortality are much more limited. Most of such studies come from developed countries. Scanty literature on this topic in the developing world includes some studies from India and one study from Bangladesh. Several studies from north India suggested significant association between lifetime IPV and infant mortality risks [1, 2, 19, 23]. A population-based study from rural Bangladesh convincingly showed association between IPV and child mortality [5].

Studies in Bangladesh convincingly showed that children of women exposed to IPV have greater exposure to potentially dangerous conditions like diarrhea and Acute Respiratory Infection (ARI) [4, 36]. Impact of IPV on child nutrition has also been demonstrated by a few studies [3, 40].

The current study builds upon the existing literature and explores association between IPV and childhood morbidity expanding the study beyond a single country to include three neighboring countries in South Asia, i.e., Bangladesh, India and Nepal.

* Correspondence: elma@juniv.edu
Department of Statistics, Jahangirnagar University, Savar, Dhaka

Methods
Study population and sampling procedure
The study uses three datasets [16]– Bangladesh Demo-graphic and Health Survey (DHS) 2007, India National Family and Health Survey (NFHS) – 2005–06 and Nepal DHS 2011. Both DHS and NFHS are nationally-representative household surveys on population, health, and nutrition. These surveys employed a two stage sampling procedure with the first stage involving the selection of primary sampling units (PSUs); these were probability proportional to the size and represent the number of households within the PSU. The second stage used a systematic technique to sample households from each of the selected PSUs. The details of the methods and procedures used in data collection in DHS and NFHS surveys are provided in the respective DHS and NFHS reports [18, 27, 29]. Informed consent was obtained from the study participants. All these three surveys have similar modules on violence. These questions were administered to a sub-sample.

This secondary analysis includes a total of 40,394 women from India, Bangladesh and Nepal. The women selected for the violence module had at least one child under the age of 5 years during the survey. We included all the children under the age of 5 years in this sample. Therefore a total number of 58,725 children of these women were included in the study.

Ethical clearance and considerations
The original survey was administrated in accordance with the WHO ethical and safety guidelines for research on IPV. The institution review board of ICF Macro (formerly Macro International Inc.), an advisory, implementation, and evaluation services firm providing research-based solutions to U.S. federal government agencies in health and other areas. Reviewed and approved the surveys used in the study. The interviewers received special training to implement this module. The training focused on how to ask sensitive questions, ensure privacy, and build rapport between interviewer and respondent. Verbal Informed consent was also obtained from the respondents. Details of the informed consent statement can be found in the appendix section of the respective reports [18, 27, 29].

Exposure and outcome measures
This study considers IPV as the main exposure variable while child morbidity as the outcome of interest.

IPV
Women were asked the following questions about their experience of IPV involving their husbands over the past 12 months.

i. Has your husband pushed, shook or threw something?
ii. Has your husband slapped you?
iii. Has your husband twisted your arm or pulled your hair?
iv. Has your husband punched with fist or something harmful?
v. Has your husband kicked you, dragged you or beaten you up?
vi. Have you been threatened by a weapon or had a weapon used against you by your husband? Has your husband been choked you or burn you on purpose?
vii. Have you been physically forced to have sex or otherwise sexually abused by your husband?

A new dummy IPV variable was created based on the answer to the above questions. A positive response to any one of the first six questions was treated as indicative of physical IPV victimization and was coded as "1" and if none of the responses was positive, exposure to physical violence was coded as "0". A similar strategy was followed for deriving a variable indicating exposure or non-exposure to sexual IPV. Then two more variables were created to indicate exposure to any IPV or both IPV.

Child morbidity
Women were asked whether their child had been ill with fever, diarrhea, or a cough accompanied by short, rapid breathing in the 2 weeks prior to the surveys. Acute Respiratory Infection (ARI) was defined as the presence of cough, along with short, rapid breathing. Binary variables for Diarrhea, ARI and Fever were created which indicated the presence of each of these outcomes among the children in the past 2 weeks prior the survey. For these cases, "0" indicated absence of the symptoms while "1" indicated presence of the same.

Covariates
The study controlled for well established correlates of child morbidity such as age, religion, education, living standard, employment status and areas of residence [18, 27, 29].

Respondent's age was classified into 5 groups. The respondents were asked if they attended any educational institution and if yes then the highest level completed (primary, secondary, higher) was asked. We used the information to classify education of the mother into the following categories: (no education, primary, secondary & higher).

Respondents were asked about the main source of drinking water for their household and presented with options like piped water, tube well or borehole, dug well, spring water, surface water etc. The responses were

Table 1 Background characteristics of women and their children included in the study (pooled data)

Variables	Percent of Women ($n = 40,394$)	Variables	Percent of Children ($n = 58,725$)
Age Groups		Mother's Age	
15–19	9.5	15–19	5.2
20–24	24.8	20–24	32.3
25–29	30.4	25–29	34.6
30–39	28.6	30–39	25.4
40–49	6.8	40–49	2.5
Education Level		Mother's Education	
No Education	38.6	No Education	40.8
Primary	37.5	Primary	37.1
Secondary	15.6	Secondary	14.5
Higher	8.3	Higher	7.6
Type of residence		Type of residence	
Urban	39.6	Urban	37.8
Rural	60.4	Rural	62.2
Wealth Index		Wealth Index	
Poorest	17.5	Poorest	17.8
Poorer	17.8	Poorer	18.6
Middle	19.8	Middle	20.7
Richer	21.7	Richer	21.9
Richest	23.3	Richest	21.0
Source of Drinking Water		Source of Drinking Water	
Tube well or Borehole	32.1	Tube well or Borehole	36.6
Piped Connection	41.1	Piped Connection	38.8
Other	26.8	Other	24.6
Toilet Facility		Toilet Facility	
No Facility	41.6	No Facility	30.8
Flush	28.2	Flush	26.5
Pit latrine or other	30.2	Pit latrine or other	42.7
Exposed to IPV		Morbidity	
Physical violence	30.4	Fever	15.4
Sexual violence	8.8	Diarrhea	9.8
Both/Either	32.6	ARI	8.9

grouped into three major categories: Tube well or borehole, piped water and other sources. Women were asked about the toilet facility and the responses were classified in the groups of pit latrine, flush and no facility. Cooking fuel of the household was classified into: electricity, gas, kerosene, wood/coal and others.

We used the DHS wealth index calculated as follows: each asset was assigned a weight (factor score) generated through principal component analysis, and the resulting asset scores were standardized in relation to a normal

Table 2 Different forms of violence and child morbidity

	Fever		Diarrhea		ARI	
	No	Yes	No	Yes	No	Yes
Sexual Only						
No	85.7 %	14.3 %	91.7 %	8.3 %	86.8 %	13.2 %
Yes	77.4 %	22.6 %	85.1 %	14.9 %	82.0 %	18.0 %
p value	<0.001		<0.001		<0.001	
Physical Only						
No	86.9 %	13.1 %	92.4 %	7.6 %	90.9 %	9.1 %
Yes	80.6 %	19.4 %	88.3 %	11.7 %	76.1 %	23.9 %
p value	<0.001		<0.001		<0.001	
Both						
No	85.6 %	14.4 %	91.6 %	8.4 %	88.2 %	11.8 %
Yes	76.5 %	23.5 %	84.4 %	15.6 %	60.7 %	39.3 %
p value	<0.001		<0.001		<0.001	

distribution with a mean of zero and standard deviation of one. Each household was then assigned a score for each asset, and the scores were summed for each household; individuals were ranked according to the total score of the household in which they resided. The sample was then divided into quintiles from one (lowest) to five (highest).

Statistical analysis
We calculated descriptive statistics for socio-demographic and morbidity characteristics for our selected sample individuals. The relationhip between morbidity and selected demographic and socio-economic factors were examined first using chi-square test. Then we used logistic regression models for exploring the relationship between IPV and different child morbidity outcomes. After this step we ran multiple logistic regression analysis. We calculated the

Table 3 Adjusted odds ratios and 95 % confidence intervals for associations between different forms of maternal IPV and under-five child morbidity (pooled data)*

	Fever	Diarrhea	ARI
Physical IPV only			
No	1.00	1.00	1.00
Yes	1.46 (1.37, 1.55)	1.55 (1.46, 1.64)	1.53 (1.42, 1.64)
Sexual IPV only			
No	1.00	1.00	1.00
Yes	1.67 (1.59, 1.75)	1.79 (1.62, 1.98)	1.72 (1.59, 1.87)
Both physical and sexual IPV			
No	1.00	1.00	1.00
Yes	1.64 (1.49, 1.81)	1.66 (1.49, 1.81)	1.76 (1.61, 1.92)
Physical or sexual IPV			
No	1.00	1.00	1.00
Yes	1.44 (1.35, 1.54)	1.56 (1.44, 1.69)	1.57 (1.48, 1.67)

*Adjusted for maternal age, maternal education, type of residence, types of cooking fuel, wealth index, toilet facility, and source of drinking water

Table 4 Adjusted and unadjusted odds ratios and 95 % confidence intervals any IPV and covariates

Variables	Fever Unadjusted OR	CI	Fever Adjusted OR	CI	Diarrhea Unadjusted OR	CI	Diarrhea Adjusted OR	CI	ARI Unadjusted OR	CI	ARI Adjusted OR	CI
Any IPV												
No (Reference)	1		1		1		1		1		1	
Yes	1.61	1.51 1.71	1.44	1.35 1.54	1.75	1.62 1.88	1.56	1.44 1.69	1.74	1.64 1.84	1.57	1.48 1.67
Mother's Age												
15–19 (Reference)	1		1		1		1		1		1	
20–24	1.95	1.74 2.19	1.94	1.73 2.18	1.88	1.65 2.19	1.82	1.58 2.11	1.93	1.73 2.14	1.9	1.71 2.12
25–29	1.71	1.53 1.91	1.76	1.57 1.98	1.55	1.35 1.78	1.52	1.32 1.76	1.64	1.48 1.83	1.68	1.51 1.88
30–39	1.43	1.26 1.61	1.48	1.31 1.67	1.27	1.09 1.47	1.27	1.09 1.48	1.27	1.13 1.41	1.31	1.17 1.47
40–49	1.14	0.98 1.31	1.15	0.99 1.33	0.90	0.78 1.09	0.89	0.73 1.07	0.97	0.85 1.12	0.99	0.86 1.14
Mother's highest education level												
No Education (Reference)	1		1		1		1		1		1	
Primary	1.14	1.06 1.24	1.08	1.00 1.18	0.95	0.86 1.05	0.93	0.84 1.03	1.22	1.13 1.31	1.12	1.04 1.20
Secondary	0.98	0.92 1.05	1.04	0.97 1.12	0.92	0.85 1.00	0.99	0.90 1.08	1.05	0.99 1.12	1.09	0.96 1.24
Higher	0.77	0.69 0.86	0.98	0.85 1.12	0.60	0.51 0.69	0.78	0.65 0.94	0.82	0.74 0.91	0.95	0.88 1.02
Type of Residence												
Urban (Reference)	1		1		1		1		1		1	
Rural	1.15	1.09 1.22	1.03	0.95 1.14	1.12	1.04 1.20	1.06	0.93 1.18	1.10	1.04 1.16	1.16	1.07 1.25
Wealth Index												
Poorest (Reference)	1		1		1		1		1		1	
Poorer	1.05	0.96 1.14	0.99	0.91 1.09	0.95	0.85 1.06	0.95	0.85 1.07	1.05	0.97 1.14	0.99	0.91 1.08
Middle	0.91	0.84 1.00	0.88	0.80 0.97	0.94	0.85 1.05	0.96	0.86 1.08	0.98	0.90 1.06	0.92	0.83 1.00
Richer	0.87	0.80 0.95	0.91	0.81 1.02	0.84	0.75 0.93	0.89	0.77 1.02	0.90	0.83 0.98	0.86	0.77 0.96
Richest	0.70	0.64 0.76	0.86	0.75 1.00	0.62	0.56 0.70	0.74	0.62 0.89	0.71	0.66 0.77	0.78	0.68 0.89
Source of Drinking water												
Tube well/ Borehole (Reference)	1		1		1		1		1		1	
Piped Water	0.98	0.92 1.05	0.80	0.68 0.94	0.78	0.72 0.85	0.98	0.90 1.07	1.03	0.96 1.10	0.91	0.77 1.07
Other	1.51	1.41 1.62	1.45	1.34 1.56	1.49	1.39 1.58	1.32	0.70 2.47	1.05	0.96 1.14	1.43	1.33 1.53

Table 4 Adjusted and unadjusted odds ratios and 95 % confidence intervals any IPV and covariates (Continued)

Type of Toilet Facility												
Pit Latrine (Reference)	1		1		1		1		1		1	
Flush	0.95	0.90	0.95	0.74	0.79	0.73	0.83	0.68	0.97	0.92	0.91	0.57
		1.01		1.20		0.85		1.02		1.03		1.44
No facility	1.56	1.45	1.79	1.50	1.69	1.56	1.63	1.19	1.03	0.93	0.94	0.74
		1.69		2.13		1.80		2.24		1.15		1.19
Type of Cooking fuel												
Electricity (Reference)	1		1		1		1		1		1	
Gas	1.33	1.00	0.80	0.60	1.29	0.70	1.05	0.95	1.32	0.84	0.86	0.65
		1.77		1.08		2.40		1.17		2.07		1.13
Kerosene	1.39	1.09	1.27	0.99	1.36	1.01	1.10	0.88	1.31	1.05	1.19	0.95
		1.76		1.62		1.83		1.37		1.63		1.49
Wood/Coal	1.73	1.1	1.14	0.71	1.45	1.02	1.26	0.87	1.43	1.10	1.6	1.47
		2.74		1.81		2.06		1.82		1.85		1.73
Other	1.96	1.55	1.75	1.61	1.78	1.32	1.61	1.19	1.78	1.44	1.58	1.34
		2.48		1.90		2.38		2.18		2.21		1.89

adjusted odds ratio to measure the strength of associations. SPSS version 17 was used for the analysis.

Results

Background characteristics of the women and their children are presented in Table 1. Most of the women were aged between 20 and 30 years and around 40 % of them had no formal education. Approximately one third of these women reported experience of IPV.

In Table 2, presents the results of cross tabulation between different form of violence against women and the three diseases of interest. Across board a higher proportion of the children of abused mothers experienced the illnesses. Mothers exposed to sexual violence reported more incidents of child fever, diarrhea or ARI which are 22.6, 14.9 and 18.0 % respectively compared to children of sexually non- abused mothers 14.3, 8.3 and 13.2 % respectively ($p < 0.001$).

Table 3 shows the results of multivariate logistic regression analysis controlled for mothers' age, education, and wealth index, type of residence, source of drinking water, toilet facility and type of cooking fuel as covariates. Table 4 shows adjusted and unadjusted result for each of the controlling variables.

The results show that Maternal experience of physical IPV increased the likelihood of child fever by 46 % (AOR: 1.46, 95 % CI: 1.37–1.55), sexual IPV by 67 % (AOR: 1.67, 95 % CI: 1.59–1.87), and both physical and sexual IPV by 64 % (AOR: 1.64, 95 % CI: 1.49–1.81).

Maternal exposure to physical IPV increased the risks of diarrhea of the child by 55 % (AOR: 1.55, 95 % CI: 1.46–1.64), sexual IPV by 79 % (AOR: 1.79, 95 % CI: 1.62–1.98) and both physical and sexual IPV by 66 % (AOR: 1.66, 95 % CI: 1.49–1.81).

Maternal experience of physical IPV increased the likelihood of child's ARI by 53 % (AOR: 1.53, 95 % CI: 1.42–1.64) sexual IPV by 72 % (AOR: 1.72, 95 % CI: 1.59–1.87) and both physical and sexual IPV by 76 % (AOR: 1.76, 95 % CI: 1.61–1.92).

Discussion

The central aim of this study was to investigate the association between Intimate Partner Violence against women and child morbidity in South. The results of the study provide evidence of an association between IPV and child morbidity in these three countries of South Asia. The results are in line with previous findings [1, 2, 5, 15, 19, 21, 23, 33, 35, 36]. We found that a higher proportion of the children of IPV survivors reported fever, diarrhea or ARI compared to the non abused mothers irrespective of the form of violence. There may be several approaches to explain the association between IPV and child morbidity. We offer the following three classes among them:

– Poor mental health of the mother: Women who experience IPV tend to have higher level of psychological stress [10, 26] which may impede their capacity to provide adequate child care. There are physiological reasons for psychological stress is associated to anemia. Psychological stress is a risk factor for oxidative stress [9, 13], that produce free radicals and other organic molecules capable of damaging living tissue and can destroy red blood cells prematurely that results in a potential cause of hemolytic anemia. Additionally chronic stress has been found to result in long term reduction of hemoglobin suggesting that stress interferes with protein synthesis required to create new red blood cells. Conditions like anemia can weaken a person and lowers a person's productivity through a decreased ability to work [37]. These physical conditions contribute poor child caring ability of a woman.

- Lack of empowerment: Intimate partner violence is often used as a tool for controlling women [32]. Thus IPV is also strongly associated with inability of a woman to make decision for herself and for her children [34] with obvious implications for her own health and nutrition and that of her children. Lack of empowerment also limits mother's ability to access household resources, health care services and participation in common health care activities [32, 34] which in turn lowers their ability to provide appropriate care to their children.

- Poor physical condition of the mother: In case of extreme IPV often the victims become physically unfit to give proper care to their children.

Besides, the children who witness IPV themselves tend to experience psychological stress; which in turn result in poor physiological conditions making the children vulnerable to morbidity [7, 11, 22]. Investigation of the specific pathways through which IPV might influence child health and morbidity should be a high priority for future research.

Limitation

The cross sectional study design represents a limitation of this study. Though there may be some concern regarding the temporal ordering of IPV and child morbidity in cross sectional studies, previous research shows that IPV in this subcontinent is a relatively stable phenomenon that has its root in patriarchal structures and community norms of high acceptability of wife beating [24].

Another limitation of the study is that both the outcome and the exposure variables are measured through self reports. Although in the DHS much care and preparation is taken into the design and execution of the interviews to create a safe atmosphere in which respondents would feel comfortable discussing the IPV, high stake in disclosure may always cause under reporting.

Conclusion

The study shows that IPV negatively affects child's health not only in individual countries, but also in the South Asia region. The children of an abused mother are more likely to experience diseases like fever, diarrhea and ARI compared to the children of non-abused mothers. IPV should be considered as a major health problem affecting not only women, but also their children in South Asia. Although it seems IPV is most strongly associated with socioeconomic

demographic and contextual disadvantages, incidents of IPV among socially marginalized groups may aggravate the negative effects of cumulative disadvantages of poor child health outcomes. The health sector in these countries needs to take action to eliminate IPV for improving child health. Future studies should investigate the influence of potential mechanisms mediating the association of IPV and child morbidity.

Competing interests
The authors declare that they have no competing interests.

Authors' contributions
EZF analyzed and interpreted the data and wrote the initial draft of the manuscript. MAM provided guidance in data analyses and interpretation of results. Both authors read and approved the final version of the manuscript.

Acknowledgement
The authors are grateful to DHS Program and ICF International of Calverton for providing the datasets.

References
1.   Ackerson SL, Subramanian SV. Intimate partner violence and death among infants and children in India. Pediatrics. 2009;124:878–89.
2.   Ahmed S, Koenig MA, Stephenson RB. Effect of domestic violence on early childhood mortality: evidence from North India. Am J Pub Health. 2006;96:1423–8.
3.   Asling-Monemi K, Naved RT, Persson LA. Violence against women and the risk of fetal and early childhood growth impairment: a cohort study in rural Bangladesh. Arch Dis Child. 2009;94:775–9.
4.   Asling-Monemi K, Naved RT, Persson LA. Violence against women and increases in the risk of diarrheal disease and respiratory tract infections in infancy: a prospective cohort study in Bangladesh. Arch Pediatr Adolesc Med. 2009;163(10):931–6.
5.   Asling-Monemi K, Tabassum NR, Persson LA. Violence against women and the risk of under five mortality: analysis of community-based data from rural Bangladesh. Acta Paediatr. 2008;97:226–32.
6.   Campbell JC. Health consequences of intimate partner violence. Lancet. 2002;359:1331–6.
7.   Campbell JC, Lewandowski LA. Mental and physical health effects of intimate partner violence on women and children. Psychiatr Clin North Am. 1997;20:353–74.
8.   Ellsberg M, Caldera T, Herrera A, Winkvist A, Kullgren G. Domestic violence and emotional distress among Nicaraguan women: results from a population-based study. Am Psychologist. 1999;54:30–6.
9.   Epel ES, Blackburn EH, Lin J, Dhabhar FS, Adler NE, Morrow JD, et al. Accelerated telomere shortening in response to life stress. Proc Natl Acad Sci U S A. 2004;101:17312–5.
10. Fikree FF, Bhatti LI. Domestic violence and health of Pakistani women. Int J Gynaecol Obstet. 1999;65:195–201.
11. Finkelstein J, Yates JK. Traumatic symptomatology in children who witness marital violence. Int J Emerg Ment Health. 2001;3:107–14.
12. Garcia-Moreno C, Jansen HAFM, Ellsberg M, Heise L, Watts CH. Prevalence of intimate partner violence: findings from the WHO multi-country study on women's health and domestic violence. Lancet. 2006;368:1260–9.
13. Hapuarachchi JR, Chalmers AH, Winefield AH, Blake-Mortimer JS. Changes in clinically relevant metabolites with psychological stress parameters. Behav Med. 2003;29:52–9.
14. Heise L, Pitanguy J, Germain A. Violence against women: The hidden health burden. World Bank Discussion Paper 1994; no. WDP 255.
15. Holt S, Buckley H, Whelan S. The impact of exposure to domestic violence on children and young people. Child Abuse Negl. 2008;32:797–810.
16. ICF International, USAID. Demographic and Health Surveys (various) [Datasets]. Available from <http://dhsprogram.com/data/available-datasets.cfm> [July, 2012]

17. International Institute for Population Sciences (IIPS) and Macro International. National Family Health Survey (NFHS-3), 2005–06. India: Volume I. Mumbai: IIPS; 2007.

18. International Institute for Population Sciences (IIPS) and Macro International. National Family Health Survey (NFHS-3), 2005–06. India: Volume I and II. Mumbai: IIPS; 2007.

19. Jejeebhoy SJ. Associations between wife-beating and fetal and infant death: impressions from a survey in rural India. Stud Fam Plann. 1998;29:300–8.

20. Jejeebhoy SJ, Cook RJ. State accountability for wife-beating: the Indian challenge. Lancet. 1997;349:SI10–2.

21. Jejeebhoy SJ, Santhya KG, Acharya R. Health and social consequences of marital violence: a synthesis of evidence from India. New Delhi: Population Council and UNFPA; 2010.

22. Kitzmann KM, Gaylord NK, Holt AR, Kenny ED. Child witnesses to domestic violence: a meta-analytic review. J Consult Clin Psychol. 2003;71:339–52.

23. Koenig MA, Stephenson R, Acharya R, Barrick L, Ahmed S, Hindin M. Domestic violence and early childhood mortality in rural India: evidence from prospective data, Int. J. Epidemiol. 2010;39:825–83.

24. Koenig MA, Stephenson R, Ahmed S, Jejeebhoy SJ, Campbell J. Individual and contextual determinants of domestic violence in North India. Am J Public Health. 2006;96(1):132–8.

25. Krug EG, Mercy JA, Dahlberg LL, Zwi AB. The world report on violence and health. Lancet. 2002;360:1083–8.

26. Kumar S, Jeyaseelan L, Suresh S, Ahuja RC. Domestic violence and its mental health correlates in Indian women. Br J Psychiatry. 2005;187:62–7.

27. Ministry of Health and Population (MOHP) [Nepal], New ERA, and ICF International Inc. Nepal demographic and health survey 2011. Kathmandu, Nepal: Ministry of Health and Population, New ERA, and ICF International, Calverton, Maryland; 2012.

28. Mullen PE, Romans Clarkson SE, Walton VA, Herbison GP. Impact of sexual and physical abuse on women's mental health. Lancet. 1988;8590:841–5.

29. National Institute of Population Research and Training (NIPORT), Mitra and Associates, and Macro International. Bangladesh demographic and health survey 2007. Dhaka, Bangladesh and Calverton, Maryland, USA: National Institute of Population Research and Training, Mitra and Associates, and Macro International; 2009.

30. Naved RT, Persson LA. Factors associated with spousal physical violence against women in Bangladesh. Stud Fam Plann. 2005;36:289–300.

31. Newberger EH, Barkan SE, Lieberman ES, McCormick MC, Yllo K, Gary LT. Abuse of pregnant women and adverse birth outcome: current knowledge and implications for practice. JAMA. 1992;267:2370–2.

32. Pence E, McDonnell C. Duluth, MN, Power and control wheel. Domestic Abuse Intervention Project 1984.

33. Rico E, Fenn B, Abramsky T, Watts C. Associations between maternal experiences of intimate partner violence and child nutrition and mortality: findings from Demographic and Health surveys in Egypt, Honduras, Kenya, Malawi and Rwanda. J Epidemiol Comm Health. 2011;65:360–7.

34. Sethuraman K, Lansdown R, Sullivan K. Women's empowerment and domestic violence: the role of sociocultural determinants in maternal and child undernutrition in tribal and rural communities in South India. Food Nutr Bull. 2006;27:128–43.

35. Silverman JG, Decker MR, Cheng DM, Wirth K, Saggurti N, RAj A, et al. Gender-based disparities in infant and child mortality based on maternal exposure to spousal violence: the heavy burden borne by Indian girls. Arch Pediatr Adolesc Med. 2011;165:22–7.

36. Silverman JG, Decker MR, Gupta J, Kapur N, Raj A, Naved RT. Maternal experiences of intimate partner violence and child morbidity in bangladesh: evidence from a national Bangladeshi sample. Arch Pediatr Adolesc Med. 2009;163(8):700–5.

37. Smith Jr RE. The clinical and economic burden of anemia. Am J Manag Care. 2010;16(supp):S59–66.

38. Valladares E, Ellsberg M, Pena R, Hogberg U, Persson LA. Physical partner abuse during pregnancy: a risk factor for low birth weight in Nicaragua. Obstet Gynecol. 2002;100:700–5.

39. World Health Organization. Global and regional estimates of violence against women: prevalence and health effects of intimate partner violence and non-partner sexual violence. Switzerland: World Health Organ; 2013.

40. Ziaei S, Naved RT, Ekström EC. Women's exposure to intimate partner violence and child malnutrition: findings from demographic and health surveys in Bangladesh. Matern Child Nutr. 2014;10(3):347–59.

Water use practices, water quality, and households' diarrheal encounters in communities along the Boro-Thamalakane-Boteti river system, Northern Botswana

G. Tubatsi[*], M. C. Bonyongo and M. Gondwe

Abstract

Background: Some rural African communities residing along rivers use the untreated river water for domestic purposes, making them vulnerable to waterborne diseases such as diarrhea.

Methods: We determined water use practices and water quality, relating them to prevalence of diarrhea in communities along the Boro-Thamalakane-Boteti river system, northern Botswana. A total of 452 households were interviewed and 196 water samples collected show during February, May, September, and December 2012 in settlements of Boro, Maun, Xobe, Samedupi, Chanoga, and Motopi. Information was sought on water use practices (collection, storage, and handling) and diarrheal experience using questionnaires. Water quality was assessed for physicochemical and microbiological parameters using portable field meters and laboratory analysis, respectively.

Results: All (100 %) of the river water samples collected were fecally contaminated and unsuitable for domestic use without prior treatment. Samples had Escherichia coli (*E.coli*) and fecal streptococci levels reaching up to 186 and 140 CFU/100 ml, respectively. Study revealed high dependence on the fecally contaminated river water with low uptake of water treatment techniques. Up to 48 % of households indicated that they experience diarrhea, with most cases occurring during the early flooding season (May). Nonetheless, there was no significant relationship between river water quality and households' diarrheal experience across studied settlements ($p > 0.05$). Failure to treat river water before use was a significant predictor of diarrhea ($p = 0.028$).

Conclusions: Even though the river water was unsafe for domestic use, results imply further recontamination of water at household level highlighting the need for simple and affordable household water treatment techniques.

Keywords: Household, Hygiene, Ngamiland, Okavango Delta, Water storage, Water treatment, Waterborne diseases

Background

Diarrhea remains one of the leading causes of morbidity and mortality worldwide [1–3] despite improved health technologies, management, and increased use of oral rehydration therapy [4, 5]. Worldwide, about two billion cases of diarrheal diseases are registered annually, out of which 1.9 million children under the age of 5 die particularly in developing countries. Diarrheal diseases display distinct geographical variation and seasonality [5–8] due to varying occurrence of their etiological

agents in the environment [9]. Several authors [10–13] attributed the burden of diarrheal diseases to the environment and associated risk factors, particularly unsafe drinking water from open water sources, poor sanitation, and poor hygiene. While causes of diarrheal diseases are multi factorial, the use of untreated water harboring diarrheal pathogens [10] remains a significant contributor to most outbreaks [11, 12].

Rotavirus and *Escherichia coli* have been implicated for most diarrheal outbreaks in developing countries [6, 13, 14] where some communities use water of quality lower than the recommended standards. When contaminated water is ingested, pathogens invade the

* Correspondence: gosatubs@gmail.com
Okavango Research Institute, University of Botswana, Private Bag 285, Maun, Botswana

intestines' epithermal walls, disturbing mechanisms that transport water and electrolytes and causing diarrhea [15]. Therefore, higher microbial concentrations in water increase chances of invasion hence diarrhea.

The revised standards [16] for drinking water recommend that the water should be free from pathogens and microbial indicators, pH between 6 and 8, turbidity less than 5 nephelometric turbidity units (NTU), and conductivity less than 1000 μS/cm. Microbial water quality indicators such as coliforms, fecal streptococci, and *E. coli* are often used to assess water quality despite the fact that they are not responsible for causing diarrhea. In addition to the quality of water at source point, the safety of drinking water and the health risks associated with its use thereof can further be influenced by hygiene practices during transportation, storage, and handling leading to microbiological contamination [4, 17–19]. Recent studies demonstrated that uptake of water treatment techniques at household level such as boiling, chlorination, and filtration could improve drinking water quality and significantly reduce the burden of diarrhea [1, 20, 21].

Like in other sub-Saharan countries, diarrhea remains a major public health concern in Botswana, particularly among children [22] despite strengthened surveillance and launching of programs such as Integrated Management of Childhood Illnesses (IMCI). Although 95 % of Botswana's population is reported to have access to treated safe water supply [23], dependency on untreated open water sources in ungazetted rural communities presents serious health risks. Unlike in gazette settlements where the government provides most of the services, water supply and many other services in ungazetted settlements are the responsibility of individual households. As such, outbreaks of water-related diseases like diarrhea are rampant mostly in the Ngamiland district in the northern part of the country, where many settlements are ungazetted and have ample access to open surface water from the Okavango Delta and its associated tributaries. For example, records at Letsholathebe II referral hospital in Maun, the capital town of Ngamiland district, show that 120 cases of diarrhea were registered over a 2-week period in June 2012. On the other hand, some landuse activities along the Thamalakane-Boteti river such as residential areas, lodges, hotels, and grazing have been reported to negatively impact on the water quality [24, 25], further pointing out to the potential health risks associated with water in these river systems.

Currently, the level of dependency on water from open sources, water use practices, and degree to which the quality of water contributes to diarrheal prevalence in Botswana has not been explored extensively. We assessed river water quality and water use patterns in selected communities along the Boro-Thamalakane-Boteti river system, an outlet of the Okavango Delta in the northern Botswana to establish their potential contribution to the prevalence of diarrheal diseases. Specifically, we (i) established the water use practices of selected respondents, (ii) related the occurrence of diarrheal diseases outbreaks to water use practice in the selected communities at different flooding seasons, and (iii) relate the occurrence of diarrheal diseases to selected water quality indicators. We hypothesized that (i) the occurrence of diarrhea will increase with increased dependency on river water, (ii) the occurrence of diarrhea will increase with low uptake of water treatment in households, and (iii) the occurrence of diarrhea in a settlement will increase as river water quality declines.

Methods

Study sites

Botswana (582,000 km^2) is a semi-arid, land-locked country in southern Africa. Rainfall occurs mostly between November and March and is highly unreliable, ranging from 310 to about 580 mm year^{-1}. The current study was conducted in settlements of Boro, Maun, Xobe, Samedupi, Chanoga, and Motopi along a 100-km stretch on the Boro-Thamalakane-Boteti (BTB) river system between the Okavango Delta and Makgadikgadi Pans (Fig. 1). Boro and Thamalakane rivers which drain the opposite sides of the Chief's Island in the Delta join a few kilometers upstream of Maun but bifurcate further downstream to form the Nhabe and Boteti rivers which drain into Lake Ngami on the south-west and the Makgadikgadi salt Pans to the south-east, respectively (Fig. 1). Livelihood activities in the study settlements are diverse and vary seasonally and include livestock and arable farming, fishing, safari (especially Mokolo poling at Boro), and sale of crafts and natural products or veld products [26]. A few residents work in government facilities, safari companies, and trusts or employed under the government funded "Ipelegeng" (*self-reliance*) scheme (Table 1).

Sampling

The study was conducted in 2012 during four distinct flooding seasons in the BTB river system; the late flood recession season (February), early flooding season (May), peak flooding season (September), and early flood recession season (December). A semi-structured questionnaire was developed, pre-tested in Matlapaneng (a ward in Maun) and Xobe, and rectified accordingly. The questionnaire was administered through face-to-face interviews in the local language (Setswana). We collected information from a total of 452 randomly selected households in the selected settlements on sources of water for domestic chores, household dependence on river water, uses of river water, their water storage

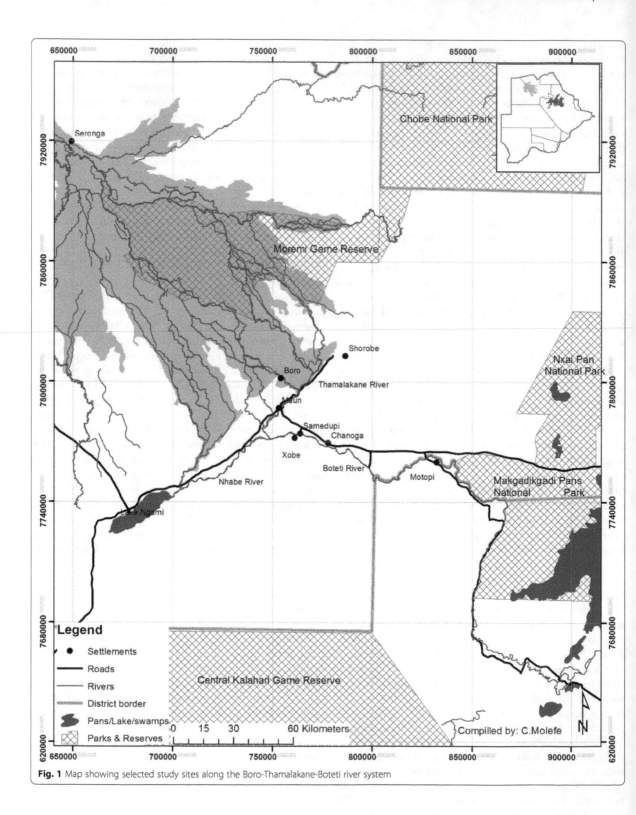

Fig. 1 Map showing selected study sites along the Boro-Thamalakane-Boteti river system

Table 1 Characteristics of settlements sampled for the study. Number of households was estimated by dividing total population of each settlement by the average household size of 5.4 reported by CSO (2010) for the Ngamiland district

Settlement	Distance (km)	Population	Number of households	Type of settlement
Boro	−11	393	73	Ungazetted
Maun	0	2053[a]	380	Gazetted
Xobe	13	260	48	Ungazetted
Samedupi	20	471	87	Ungazetted
Chanoga	30	347	64	Ungazetted
Motopi	87	3591	248	Gazetted

[a]Note that the population for Maun indicated here is only for Shashe ward and Matlapana which were sampled for this study. The total population of Maun is 60, 273 (CSO, 2012)

practices, and water treatment techniques known and/or used in their households. Respondents were also asked about their encounters and experiences with diarrhea in their households. Diarrhea was defined to each respondent as passing out three or more watery stools within a period of 24 h. Respondents were those members of households who were responsible for general household chores including fetching water.

Socio-economic characteristics of respondents
Majority (405) of the respondents were females, while only few (47) were males. A quarter (113) of respondents were aged below 30 years; while almost half (242) were between 31 and 45 years, 81 respondents were between 46 and 65 years, and just a small number (16) aged over 65 years. Majority (316) of the respondents were not employed, 52 employed in the government sector, and 84 were self-employed or in non-governmental employment. Only 86 of the respondents reported a monthly income over P500, and majority (366) were earning P500 or less per month. Almost a third (127) of the total respondents did not have formal education. Majority had attained primary (128) and Junior Secondary (134) education. Thirty six (36) have attained senior secondary education. Very few respondents (13) have attained up to tertiary education level.

Ethical considerations
A written ethical clearance to conduct the study was obtained from the Health Research and Development Division, Ministry of Health (Gaborone, Botswana). Participation by respondents in the study was entirely on voluntary basis. The study objectives, procedure, and benefits were clearly defined to potential respondents; after which, those who agreed to participate in the study were asked to sign the informed consent which was sought before participants took part in the study.

Participation was entirely on voluntary basis. Participants who were not willing to take part in the study were allowed to do so without giving any reasons for their decisions. Information obtained during interviews was kept confidential and anonymous and was used only in this study.

Water quality analysis
All the six study settlements were sampled once in February, May, September, and December 2012. These months corresponded to different seasons in relation to flooding (February is late flood recession season; May is early flooding season; September is peak flooding season and December is early flood recession). At each sampling point, in situ water temperature (°C), pH, dissolved oxygen (DO, mg l^{-1}), electrical conductivity (EC, $\mu S\ cm^{-1}$), and turbidity (NTU) were measured using WTW pH 330i, WTW OXi 330i, WTW Cond 720, and TN-100 portable Turbidimeter meters, respectively.

A total of 196 water samples were collected in 250-ml borosilicate glass bottles sterilized at 121 °C for 15 min. The samples were transported to the laboratory at the Department of Water Affairs in Maun in cooler boxes with ice. At the laboratory, water samples were analyzed for fecal coliforms, E. coli, and fecal streptococci using membrane filter technique as described in [27]. Aliquots of the water samples (100 ml) were filtered through sterile 0.45-μm membrane filter papers which were incubated in agar plates at 37 °C for coliforms; E. coli was incubated at 35 °C and fecal streptococci at 44.5 °C. Oxoid CM 1031 Membrane Lactose Glucoronide Agar (MLGA) was used for identification and enumeration of E. coli and coliforms while Oxoid CM 0377 Slanetz & Bartley medium was used for isolation of fecal streptococci.

Data analyses
Data were captured using Statistical Package for Social Scientists (SPSS) version 20.0. Frequencies and percentages were used for determining water use practices and households' diarrheal encounters. Analysis of variance (ANOVA) was used to compare households' diarrheal encounters' means across study sites and seasons. Pair wise comparisons of households' diarrheal encounters between sites and seasons were computed using Turkey's honest significant difference (HSD) test. Correlations between water use practices, water quality, and households' diarrheal encounters were measured before regression analysis was done. Multiple regression analyses were used to measure associations at 95 % confidence level. Further analyses were computed using SYSTAT 13 statistical software (SYSTAT Inc.).

Results

Water sources

All (100 %) respondents in the ungazetted settlements of Xobe and Samedupi fetched their water from the river for all domestic purposes. In contrast, settlements of gazetted Boro, Maun, Chanoga, and Motopi had safe water supply systems providing potable water to residents. All (100 %) interviewed households in Boro, Chanoga, and Motopi, and 70 % in Maun, indicated they sometimes get water from the river at least once in a week for domestic purposes despite available connections to treated water supplies through private and communal standpipes.

Only a few respondents (1.7 % in Motopi) indicated harvesting rain water from corrugated roofs during the rainy season. The low application of rainwater harvesting technique was confirmed by a quick survey of the houses in the settlements which showed high numbers of traditional grass thatched huts particularly in all the studied settlements except Maun. None of the respondents in Maun had indicated ever harvesting rain water.

Water collection and storage

Almost two thirds (63 %) of interviewed households in Maun had piped/tapped water connections in their homes (Fig. 2). The percentages were lower for Motopi (36.7 %) and Chanoga (13 %). Those without water connections at home use communal standpipes, which are centrally located to be used by all residents and supplied by the government through the Department of Water Affairs. Boro, Xobe, and Samedupi did not have access to treated water supply altogether and collected their water from the river.

Water fetching patterns were observed to be similar in all the study settlements from sources (river, taps) which

were generally less than 2 km from households and stored in containers of various sizes such as buckets, 25-l jerry cans (locally called "Dikupu"), 200-l drums, and 260-l or more polyethylene tanks manufactured by JOJO Tanks (Pty) Ltd, South Africa (Fig. 5). While households in gazetted settlements are generally within 400 m from communal water standpipes, residents in gazetted settlements had to travel longer distances to fetch water. Water from source was transported home either on the head by female individuals, donkey carts, and cars by male household members (Fig. 3). Because large storage containers were usually used and water was sparely used by household members, the stored water took a several days to finish, and as result, the containers were not regularly cleaned before refilling. It was also observed that not all containers had lids, and in some instances, the lids were not of the right size and therefore did not fit properly.

River water usage

The river water was used for drinking and non-drinking purposes such as cooking, washing, bathing, and watering gardens. Almost all of respondents (>90 %) in Xobe, Samedupi, and Chanoga indicated using river water for all domestic purposes including drinking compared to 30 % in Maun and slightly above half (53.3 %) of the households interviewed in Boro and Motopi (Fig. 4).

Water treatment

Boiling was the only form of water treatment known by most respondents, especially for drinking water. However, few respondents reported boiling river water for drinking in Boro (12.8 %), Maun (20.4 %), Xobe (14.9 %), Samedupi (15.0 %), Chanoga (24.4 %), and Motopi (25.9 %). Respondents further indicated that they boiled drinking water particularly for children below the age of 5 only. The rest of the household members frequently consumed untreated river water. Some of the reasons given for not treating river water before drinking included (i) water loses taste or tastes unpalatable after boiling, (ii) it takes time to boil and cool water for drinking while one is thirsty, (iii) boiling reduces the amount of water, (iv) boiling water for large families is tedious (iv), the river water is generally perceived to be clean and with minimal health risks to consumers, and (v) residents feel they have gained immunity against waterborne diseases (including diarrhea) associated with the consumption of river water.

Physicochemical and microbiological quality of the river water

The quality of water in the Boro-Thamalakane-Boteti river system reflected by physicochemical and microbiological parameters was unsuitable for domestic use as

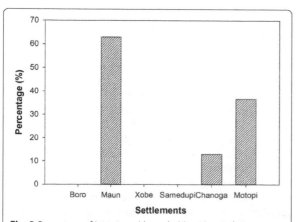

Fig. 2 Percentage of interviewed households with standpipes at home in settlements along the Boro-Thamalakane-Boteti river system

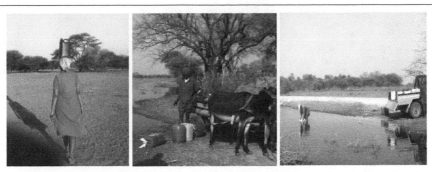

Fig. 3 Some of the water fetching practices in selected settlements along the Boro-Thamalakane-Boteti river system, Ngamiland District, Botswana

turbidity, *E. coli*, and fecal streptococci concentrations exceeded recommended limits for drinking water set by the Botswana Bureau of Standards (Table 2). We noted a significant decline in water quality from settlements upstream of urban Maun (Boro) towards downstream (Xobe, Samedupi, Chanoga, and Motopi). The quality of water in the river system improved as the water level in the system increased during the peak flooding season (September) and declined subsequently thereafter.

Households' diarrheal encounters
Diarrhea cases varied across settlements (Fig. 5). Generally, respondents in Boro (upstream settlement of Maun) and Maun residents reported less diarrhea cases than downstream settlements of Xobe, Samedupi, Chanoga, and Motopi. During the early flooding season (May),

about 33 % of the respondents in Boro reported diarrhea cases compared to 38–66 % settlements downstream of Maun reported cases of diarrhea (Fig. 5b). A similar pattern where upstream had less prevalence than downstream settlements was noted again during the peak flood season (September) (Fig. 5c). Prevalence recorded in Maun during the early (18 %) and late (13 %) flood recession seasons was lower compared to what was recorded in downstream settlements of Xobe, Samedupi, Chanoga, and Motopi (Fig. 5a, d). Downstream settlements recorded in 27–38 % and 20–27 % of the interviewed households during the early and late flood recession seasons, respectively. A similar pattern where prevalence increased in downstream settlements was observed again during the peak flooding season (September) (Fig. 5c).

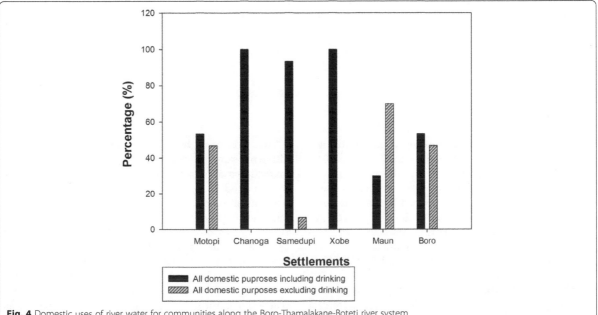

Fig. 4 Domestic uses of river water for communities along the Boro-Thamalakane-Boteti river system

Table 2 Water quality indicators (mean ± sd) for LFR, EF, PF, and EFR seasons in the BTB river system

| | Settlements | | | | | | |
	Boro	Maun	Xobe	Samedupi	Chanoga	Motopi	BOBS
Temperature (°C)							
LFR	26.5 ± 0.1	30.3 ± 0.0	32.0 ± 0.1	28.8 ± 0.1	32.1 ± 0.0	30.6 ± 0.0	N/A
EF	19.5 ± 0.2	20.6 ± 0.0	17.8 ± 0.0	19.5 ± 0.0	19.2 ± 0.0	18.8 ± 0.0	
PF	20.9 ± 0.0	23.2 ± 0.0	21.8 ± 0.1	21.5 ± 0.0	24.2 ± 0.0	22.8 ± 0.0	
EFR	26.4 ± 0.0	27.5 ± 0.1	23.7 ± 0.0	24.6 ± 0.2	29.2 ± 0.1	28.4 ± 0.0	
Conductivity ($\mu S\ cm^{-1}$)							
LFR	118.2 ± 0.6	123.0 ± 0.7	123.2 ± 0.8	127.4 ± 0.1	134.0 ± 0.0	131.1 ± 0.1	<1000
EF	104.0 ± 1.2	121.6 ± 9.3	124.1 ± 0.3	126.4 ± 0.1	133.0 ± 0.0	152.7 ± 0.8	
PF	92.1 ± 0.8	113.3 ± 1.8	104.1 ± 0.0	110.0 ± 0.1	106.6 ± 2.2	112.8 ± 7.9	
EFR	113.8 ± 0.5	122.1 ± 0.1	126.1 ± 1.0	127.8 ± 0.0	128.3 ± 0.1	119.4 ± 0.1	
pH							
LFR	6.7 ± 0.0	7.2 ± 0.1	7.8 ± 0.4	7.4 ± 0.0	8.1 ± 0.0	7.6 ± 0.2	6.5–8
EF	6.8 ± 0.0	7.4 ± 0.3	7.2 ± 0.1	7.5 ± 0.1	7.6 ± 0.0	7.6 ± 0.0	
PF	7.3 ± 0.0	7.4 ± 0.2	7.5 ± 0.1	7.3 ± 0.0	7.7 ± 0.1	7.4 ± 0.0	
EFR	7.0 ± 0.0	7.1 ± 0.0	7.5 ± 0.2	7.3 ± 0.0	7.8 ± 0.0	6.6 ± 0.1	
Turbidity (NTU)							
LFR	2.4 ± 0.2	6.8 ± 0.2	11.4 ± 0.20	4.1 ± 0.2	4.4 ± 0.4	8.8 ± 0.2	5
EF	0.8 ± 0.0	3.0 ± 0.2	4.9 ± 0.7	4.8 ± 0.2	3.3 ± 0.4	10.0 ± 0.5	
PF	1.7 ± 0.2	3.3 ± 0.6	8.0 ± 0.2	3.8 ± 0.2	8.0 ± 0.6	9.0 ± 0.1	
EFR	1.3 ± 0.0	6.3 ± 0.2	3.7 ± 0.7	1.9 ± 0.2	2.9 ± 0.2	8.1 ± 0.7	
E. coli (CFU/100 ml)							
LFR	54 ± 1	126 ± 0	127 ± 2	64 ± 4	82 ± 5	98 ± 15	0
EF	6 ± 3	168 ± 1	93 ± 2	186 ± 5	77 ± 2	139 ± 4	
PF	22 ± 0	102 ± 1	70 ± 1	106 ± 3	43 ± 3	32 ± 1	
EFR	20 ± 1	123 ± 1	56 ± 1	84 ± 2	40 ± 4	104 ± 9	
Fecal streptococci (CFU/100 ml)							
LFR	67 ± 8	140 ± 11	76 ± 6	93 ± 6	89 ± 3	26 ± 1	0
EF	2 ± 0	66 ± 8	30 ± 4	80 ± 1	21 ± 0	46 ± 2	
PF	12 ± 0	47 ± 1	4 ± 1	21 ± 0	47 ± 2	21 ± 2	
EFR	6 ± 0	53 ± 2	21 ± 4	37 ± 1	54 ± 8	32 ± 1	

A comparison of diarrhea cases within each settlement for the entire study period (February to December 2012) revealed a similar pattern (Fig. 6). All settlements recorded the highest number of cases during the early flooding season (May) which dropped in the subsequent seasons. However, respondents in Boro reported little variation in the number of diarrhea cases across seasons with a range of 5.9 % (SD = 2.93) compared to Maun and downstream settlements; Maun (30.3 %, SD = 13.6), Xobe (29.5 %, SD = 13.6), Samedupi (18.4 %, SD = 7.82), Chanoga (19.5 %, SD = 8.20), and Motopi (25.0 %, SD = 12.9) (Fig. 6a–f). Changes in prevalence were more profound in Maun.

Comparisons of households' diarrheal encounters for different sampled seasons using ANOVA revealed a marked variation in diarrheal prevalence during the study period ($F_{(3, 20)} = 11.02$, $p = 0.000$). Post hoc comparisons showed that prevalence during the early flooding season (May) was significantly higher than the flood recession seasons (February ($p = 0.03$) and December ($p = 0.000$)) but less than during the peak flooding season (September). Diarrhea cases during peak flooding season (September) was significantly higher than during late flood 41 recession season (December, $p = 0.007$) (Fig. 7a). Diarrhea cases during the peak and flood recession seasons was not significantly different ($p > 0.05$). Even

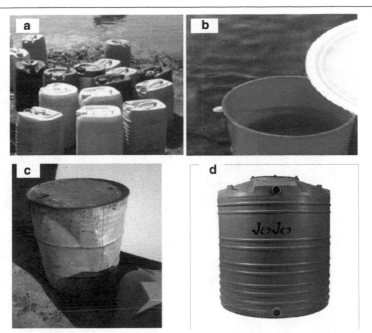

Fig. 5 Some of the containers used by residents in the selected settlements to fetch and store water in households for their domestic uses—**a** jerry cans, **b** bucket, **c** drums, **d** polyethylene containers (Jojo)

though Boro and Maun tended to record slightly less diarrhea cases than downstream settlements of Xobe, Samedupi, Chanoga, and Motopi during different seasons (Fig. 7b), spatial variation was not statistically significant ($F_{(5, 18)} = 0.555$, $p = 0.733$).

Households' diarrheal encounters and water use practices

The practice of boiling water for domestic purposes was a significant predictor of households' diarrheal encounters ($p = 0.028$). However, there was no significant relationship between prevalence of diarrhea and whether residents used river water for all household purposes including drinking (Table 3). There was no significant association between the number of households with standpipes and households' diarrheal encounters in the study settlements ($p > 0.05$).

Households' diarrheal encounters and river water quality

E. coli and fecal streptococci concentrations were found to be significant predictors ($p = 0.0394$ and $p = 0.040$, respectively) of households' diarrheal encounters only during the early flooding season around May, while turbidity was a significant ($p = 0.045$) predictor of household diarrheal encounters during the peak flooding season in September (Table 4). The conductivity, pH, and dissolved oxygen did not show any significant relationship ($p > 0.05$) between water quality and households' diarrheal encounters in the study settlements.

Discussion

Many communities worldwide are dependent on rivers in their vicinity for livelihoods despite high pollution of such water sources [28–30]. Similarly, we observed high dependency on the contaminated Boro-Thamalakane-Boteti river system for domestic purposes, even in the gazetted settlements of Maun, Chanoga, and Motopi which are supposedly provided with treated piped water by the government through the Department of Water Affairs and Water Utilities with treated water supplies. Lack of treated piped water supplies explains high household dependency on river water in ungazetted settlements of Xobe and Samedupi. In contrast, residents in gazetted settlements of Boro, Maun, Chanoga, and Motopi have been compelled to use untreated surface water from the Boro-Thamalakane-Boteti river system by the unreliability and unpredictability and poor taste (due to high salinity, color, and microbial concentrations) of the piped water supply [31]. Furthermore, 51 % of households in Maun reported acute water shortage and no water flow from pipes [32].

Furthermore, very few communal standpipes have been reported to be functional in Maun and other settlements due to frequent breakdowns of boreholes caused by floods and lack of spares [30]. Tubatsi et al. (2014) [25] reported that although the surface water is not saline (i.e., its freshwater), it was also unsuitable for domestic use as it contained high *E. coli* and fecal

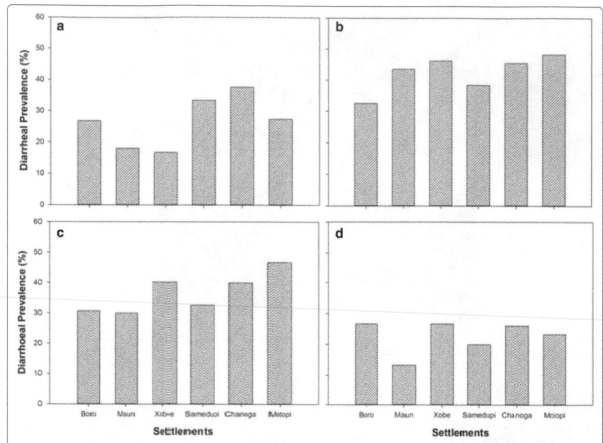

Fig. 6 Spatial variation of diarrheal for **a** late flood recession season, **b** early flooding season, **c** peak flooding season, and **d** early flooding season among 160 communities along the Boro-Thamalakane-Boteti river system. Seasons *LFR* late flooding recession, *EF* early flooding, *PF* peak flooding, *EFR* early flood recession

streptococci concentrations and turbidity levels which exceeded the Botswana Bureau of Standards recommended limits for drinking water. The high *E. coli* and fecal streptococci concentrations in the river water are probably from fecal contamination by animals since most people in the studied settlements using the same water sources for watering their livestock and wild animals [31].

Even though the use of polluted surface water sources has been implicated for diarrheal outbreaks in other studies [28, 29, 33], our results seem to suggest that river water quality at source may not be the only predictor of households' diarrheal encounters in our study settlements. Although some respondents interviewed by Kaluli et al. (2011) [34] associated diarrhea and skin rash diseases with use of untreated surface water in settlements around the Okavango Delta, we were unable to demonstrate any significant relationship between water quality in the Boro-Thamalakane-Boteti river system and households' diarrheal encounters in our study settlements during the

LFR, PF, and EFR seasons. River water quality was only significantly related to households' diarrheal encounters during the early flooding (EF) season around May when *E. coli* and fecal streptococci counts in the river water (CFU/100 ml) and households' diarrhea cases in the study settlements were highest. A similar lack of association between river water quality and diarrheal prevalence has previously been reported in Ethiopia [33]. Perhaps the pollution of water in the river system during the rest of the seasons was moderate enough not to pose a significant health risk as argued by [35] who advocated for a threshold effect of indicator density for diarrheal risk.

Even though isolation of rotavirus was beyond the scope of this study, it might have been the main etiological agent responsible for the highest diarrheal prevalence during cold and dry early flooding season (May). Rotavirus, which has been associated with most diarrheal outbreaks in the sub Sahara region [36–38], occurs mostly during cold dry seasons of the year [34, 36, 39].

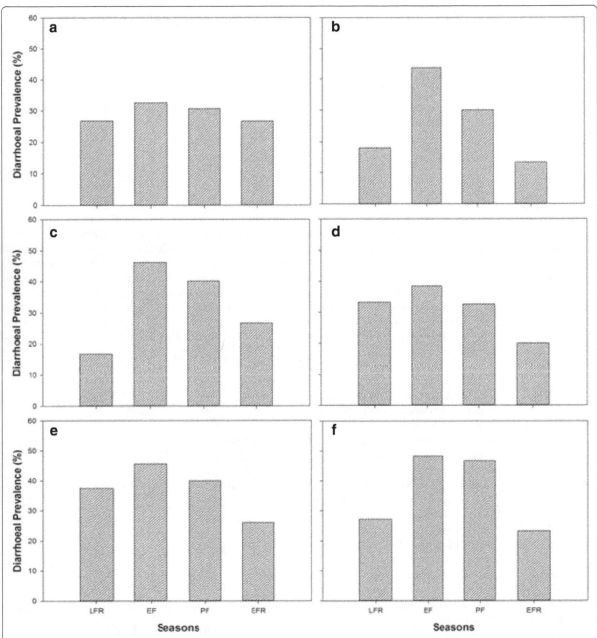

Fig. 7 Temporal variation of households' diarrheal encounters within settlements of **a** Boro, **b** Maun, **c** Xobe, **d** Samedupi, **e** Chanoga, and **f** Motopi along the Boro-Thamalakane-Boteti river system. Seasons *LFR* late flooding recession, *EF* early flooding, *PF* peak flooding, *EFR* early flood recession

Table 3 Multiple regression coefficients where households' diarrheal encounters was the dependent variable

Independent variables	Coefficient	Standard error	t value	p value
RW treated before use	0.643	0.162	3.967	0.028[a]
RW used for drinking	0.007	0.067	0.108	0.921

RW river water
[a]Significant

Results are suggestive of other possible diarrheal risk factors other than source water quality. Even though some have argued that post-source contamination present little and insignificant health risk [40, 41], our results question the strength of this argument. Lending support from previous research where unhygienic storage conditions were underlined to contribute to declining of water quality in

Table 4 Multiple regression coefficients of selected water quality parameters during various seasons where households' diarrheal encounters was the dependent variable

Independent variables	Seasons											
	LFR			EF			PF			EFR		
	(β)	t	p	(β)	t	p	(β)	t	p	(β)	t	p
	$R^2 = 0.559$			$R^2 = 0.953$			$R^2 = 0.930$			$R^2 = 0.857$		
Escherichia coli	−0.118	−0.241	0.832	0.451	4.865	0.0394**	−0.042	−1.089	0.390	−0.164	−2.558	0.1249
Fecal streptococci	−0.033	−0.154	0.982	−0.960	−4.825	0.040[a]	−0.0343	−0.446	0.699	−0.0352	−0.387	0.736
Turbidity	−0.0737	−0.167	0.883	−0.343	−0.803	0.506	2.037	4.536	0.0453[a]	1.144	1.338	0.313

Seasons—*LFR* late flooding recession, *EF* early flooding, *PF* peak flooding, *EFR* early flood recession, β regression coefficient
**Significant

households [40–43], we argue that the unhygienic storage conditions observed during the survey, such as inadequate care for and washing of storage containers and storage vessels with no lids or lids not fitting properly, might have possibly led to further decline of water quality in households. Further contamination might have also occurred during transportation from water source as most surveyed households lacked on-plot water connections. On a similar note, Hamer et al. (1998) [44] positively correlated water availability in a household with good hygiene behavior while [45] associated distance from house to source with diarrhea.

This study also reaffirms the benefits of boiling water in households. As expected, settlements where more households boiled water experienced significantly less diarrhea prevalence than their counterparts. Studies elsewhere have shown that adoption of measures such as boiling to improve drinking water quality at home effectively reduces diarrheal risks [20, 21, 45]. The high boiling temperatures denatures bacterial proteins needed to function and reproduce, rendering the bacteria nonviable and making the water safer.

We acknowledge the complexity of factors driving prevalence of diarrhea making prediction of their contribution to a high degree of accuracy relatively difficult. This study only focused on water use practices and water quality, but other factors such as sanitation, individuals' natural immunity, HIV/AIDS, malnutrition, and other infections can limit individuals' response to diarrhea [37]. As put forward by Trevett et al. (2004) [39], it is also possible that these communities' farming activities such as animal keeping contributed to some cases of diarrhea. Some residents were observed bathing in the river, an activity which has been linked with diarrhea in other studies [46–47] and could have possibly contributed to some diarrhea cases in communities along the Boro-Thamalakane-Boteti river system. Further research is therefore necessary to elucidate other factors. Further research can also be done to evaluate the effectiveness and adoption of different water treatment techniques.

Conclusions
This study has provided evidence that although provision of safe water is essential for reducing diarrheal burden, as a single effort, it is not sufficient. The quality of water and how the water is stored at home may contribute to increased diarrheal diseases burden. Therefore, integrated control programs focusing on improving quality of water both at source and point of use will be more effective. Specifically, promotion of good hygiene practices is essential.

Competing interests
The authors declare that they have no competing interests.

Authors' contributions
GT collected data, analysed samples and did data analysis. MG was involved in data collection and analysis. MCB was involved in data analysis. All authors drafted the manuscript. All authors read and approved the final manuscript.

Acknowledgements
We would like to extend special thanks to CARNEGIE-RISE for financially supporting this project and the Office of Research and Development (ORD) of the University of Botswana for providing additional funding. We are also particularly grateful to the Department of Water Affairs for offering us space and other resources to do water analysis, as well as all the technical assistance they offered. We greatly acknowledge the assistance provided by field technicians and research assistants during data collection.

References
1. Fewtrell L, Kaufmann RB, Kay D, Enanoria W, Haller L, Colford Jr JM. Water, sanitation, and hygiene interventions to reduce diarrhoea in less developed countries: a systematic review and meta-analysis. Lancet Infect Dis. 2005;5:42–52.
2. Mandomando ICM, Macete EBV, Ruiz J, Sanz S, Abacassamo F, Vallès X, et al. Etiology of diarrhea in children younger than 5 years of age admitted in a rural hospital of southern Mozambique. Am J Trop Med Hyg. 2007;76:522–7.
3. Yilgwan CS, Okolo SN. Prevalence of diarrhea disease and risk factors in Jos University teaching hospital, Nigeria. Annal Afr Med. 2012;11(4):217–21.
4. Gyimah S O. Interaction effects of maternal education and household facilities on childhood diarrhea in sub-Saharan Africa: the case of Ghana. J Health Popul Dev Countries 2003;13:1-17.
5. Boschi-Pinto C, Lanata CF, Mendoza W, Habte D. Diarrheal diseases. In: Jamison DT, Feachem RG, Makgoba MW, Bos ER, Baingana FK, Hofman KJ, Rogo KO, editors. Diseases and mortality in sub-Saharan Africa. Washington DC: Oxford University Press for the World Bank; 2006. p. 107–24.
6. Cooke ML. Causes and management of diarrhoea in children in a clinical setting. S Afr J Clin Nutr. 2010;23(1):S42–6.
7. Sastry N, Burgard S. The prevalence of diarrheal disease among Brazilian children: trends and differentials from 1986 to 1996. Soc Sci Med. 2005;60(5):923–35.

8. Alexander KA, Herbein J, Zajac A. The occurrence of cryptosporidium and giardia infections among patients reporting diarrheal disease in Chobe District, Botswana. Advance Infect Dis. 2012;2:143.

9. Walker CLF, Perin J, Aryee MJ, Boschi-Pinto C, Black RE. Diarrhea incidence in low-and middle-income countries in 1990 and 2010: a systematic review. BMC Public Health. 2012;12(1):212–20.

10. Obi CN, Okocha CO. Microbiological and physico-chemical analysis of selected borehole waters in World Bank Housing Estate, Umuahia, Abia State, Nigeria. J Eng Appl Sci. 2007;2(5):920–5.

11. Preez M, Conroy RM, Wright JA, Moyo S, Potgieter N, Gundry SW. Use of ceramic water filtration in the prevention of diarrheal disease: a randomized controlled trial in rural South Africa and Zimbabwe. Am J Trop Med Hyg. 2008;79(5):696–701.

12. Regassa G, Birke W, Deboch B, Belachew T. Environmental determinants of diarrhea among under-five children in Nekemte town, western Ethiopia. Ethiop J Health Sci. 2008;18:39-45.

13. Guerrant RL, Hughes JM, Lima NL, Crane J. Diarrhea in developed and developing countries: magnitude, special settings, and etiologies. Rev Infect Dis. 1990;12(1):S41–50.

14. Parashar UD, Gibson CJ, Bresee JS, Glass RI. Rotavirus and severe childhood diarrhea. Emerg Infect Dis. 2006;12(2):304–6.

15. Low-Beer TS, Read AE. Diarrhoea: mechanisms and treatment. Gut. 1971;12(12):1021–36.

16. Botswana Bureau of Standards (BOBS). Water quality: drinking water. BOS. 2009;32:2009.

17. Pokhrel D, Viraraghavan T. Diarrhoeal diseases in Nepal vis-à-vis water supply and sanitation status. J Water Health. 2004;2:71–81.

18. Wright J, Gundry S, Conroy R. Household drinking water in developing countries: a systematic review of microbiological contamination between source and point of use. Tropical Med Int Health. 2004;9(1):106–17.

19. Pande S, Keyzer MA, Arouna A, Sonneveld BGJS. Addressing diarrhea prevalence in the west african middle belt: Social and geographic dimensions in a case study in Benin. Int J Health Geogr. 2008;7:17.

20. Nath KJ, Bloomfield S, Jones M. Household water storage, handling and point of use treatment: a review commissioned by International Scientific Forum on Home Hygiene (IFH). 2006. Available at http://www.ifh-homehygiene.org. Accessed 10 July 2012.

21. Thompson T, Sobsey M, Bartram J. Providing clean water, keeping water clean: an integrated approach. Int J Environ Health Res. 2003;13(S1):S89–94.

22. Central Statistics Office (CSO). Botswana causes of mortality 2008. Botswana: Government of Botswana; 2010.

23. Central Statistics Office (CSO). Botswana population and housing census. Botswana: Government of Botswana; 2011.

24. Masamba WRL, Mazvimavi D. Impact on water quality of land uses along Thamalakane-Boteti River: an outlet of the Okavango Delta. Phys Chem Earth. 2008;33(8):687–94.

25. Tubatsi G, Bonyongo MC, Gondwe M. The dynamics of water quality in the Boro-Thamalakane-Boteti river system, northern Botswana. Afr J Aqua Sci. 2014;39(4):351–60.

26. Mazvimavi D, Mmopelwa G. Access to water in gazetted and ungazetted rural settlements in Ngamiland, Botswana. Physics and Chemistry of the Earth. Parts A/B/C. 2006;31(15):713–722.

27. Apha, A. WPCF, 1998. Standard methods for the examination of water and wastewater, 1998: 20.

28. Nwidu LL, Oven B, Okoriye T, Vaikosen NA. Assessment of the water quality and prevalence of waterborne diseases in Amassoma, Niger Delta, Nigeria. Afr J Biotechnol. 2008;7(17):2993–7.

29. Kujinga K, Vanderpost C, Mmopelwa G, Wolski P. An analysis of factors contributing to household water security problems and threats in different settlement categories of Ngamiland, Botswana. Physics and Chemistry of the Earth, 2014; Parts A/B/C, 67:187–201.

30. Kaluli JW, Githuku C, Home P, Mwangi BM. Towards a national policy on wastewater reuse in Kenya. J Agricult Sci Technol. 2011;13(1):115–125.

31. Teklemariam S, Getaneh T, Bekele F. Environmental determinants of diarrheal morbidity in under-five children, Keffa-Sheka zone, south west Ethiopia. Ethiop Med J. 2000;38(1):27–34.

32. Ashbolt NJ, Grabow WOK, Snozzi M. Indicators of microbial water quality. In: Fewtrell L, Bartram J, editors. Water quality: guidelines, standards and health. Risk assessment and management for water-related infectious disease, vol. Chapter 13. London: IWA Publishing; 2001. p. 289–315.

33. Hanlon P, Marsh V, Shenton F, Jobe O, Hayes R, Whittle HC, et al. Trial of an attenuated bovine rotavirus vaccine (RIT 4237) in Gambian infants. Lancet. 1987;329(8546):1342–5.

34. Moe CL, Sobsey MD, Samsa GP, Mesolo V. Bacterial indicators of risk of diarrhoeal disease from drinking-water in the Philippines. Bull World Health Organ. 1991;69(3):305.

35. Bern C, Glass RI. Impact of diarrheal diseases worldwide, vol. 1. New York: Marcel Dekker; 1994.

36. Steele AD, Ivanoff B. Rotavirus strains circulating in Africa during 1996–1999: emergence of G9 strains and P [6] strains. Vaccine. 2003;21(5):361–7.

37. Molbak K, Jensen H, Ingholt L, Aaby P. Risk factors for diarrheal disease incidence in early childhood: a community cohort study from Guinea-Bissau. Am J Epidemiol. 1997;146(3):273–82.

38. Feachem RG. Water, health and development. An interdisciplinary evaluation. London: Trime Books; 1978.

39. Trevett AF, Carter RC, Tyrrel SF. Water quality deterioration: a study of household drinking water quality in rural Hondus. Int J Environ Health Res. 2004;14(4):273–83.

40. Jagals P, Jagals C, Bokako TC. The effect of container biofilm on the microbiological quality of water used from plastic household containers. J Water Health. 2003;1(3):101–8.

41. Momba MN, Kaleni P. Regrowth and survival of indicator microorganisms on the surfaces of household containers for the storage of drinking water in rural communities of South Africa. Water Resour. 2002;36(12):3023–8.

42. Pickering AJ, Davis J. Freshwater availability and water fetching distance affect child health in sub-Saharan Africa. Environ Sci Technol. 2012;46(4):2391–7.

43. Gascon J, Vargas M, Schellenberg D, Urassa H, Casals C, Kahigwa E, et al. Diarrhea in children under 5 years of age from Ifakara, Tanzania: a case-control study. J Clin Microbiol. 2000;38(12):4459–62.

44. Hamer DH, Simon J, Thea D, Keusch GT. Childhood diarrhea in sub Saharan Africa. Washington DC, United States Agency for International Development 2. Child Health Res Project Special Rep 1998. http://www.bu.edu/cghd/files/2010/10/Hamer-Simon-Thea-Keusch-1998-Childhood-diarrhea in-sub-Saharan-Africa.pdf.

45. Kausar S, Asghar K, Anwar SM, Shaukat F, Kausar R. Factors affecting drinking water quality and human health at household level in Punjab, Pakistan. Life Soc Sci. 2011;9(1):33–7.

46. Alexander LM, Heaven A, Tennant A, Morris R. Symptomatology of children in contact with sea water contaminated with sewage. J Epidemiol Community Health. 1992;46(4):340–4.

47. Wade TJ, Calderon RL, Sams E, Beach M, Brenner KP, Williams AH, et al. Rapidly measured indicators of recreational water quality are predictive of swimming-associated gastrointestinal illness. Environ Health Perspect. 2006;114(1):24.

From home deliveries to health care facilities: establishing a traditional birth attendant referral program in Kenya

Angelo Tomedi[1,2*], Sophia R. Stroud[1], Tania Ruiz Maya[1], Christopher R. Plaman[1] and Mutuku A. Mwanthi[3]

Abstract

Objective: To assess the effectiveness of a traditional birth attendant (TBA) referral program on increasing the number of deliveries overseen by skilled birth attendants (SBA) in rural Kenyan health facilities before and after the implementation of a free maternity care policy.

Methods: In a rural region of Kenya, TBAs were recruited to educate pregnant women about the importance of delivering in healthcare facilities and were offered a stipend for every pregnant woman whom they brought to the healthcare facility. We evaluated the percentage of prenatal care (PNC) patients who delivered at the intervention site compared with the percentage of PNC patients who delivered at rural control facilities, before and after the referral program was implemented, and before and after the Kenya government implemented a policy of free maternity care. The window period of the study was from July of 2011 through September 2013, with a TBA referral intervention conducted from March to September 2013.

Results: The absolute increases from the pre-intervention period to the TBA referral intervention period in SBA deliveries were 5.7 and 24.0 % in the control and intervention groups, respectively ($p < 0.001$). The absolute increases in SBA delivery rates from the pre-intervention period to the intervention period before the implementation of the free maternity care policy were 4.7 and 17.2 % in the control and intervention groups, respectively ($p < 0.001$). After the policy implementation the absolute increases from pre-intervention to post-intervention were 1.8 and 11.6 % in the control and intervention groups, respectively ($p < 0.001$).

Conclusion: The percentage of SBA deliveries at the intervention health facility significantly increased compared to control health facilities when TBAs educated women about the need to deliver with a SBA and when TBAs received a stipend for bringing women to local health facilities to deliver. Furthermore, this TBA referral program proved to be far more effective in the target region of Kenya than a policy change to provide free obstetric care.

Keywords: Skilled birth attendants, Traditional birth attendants, Midwifery, Maternal health, Kenya, Childbirth, Maternal health services

Background

Modern obstetric care and hygienic childbirth practices have been heralded as the main reasons for the decrease in the neonatal mortality rate during the 20th century [1]. This remarkable decline does not extend to developing countries to the same extent [2], where skilled birth attendants (SBAs) preside over fewer than half of deliveries, and where 60 million births occur outside health facilities each year [3]. The lack of appropriate health services during childbirth is also responsible for high maternal mortality rates with at least 42 % of the annual estimated 352,000 maternal deaths occurring during labor and the first 2 days after birth [4]. A large number of maternal deaths and one million neonate stillbirths could be prevented with intrapartum interventions [5]. Most maternal deaths occur during labor, delivery and the immediate postpartum period. The main direct cause is obstetric hemorrhage accounting for

* Correspondence: atomedi@salud.unm.edu
[1]School of Medicine, MSC09 5040, 1 University of New Mexico, Albuquerque, NM 87131, USA
[2]Department of Family and Community Medicine, School of Medicine, Albuquerque, NM, USA
Full list of author information is available at the end of the article

25 % of maternal deaths, infections (15 %), unsafe abortion (13 %), eclampsia (12 %), and obstructed labor (8 %) [6]. These complications are preventable with adequate medical care during and after delivery. It is therefore logical that measures should be taken to increase the number of women who utilize healthcare facilities and SBAs during childbirth.

Maternal and newborn mortality are frequent in Kenya where a high number of deliveries occur at home, often under the supervision of a traditional birth attendant (TBA) [7]. A TBA is defined by World Health Organization as a person who "assists the mother during childbirth and who initially acquired her skills by delivering babies herself or through an apprenticeship to other TBAs" [7].

It is interesting to note that increased training of TBAs has not been shown to reduce maternal mortality during childbirth. A systematic review by Wilson et al. found that the strategy of training and support of traditional birth attendants reduced perinatal and neonatal deaths but had no significant effect on maternal mortality [8]. A joint statement by the World Health Organization, the International Confederation of Midwives (ICM), and the International Federation of Gynecology and Obstetrics (FIGO) also stated "Research indicates that training of TBAs has not contributed to reduction of maternal mortality" [9]. This has led to a call for a concerted effort to replace TBA-attended home births with a health center intrapartum care strategy [10]. Therefore, it is important to create programs that focus on increasing the number, accessibility, and utilization of SBAs [11].

Although TBAs are not as effective as SBAs at reducing childbirth morbidity and mortality, they continue to play an important role in women's health. In the 1990's, WHO, UNICEF, and UNFPA described the role of TBA programs in promoting global reproductive health as: a) enhancing the links between modern health care and communities; and b) increasing the number of births attended by trained birth attendants [12]. The ubiquitous presence and availability of TBAs in many rural regions of Africa provides a potential means for contact of pregnant women with the health care system and early referral to health facilities.

According to the 2008–2009 Kenya Demographic and Health Survey, over 92 % of Kenyan women are seen at least once per pregnancy at an antenatal clinic, but only 44 % of deliveries are attended by SBAs. This rate has only improved by 3 % since the previous demographic study conducted in 2003. Additionally, there are regional discrepancies in care during delivery. For example, data collected in 2003 from Western Province revealed that SBAs delivered only 28 % of births. In contrast, in Central Province, the most urban of all provinces, 70 % of women delivered with a SBA [11]. These figures illustrate the minimal improvement in the rate of deliveries attended by

SBAs despite efforts made throughout a 5 year period by the Kenya Ministry of Health.

The available data from 2008 show that deliveries assisted by SBAs in Eastern Province were 42.8 % [13]. In contrast to the number for this large area, the Yatta sub-county of Machakos county in eastern Kenya had a much lower rate, showing a need for an intervention program targeted at increasing the rate of childbirths in health facilities with SBAs [14]. According to a recent annual report, the Yatta District SBA rate is only 7 % [15]. Data collected by Tomedi et al. elucidate the beneficial effect of an intervention program targeted at increasing the rate of childbirths in facilities with SBAs in this rural area of eastern Kenya. The study found that a TBA referral system resulted in a large increase in the rate of deliveries in two healthcare facilities [16].

On June 1, 2013 the Kenyan government abolished all fees for maternity services in public facilities with the expressed purpose of increasing SBA deliveries. The purposes of our study were to assess an expansion of the previously studied TBA referral system to a health facility in Yatta sub-county, and to further determine if the TBA referral program increased the SBA delivery rate beyond the effect of the abolishment of fees for services.

Materials and methods

We conducted a non-randomized controlled trial to investigate if women's exposure to TBA referrals and a community education program changed their medical facility/SBA-seeking behavior for delivery. We hypothesized that enlisting the support of TBA referrals would significantly increase the number of women who choose to give birth in a health facility with a SBA present.

The site of the study is in southeastern Kenya, in Yatta sub-county of Machakos County. The region is part of the arid and semi-arid lands of Kenya, populated by the Kamba tribe. Dry land rain-fed agriculture and small-scale animal husbandry are the primary source of livelihood for the non-urban population that is included in this study. Extreme poverty and geographic isolation of the population limit access to health care and contribute to a high child and neonatal mortality. The intervention facility was chosen because of its remarkably low percentage (2.4 %) of deliveries of antenatal care patients occurring in a facility with a SBA [16]. The Yatta sub-county has a female population of 141,075 and a total population of 273,519 [17]. A planning meeting was held with the Kisiiki Health Center staff in which the purpose and methods of the intervention were presented. After gaining the support of the clinical staff, they contacted TBAs known to them and recruited the assistance of the chief and the local community health workers to contact other TBAs who were active in the catchment area of the health center. The TBAs who were contacted were asked to attend a meeting with the investigators to discuss the project and request their participation and consent.

In February 2013, we held a meeting with TBAs from the area surrounding the Kisiiki healthcare facility in Yatta sub-county to recruit them into the TBA referral program in order to expand the work of Tomedi et al. [16]. We met with the TBAs and encouraged them to educate or inform their clients about the potential complications that can occur for the mother and newborn at the time of delivery (with examples solicited from experienced TBAs), and why it is important to deliver at a health facility that can handle the complications or provide transport to a higher level of care (e.g. blood transfusion, C-section). Enrolled TBAs were told that they would be compensated with a per diem of KSH 200 (approximately $2.50 USD) for each pregnant woman that the TBAs referred to a facility for an SBA delivery.

The Kenya government/Ministry of Health has emphasized the importance of health facility deliveries and that TBAs are not legitimate providers of health care (e.g. they are practicing without a license). The TBAs are aware of that, but in this and other meetings have stated that pregnant women continue to come to them requesting their assistance, and they feel an obligation to help. The lead author was told in preliminary meetings with TBAs (before the study was started) that they do not charge a fee for their services, but other community sources (e.g. the chief of some of the villages, local health staff) have said that they are paid by the client's family, an amount that could range from KSH 200 to 500. Because of the government's stated position regarding TBAs, they have been reluctant to refer the client when complications occur. The pregnant women, when asked about barriers to facility birth, have expressed a fear that they might deliver while traveling the long distance to a health facility. Therefore, in addition to providing the TBAs with an educational message for them to deliver to their clients, the meeting addressed other concerns and barriers. A Ministry of Health official in charge of maternity services for the district spoke of the important role of the TBAs to educate their clients and improve maternal outcomes. She and the hospital staff welcomed and encouraged the involvement of TBAs (up to the point of delivery). It was recognized that the TBAs would continue to be consulted by many families. They are asked to assess if a woman is in active labor, and if there likely is adequate time for the trip to the health facility. The TBA then accompanies the woman in case delivery should occur en route. The stipend paid to the TBA is considered a "per diem" to defray her personal expenses for the trip to the health facility. The amount of the stipend was chosen because the volunteer community health workers (CHWs) in the target area of the non-governmental organization that supports this project are paid a "per diem" of KSH 200 per day of work.

The number of TBAs participating in the referral program was 38.

The number of births from the Kisiiki area, which was estimated by the number of new PNC patients, was compared to the rural control facilities in the Yatta sub-county. Data from the Ministry of Public Health and Sanitation (MOPHS) facilities' records was used to determine PNC visits and pregnant women who delivered at a rural health facility with or without a TBA.

The control facilities consisted of 28 rural dispensaries and health centers within the Yatta sub-county that did not participate in the TBA referral program. The two intervention facilities for which results were reported in the previous study [16] were excluded from this analysis because we did not have data from them for each time interval. The two urban hospitals were also excluded, since the focus of this study is on rural health facilities. The number of first visits of PNC patients was used to estimate the number of pregnancies because the actual number of pregnancies cannot be determined from the available government statistics. Over 90 % of pregnant women are seen for at least one PNC visit, so the number of first PNC patient visits approximates the number of viable pregnancies. Informed consent was obtained from the participating TBAs.

Table 1 Pre intervention percent of PNC patients with SBA deliveries

	MOPHS Facility Intervention site		
	Deliveries	New PNC patients	% Deliveries/ PNC
Kisiiki	12	334	3.6
	Control Yatta District Facilities		
	Deliveries	New PNC patients	% Deliveries/ PNC
TOTAL	218	2112	10.3
Ikombe	61	181	33.7
Kauthulini	3	104	2.9
Kikesa	25	333	7.5
Kinyaata	15	213	7.0
Kitheuni	27	157	17.2
Kithimani	38	360	10.6
Kwamwatu	5	51	9.8
Kyanzavi	0	3	0.0
Kyasioni	11	150	7.3
Mamba	0	83	0.0
Mbembani	2	34	5.9
Ndalani	7	160	4.4
Nthungululu	23	99	23.2
NYS Mavoloni	1	116	0.9
St. Kizito	0	68	0.0

July 2011- February 2013

The pre-intervention data was collected from July 2011 through February 2013. In the control facilities, the number of new PNC patients and the number of deliveries were 2112 and 218 respectively. The intervention facility (Kisiiki) recorded 334 new PNC patients and 12 deliveries during the same time period.

These pre-intervention figures were compared with post intervention data collected from March 1, 2013 through May 31, 2013 (prior to enactment of the policy where maternity services are free at health care facilities) and from June 1, 2013 through September 30, 2013 (after the enactment of the policy). Therefore, the post intervention period was divided into subintervals, one before the free maternity care policy was enacted and one after the policy went into effect. These periods were analyzed separately to assess changes in SBA-attended birth rates related to the effect of the change in the government policy.

Ethics
The University of New Mexico Human Research Protections Office and the Kenyatta National Hospital-University of Nairobi Ethics and Research Committee in Kenya approved the study.

Statistics
The SBA rate was calculated as a percentage of the prenatal care (PNC) patients who delivered at the facility, with the denominator being the number of first visit prenatal care patients and the numerator being the number of deliveries at the facility. The total number of the PNC patients and deliveries at all non-intervention rural facilities were used for the control percentages. Chi-square tests were used to test differences in percent of SBA (facility) deliveries between intervention and control groups for individual time periods: baseline rates (pre-intervention), for the rates during the entire 7-month intervention period, and for the rates during the two parts of the intervention period (before and after the implementation of the free maternity care policy). Differential changes over time between the intervention and control groups were tested using binomial regression with a term for the interaction between group and time. Statistical analyses were performed using Stata version 13 (StataCorp LP, College Station, TX, USA).

Results
During the pre-intervention (baseline) period, the percent of SBA deliveries was significantly higher in the

Table 2 Post-intervention percent of PNC patients with SBA deliveries before free obstetric care policy (i.e. prelegislation)

MOPHS Facility Intervention site			
	Deliveries	New PNC patients	% Deliveries/ PNC
Kisiiki	11	53	20.8
Control Yatta District Facilities			
	Deliveries	New PNC patients	% Deliveries/ PNC
TOTAL	54	359	15.0
Ikombe	5	35	14.3
Kauthulini	2	17	11.8
Kikesa	8	61	13.1
Kinyaata	6	38	15.8
Kitheuni	4	24	16.7
Kithimani	6	62	9.7
Kwamwatu	2	10	20.0
Kyanzavi	0	0	0.0
Kyasioni	5	18	27.8
Mamba	0	12	0.0
Mbembani	3	9	33.3
Ndalani	6	32	18.8
Nthungululu	7	13	53.8
NYS Mavoloni	0	13	0.0
St. Kizito	0	15	0.0

March 2013-May 2013

Table 3 Post-intervention Deliveries percent of PNC patients with SBA deliveries after free obstetric care policy (i.e. post legislation)

MOPHS Facility Intervention site			
	Deliveries	New PNC patients	% Deliveries/ PNC
Kisiiki	24	74	32.4
Control Yatta District Facilities			
	Deliveries	New PNC patients	% Deliveries/ PNC
TOTAL	81	483	16.8
Ikombe	8	33	24.2
Kauthulini	3	29	10.3
Kikesa	19	69	27.5
Kinyaata	4	40	10.0
Kitheuni	10	60	16.7
Kithimani	8	86	9.3
Kwamwatu	2	11	18.2
Kyanzavi	0	1	0.0
Kyasioni	5	21	23.8
Mamba	1	21	4.8
Mbembani	5	10	50.0
Ndalani	1	42	2.4
Nthungululu	15	24	62.5
NYS Mavoloni	0	22	0.0
St. Kizito	0	14	0.0

June 2013- September 2013

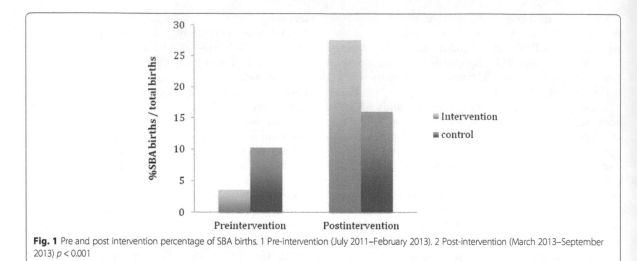

Fig. 1 Pre and post intervention percentage of SBA births. 1 Pre-intervention (July 2011–February 2013). 2 Post-intervention (March 2013–September 2013) $p < 0.001$

control facilities (10.3 %) than in the intervention facility (3.6 %) ($\chi^2 = 15.33$; $p < 0.001$) (Table 1).

During the 7-month intervention period, 16.0 % of PNC patients delivered with an SBA at the control facilities, compared to 27.6 % of PNC patients at the intervention facility (Tables 2, 3, Fig. 1). The absolute increases (from pre-intervention to post-intervention) in SBA facility deliveries were 5.7 and 24.0 % in the control and intervention groups, respectively ($z = 4.21$; $p = 0.001$).

The Kenya government implemented a policy that provided free maternity care halfway through our post intervention period. In order to assess the effect of this new policy on SBA deliveries, the 7-month intervention period was divided into two sub- periods (Table 4, Fig. 2):

1) Before the free maternity care policy (Table 2), 15.0 and 20.8 % of PNC patients had SBA deliveries at the control and intervention sites respectively. The absolute increases in SBA facility deliveries between the baseline period and the first intervention sub-period were 4.7 and 17.2 % in the control and intervention groups, respectively ($\chi^2 = 2.07$; $p = 0.04$).

2) After the free maternity care policy implementation (Table 3), 16.8 and 32.4 % of PNC patients had SBA deliveries at the control and intervention sites respectively ($\chi^2 = 10.29$; $p < 0.001$). The

Table 4 Summary of percentage of PNC patients with SBA deliveries

Pre-intervention	12/334 (3.6 %)	218/2112 (10.3 %)	$P < 0.001$
Post-intervention Before free OB care	11/53 (20.8 %)	54/359 (15.0 %)	
Post-intervention After free OB care	24/74 (32.4 %)	81/483 (16.8 %)	

absolute increases in SBA facility deliveries between the baseline period and the period with free maternity care were 1.8 and 11.6 % in the control and intervention groups, respectively ($z = 3.84$; $p < 0.001$).

In the control facilities, the SBA delivery rate increased from 15 % in the first intervention period (before the free maternity care policy) to 16.8 % after the policy implementation ($\chi^2 = 0.46$; $p = 0.50$).

Discussion

This study shows that a TBA referral and maternal education program was associated with an increase in the percentage of SBA deliveries. We found a significant increase in delivery rates in the before-after comparison at the intervention site, as well as in the comparison of the control and the intervention sites during the study period. The implementation of the Kenyan government policy of free obstetric care at hospitals was enacted with the explicit purpose of increasing the number of women who choose to deliver at health care facilities. However, there was no significant increase in SBA deliveries observed at the control sites, or any further increase in the SBA rate in the intervention facility, after the Kenya government implemented the policy of free maternity care.

Two control facilities were excluded from the statistical analysis of the results. Matuu District Hospital and Matuu Mission Hospital are located in an urban area and had high numbers of PNC patients and deliveries. We attribute these high numbers to the fact that both facilities were located in an area with accessible transportation, increased education level, and increased resources. Because our study aims at targeting rural communities, we determined that these two facilities are not appropriate control sites.

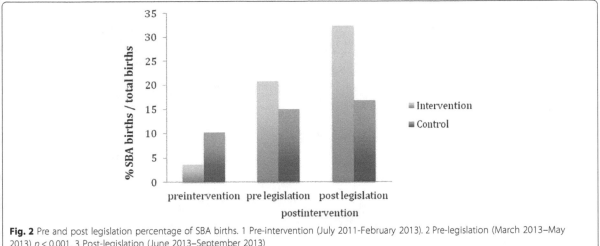

Fig. 2 Pre and post legislation percentage of SBA births. 1 Pre-intervention (July 2011-February 2013). 2 Pre-legislation (March 2013–May 2013) $p < 0.001$. 3 Post-legislation (June 2013–September 2013)

No qualitative or quantitative data were collected that would explain the reason for the increase in SBA deliveries, so the reasons are speculative. Most if not all of the TBAs are aware of potential childbirth complications, though the discussion led by respected health care professionals may have served as a reminder and helped them prepare a message for the pregnant women who consult them. However, the authors speculate, based on informal observations and feedback, that the most important components of the intervention were likely the recognition of their importance in the community and the offer from health care professionals and government officials for them to participate in an important role, at a time when they felt excluded or ostracized. The stipend was also clearly an important component, even though it may have been less than the fee they might have received from the client. Our impression from TBA interactions is that there would be far less participation if they received nothing for their effort and had to pay their own transportation costs to get to the health facility. The stipend can only be sustainable as long as the non-governmental organization (NGO) provides the funds, or the government takes over that responsibility. The amount of funds required is small relative to other costs of the health care system. Other NGOs and low-income developing country governments have decided to pay a salary to lay CHWs for community work, at greater cost than this TBA program. However, the hope is that over time the "norm" in the community will be a health facility delivery rather than a home delivery, and the TBA stipend will not be necessary.

There are recognized limitations of this quasi-experimental study. The relatively brief time period and the number of deliveries in the target facilities limit the power and strength of the conclusions. The intervention and control sites were not randomly assigned, which increases the risk of the influence of potential confounding variables. Unmeasured factors, such as improved accessibility and cultural issues or preferences may have contributed to the results, but are not likely to have influenced the outcome significantly more in the intervention region than in the control region. We did not collect qualitative or quantitative data on the population characteristics, potential confounders, and about the community's reasons for lack of response to the Kenya policy change. The restriction of the study population to one ethnic group in one district limits the generalizability of the results.

The efforts in Kenya thus far to increase SBA deliveries has met with very limited success. Our approach of involving TBAs in a referral program could offer the potential for Kenya and other sub-Saharan African countries to improve SBA facility delivery rates at a very low cost. A larger study of this approach would seem warranted in other regions and countries where TBAs play an active role in the community.

Conclusion

The percentage of SBA deliveries at the intervention health facility significantly increased compared to control health facilities when TBAs educated women about the need to deliver with a SBA and when TBAs received a stipend for bringing women to local health facilities to deliver. Furthermore, this TBA referral program proved to be far more effective in the target region of Kenya than a policy change to provide free obstetric care.

Competing interest
The authors declare that they have no competing interests.

Authors' contributions
AT developed the protocol arranged TBA meetings, and edited the manuscript. SRS, TRM, and CRP collected and compiled the data and drafted the manuscript. MAM reviewed the protocol for submission to the Kenya IRB and participated in the editing of the manuscript. All authors read and approved the final manuscript.

Authors' information
Angelo Tomedi, MD, Visiting Associate Professor, Mutuku A. Mwanthi, Ph.D., Associate Professor, Sophia Stroud BS, Medical Student, Tania Ruiz Maya BS, Medical Student, Christopher R. Plaman, BA, Medical Student.

Acknowledgements
We thank The University Of New Mexico School Of Medicine and Global Health Partnerships for supporting our study. Special thanks to Dr. Betty Skipper for her assistance with statistical analysis. Thanks to all the health care staff in Kenya that made this project possible.

Disclaimers
The views expressed in the article are the authors' own, and not an official position of the University of New Mexico.

Sources of support
University of New Mexico Health Sciences Center.

Author details
[1]School of Medicine, MSC09 5040, 1 University of New Mexico, Albuquerque, NM 87131, USA. [2]Department of Family and Community Medicine, School of Medicine, Albuquerque, NM, USA. [3]School of Public Health, University of Nairobi, Nairobi, Kenya.

References
1. Piekkala P, Erkkola R, Kero P, Tenovuo A, Sillanpaa M. Declining perinatal mortality in a region of Finland, 1968–82. Am J Public Health. 1985;75(2):156–60.
2. Lawn JE, Lee AC, Kinney M, Sibley L, Carlo WA, Paul VK, et al. Two million intrapartum-related stillbirths and neonatal deaths: where, why, and what can be done? Int J Gynaecol Obstet. 2009;107 Suppl 1:S5-18–S19.
3. UNICEF: State of the World's Children 2009. In maternal and newborn health. New York, NY: UNICEF; 2008.
4. Hogan MC, FK K, Naghavi M, Ahn SY, Wang M, Makela SM, et al. Maternal mortality for 181 countries, 1980–2008: a systematic analysis of progress towards millennium development goal 5. Lancet. 2010;375(9726):1609–23.
5. Bhutta ZA YM, Lawn JE. Stillbirths: how much difference can we make and at what cost? Lancet. 2011.
6. Wanjira C, Mwangi M, Mathenge E. Delivery practices and associated factors among mothers seeking child welfare services in selected health facilities in Nyandarua south district, Kenya. BMC Public Health. 2011;11:360.
7. WH Organization. Traditional birth attendants: a joint WHO/UNICEF/UNFPA statement. Geneva: World Health Organization; 1992.
8. Wilson A, Gallos ID, Plana N, Lissauer D, Khan KS, Zamora J, et al. Effectiveness of strategies incorporating training and support of traditional birth attendants on perinatal and maternal mortality: meta-analysis. BMJ. 2011;343:d7102. doi:10.1136/bmj.d7102.
9. Making pregnancy safer: the critical role of the skilled attendant. A joint statement by WHO, ICM and FIGO. Geneva: World Health Organization; 2004.
10. Campbell OM, Graham WJ. Lancet maternal survival series steering group. Strategies for reducing maternal mortality: getting on with what works. Lancet. 2006;368(9543):1284–99.
11. Wilson N. Liambila, Population Council. Nairobi Office, Kenya. Ministry of Health, University of Nairobi. Safe Motherhood Demonstration Project, Western Province: Final Report. Population Council, Sub-Saharan Africa Region, Nairobi Office. 2004:95–9.
12. United Nations Population Fund: office of oversight and evaluation. Support to traditional birth attendants. 1996. <http://www.unfpa.org/monitoring/pdf/n-issue7.pdf> accessed July 2012.
13. Kenya National Bureau of Statistics (KNBS) and ICF Macro (2010) Kenya Demographic and Health Survey 2008–2009. Calverton, Maryland: KNBS and ICF Macro; 2010. http://dhsprogram.com/pubs/pdf/fr229/fr229.pdf.
14. Olenja J, Godia P, Kibaru J, Egondi T. Influence of Provider Training on Quality of Emergency Obstetric Care in Kenya. 2004 Kenya Service Provision Assessment Survey. Kenya Working Papers No.3, DHS Program. http://dhsprogram.com/pubs/pdf/wpk3/wpk3.pdf.
15. Annual Operational Plan for Yatta District. Consolidated District Health Sector Plan 2011/2012. Republic of Kenya Ministry of Health, 2011. Afya House, Cathedral Road, Nairobi 00100, Kenya.
16. Tomedi A, Tucker K, Mwanthi MA. A Strategy to Increase Skilled Attendant Births in Kenya. Int J Gynaecol Obstet. 2013;120(2):152-5.
17. Kenya 2009 Census Data. Mars Group Kenya. 2012. http://www.marsgroupkenya.org/census/?data=phoudk&province=4:Eastern+Province&district=423:YATTA+District.

4

The validity of birth and pregnancy histories in rural Bangladesh

Donna Espeut* and Stan Becker

Abstract

Background: Maternity histories provide a means of estimating fertility and mortality from surveys.

Methods: The present analysis compares two types of maternity histories—birth histories and pregnancy histories—in three respects: (1) completeness of live birth and infant death reporting; (2) accuracy of the time placement of live births and infant deaths; and (3) the degree to which reported versus actual total fertility measures differ. The analysis covers a 15-year time span and is based on two data sources from Matlab, Bangladesh: the 1994 Matlab Demographic and Health Survey and, as gold standard, the vital events data from Matlab's Demographic Surveillance System.

Results: Both histories are near perfect in live-birth completeness; however, pregnancy histories do better in the completeness and time accuracy of deaths during the first year of life.

Conclusions: Birth or pregnancy histories can be used for fertility estimation, but pregnancy histories are advised for estimating infant mortality.

Keywords: Bangladesh, Birth histories, Displacement, Omission, Fertility estimation, Maternity history, Mortality estimation, Pregnancy histories, Validation

Background

Population-based surveys such as the Demographic and Health Surveys (DHS) play an important role in generating evidence for decision-making, particularly in countries where population-level data are either scarce or of poor quality. DHS always include a module known as a maternity history. A maternity history is used to gather information that is needed to estimate fertility and child mortality, as well as to identify currently living children in order to assess various aspects of child health and nutrition.

There are two types of maternity histories: birth histories and pregnancy histories. A birth history collects information from mothers on pregnancies that resulted in a live birth, whereas a pregnancy history collects information on both live births and pregnancy losses (i.e., spontaneous abortions, induced abortions, and stillbirths). Each type of history can be either backward or forward in time orientation. A backward history starts with the collection of information on a woman's most recent birth or pregnancy and goes back in time to her first birth or pregnancy. In

contrast, a forward history starts with a woman's first birth or pregnancy and ends with her most recent. In the World Fertility Survey project carried out between 1974 and 1981, pregnancy histories were collected from representative samples of women in over 40 countries [1]. More recently, the DHS project has used birth histories in over 300 surveys in over 90 developing countries [2]. Both programs have used forward histories.

Given the importance of DHS data in macro-level health planning, it is important to determine the validity of maternity history data. Two types of errors affect the validity of such data: (1) event omission and (2) event displacement in time. Event omission leads to underestimation of demographic indicators derived from the data. Event displacement occurs when the mother inaccurately reports a child's date of birth, age, or date of death. An event whose timing is incorrectly pushed further back in time than it actually occurred is called "backward displaced," whereas an event whose timing is incorrectly pushed closer to the date of the interview is called "forward displaced." Characteristics of the questionnaire, the mother (respondent), the interviewer, and the vital event itself can all contribute to the likelihood of omission or displacement [3].

* Correspondence: donna_espeut@yahoo.com
Department of Population, Family and Reproductive Health, Johns Hopkins University, Baltimore, USA

There have been a number of data-quality assessments involving birth and/or pregnancy histories [3–18]. The DHS program has documented a number of problems associated with fertility and mortality estimation from birth histories. Across 128 surveys between 1985 and 2003, an average of 11 % of births had incomplete information about date of birth, with month of birth the most common missing information [19]. There was also considerable heaping of age at death at 12 months. Another analysis of DHS data showed that missing date of birth information is a more frequent phenomenon among rural than among urban women and in cases where a translator is needed [5]. The DHS program has dealt with the problem of missing or partially recorded date information through standard data editing and imputation procedures.

Previous assessments have also documented reporting problems such as age heaping and digit preference. However, only two of these assessments [3, 8] were actual validation studies; the others were reliability studies or relied on expected patterns to detect problems in data quality. Based on the multi-decade experiences using WFS pregnancy histories and DHS birth histories, it has been argued that birth histories are adequate for estimation of fertility and infant mortality [20]. However, this claim has not been substantiated by research that included both types of maternity histories within the same study. The present study was designed to fill that gap.

Methods
Study purpose and hypotheses
In this study, we compare birth and pregnancy histories in terms of the validity of fertility and infant mortality information at the individual level. We test three hypotheses regarding the two questionnaire types—specifically that both types of histories have the same:

1. Completeness of live births, early neonatal deaths, neonatal deaths, and infant deaths
2. Differences between reported and actual "total fertility"
3. Accuracy of the time placement of live births, early neonatal deaths, neonatal deaths, and infant deaths

Testing of the first and third hypotheses is based on individual matching of a woman and her live births, early neonatal deaths, and infant deaths between two data sources described below. The second hypothesis is based on aggregate-level fertility measures.

Data sources
The analyses involve two data sources from Bangladesh: (1) census and vital event data from the Matlab Demographic Surveillance System (DSS) and (2) birth and pregnancy

history data from the 1994 Matlab Demographic and Health Survey (MDHS). Each is now described.

The Matlab DSS
Matlab, a rural sub-district in southeastern Bangladesh, is home to a DSS that has been operational since 1966. The International Centre for Diarrhoeal Disease Research, Bangladesh (ICDDR,B) manages the DSS, which covers 149 contiguous villages that are divided into two areas: (1) the Maternal and Child Health Family Planning area (henceforth referred to as the "program area"), where intensive public health interventions have been in existence since 1978 and (2) a comparison area (henceforth referred to as the "non-program area"), where villages are almost exclusively dependent upon government-sponsored programs.

The hallmark of the DSS is longitudinal surveillance of the population. At the time of the fieldwork for this study in 1994, Community Health Workers (CHWs) were visiting households bi-weekly in their assigned areas, inquiring about vital events and changes in family composition (pregnancy outcomes, deaths, marriages, divorces, or migration) and making entries in a notebook. Field supervisors made monthly visits to each household with the CHW and completed event registration forms as indicated: pregnancy outcome, death, marriage, in-migration, out-migration, and divorce [21].

In 1982, ICDDR,B created a DSS Database that consolidates all vital information on each DSS resident. A 10-digit registration number is assigned once to an individual and is permanent. There is a minimum residency of 6 months in the DSS in order to be included in the Database. Although completeness of the DSS data has not been assessed formally, it is a good assumption that vital event ascertainment is near 100 % due to the timely nature of the data collection and quality control. Thus, the DSS is a viable "gold standard" data source for validation of vital event reporting by women in the Matlab population.

The 1994 MDHS
The MDHS took place from April to May 1994, immediately after the 1993–1994 Bangladesh Demographic and Health Survey (BDHS) [22]. The rationale for conducting the MDHS was twofold: (1) to ascertain the plausibility of 1993–1994 BDHS fertility estimates (which were much lower than anticipated) and (2) to document the level of validity of birth histories versus pregnancy histories.

MDHS Sample: A stratified random sampling design was used, with each of the 149 DSS villages as a stratum and a fixed sampling fraction of 22/300 = 0.073 within each village in order to yield a desired sample size of approximately 3000 women. With this schema, 3,225 households were selected from DSS villages. Of the households selected, 3,037 were occupied dwellings and had persons present and 3009 had completed household interviews. Of 3,480 women age 15–49 in these households, 3039 had completed interviews (a 97.4 percent response rate).

Also selected were 250 households from 12 neighboring villages just outside of the DSS area. These non-DSS villages were chosen because they were comparable to the adjacent DSS villages in terms of their geographic, economic, social, and religious characteristics. The comparison of the survey data from respondents in the non-DSS villages with data from respondents in the adjacent DSS villages provides insight on the generalizability of the validation results. In particular, we wanted to test for possible biases of survey responses of DSS women since they have been asked about vital events for so long that they may give more accurate responses than would otherwise be the case. Such a bias is referred to as a 'contamination effect' below.

Questionnaires: One-half of the MDHS questionnaires contained a standard birth history module (as was used in the 1993–94 BDHS) and the other half contained a pregnancy history module. Both types of maternity history were forward histories and had similar formats, with the exception of three pregnancy history questions on non-live birth pregnancies. (See below.)

Data collection: Thirty-two of the 48 interviewers who were involved in fieldwork for the 1993–94 BDHS were engaged to conduct the interviews in the MDHS. Having the same interviewers in both the BDHS and MDHS effectively controlled for interviewer effects. Interviewers administered a birth history or pregnancy history questionnaire by random assignment within each village, i.e., about half received each type.

An area-level validation study of fertility, infant mortality, and contraceptive prevalence estimates from the MDHS compared to the DSS has been published, noting some discrepancies between MDHS- and DSS-derived estimates [8]. Survey-based TFR estimates were accurate for the 60-month period before the survey (3.18 and 4.40 for Matlab program and non-program areas, respectively) compared to corresponding DSS values for the same period (3.15 and 4.37, respectively). Also, the survey-based estimates of infant mortality were consistent with DSS estimates for the 5-year period prior to the survey. However, survey-based estimates considerably underestimated infant mortality for the 5–9-year period before the survey (MDHS estimates of 71.1 and 84.0 per 1000 live births for program and non-program areas, respectively, compared with corresponding DSS values of 89.6 and 105.0 per 1000 live births). The present study

investigates these discrepancies using individual-level data for women who met the inclusion criteria for the validation analysis.

Data processing: The original MDHS data were entered into the Integrated System for Survey Analysis (ISSA, [23]), and standard DHS range and consistency checks were done. Modifications to this original MDHS data file were needed in order to conduct the validation with individual-level matched data from the DSS. Specifically, the Bengali names of mothers and their births (as originally recorded on the paper questionnaires) were appended to the MDHS records. The mother's full name was the key variable used to match individual births in the MDHS and DSS files, followed by the sex and birth order of each of her births. (Details of the matching are available from the first author.)

For the analysis of possible contamination, first, we compared background characteristics of women in the 12 non-DSS villages with those of women in the 17 adjacent DSS villages, and another comparison was with the characteristics of all women in the DSS sample. Second, we compared levels of three indicators of data quality between the DSS and non-DSS samples. If contamination exists, we would expect data quality to be superior for women in the DSS villages. The three indicators were (1) heaping of women's ages on ages ending in 0 or 5 (e.g., 15, 20, 25, 30, etc.), (2) the percentage of women who gave a complete birth date (month and year) for all births, and (3) heaping of birth interval lengths on multiples of 12 months.

Study outcomes

Various pregnancy outcomes (live births, stillbirths, abortions) are recorded in a pregnancy history; therefore, mothers who were interviewed using a pregnancy history questionnaire were first asked: "What was the outcome of the pregnancy (live birth, stillbirth, abortion)?" The following questions further helped to classify the pregnancy outcome based on the mother's responses: "Did the baby cry or show any sign of life after its birth?" and "How many months did the pregnancy last?"

In both the pregnancy and birth history questionnaires, the interviewer identified deaths by asking the mother the following for each live birth reported: "Is (NAME) still alive?" If the mother reported that the child was not alive, the interviewer then asked: "How old was he/she when he/she died?" Deaths occurring before the second birthday were recorded in months, and deaths occurring within the first month of life were recorded in days. (Deaths at 2 years and above were recorded in years.)

The analysis focuses on four demographic outcomes: (1) live births, (2) early neonatal deaths, (3) neonatal deaths, and (4) infant deaths. We used the following definitions for the analyses:

- *Early neonatal deaths*—live births that die within the first week (0 to 6 days) of life
- *Neonatal deaths*—live births that die within the first month (0 to 29 days) of life
- *Infant deaths*—live births that die within the first year (0 to 11 months) of life

Validation indicators: The match rate, more specifically, the proportion of vital events of a certain type (i.e., live birth, early neonatal death, neonatal death, or infant death) documented in the DSS that were also reported in the MDHS, was the main indicator of the completeness of event reporting. Because the DSS was the "gold standard" data source in the analysis, the denominator was the total number of events identified in the DSS during a given time period.

The accuracy of time placement can obviously be assessed only for matched events. Date of birth was recorded in the MDHS using either the western calendar or the Bengali calendar. (Two Bengali months overlap with one English calendar month.) For each matched live birth, the date of birth was converted to the completed number of months preceding the survey (i.e., "months ago"). Time displacement was defined as the difference between the DSS date of birth/death and the MDHS date of birth/death, with both of these dates converted to "months ago". Given the slight differences in the calendars, the "correct" time placement was defined as the actual minus reported difference equal to zero or within ±1 month.

Indicators of displacement for live births were the proportion of matched live births with dates reported: (a) too early (i.e., backward displaced by more than a month), (b) correctly (i.e., within ±1 month of the actual date), and (c) too late (i.e., forward displaced more than a month). The mean number of months backward or forward displaced was also calculated. Another indicator was the mean absolute overall error in months. Key indicators pertaining to the time placement of deaths were the proportion of actual infant deaths reported to have occurred after the first year of life in the MDHS; the proportion of actual neonatal deaths reported to have occurred after the first month of life in the MDHS; and the proportion of early neonatal deaths reported to have occurred after the first week of life in the MDHS.

The phenomenon of heaping—or the tendency to report ages or dates ending in certain digits more than others—was explored by calculating the proportion of DSS infant deaths that were heaped on 12 months in the MDHS, and the proportion of DSS neonatal deaths heaped on 1 month in the MDHS. The rationale for examining those two heaping measures was that deaths heaped on 12 months or on 1 month would be excluded from the numerator when calculating infant mortality rates and neonatal mortality rates, respectively.

Reference periods: Individual-level validation indicators are presented for a 15-year reference period (i.e., June 1979 to May 1994). Aggregate-level fertility and mortality measures (as described below) are validated for a 10-year reference period (June 1984 to May 1994) and are presented in a manner comparable to that of standard DHS surveys (i.e., 5-year periods of analysis for mortality rates; 3-year periods for analysis for fertility rates).

This analysis examined both individual-level and aggregate fertility measures. As mentioned previously, our study used strict inclusion criteria (i.e., each woman included in the validation analysis had at least one birth and did not out-migrate during the reference period). Consequently, aggregate-level fertility measures have been calculated for this specific subset of women, not for all women residing in the DSS during the time frame in question. The validity of 3-year (36-month) "total fertility" estimates for this group of women was assessed by first calculating age-specific birth rates (5-year age groups) for the 36-month period before the survey, summing these and then calculating the actual (DSS) minus (MDHS) "total fertility" estimate. We also examined cumulative fertility from age 15 to age 39 for these women. The latter measure was examined because, beyond the most recent 36-month period, it was not possible to calculate age-specific rates for the entire reproductive span (15–49 years) using the MDHS data. (This is due to the classic lexis problem–that women 15–49 at the time of the survey are age 10–44 5 years earlier so information on women 45–49 is missing for that time period, and so on.) Age-specific birth rates could, however, be calculated for the age range 15–39 for each 36-month period within the 10-year study period.

Statistics

The significance of differences in event coverage and time placement was determined using independent two-sample z tests and t tests. These statistics were also used to test for differences between birth and pregnancy histories in the actual minus reported differentials for "total fertility". The significance of differences in event coverage and time placement was also determined using independent two-sample z tests and t tests. Multivariate logistic regression was used to estimate differences between birth and pregnancy histories in live birth omission while adjusting for other identified determinants of such omission. Children born to the same woman were regarded as being part of the same "cluster." As a result, the conventional regression assumption of independent observations does not hold so we used regression with generalized estimating equations (GEE) to account for the correlation of events within the same cluster. The analyses were conducted using SPSS and Stata [24, 25].

The following variables were considered for inclusion in the multivariate model:

Maternal variables: age, years of schooling, parity
Event variables: child's sex, child's survival status at the time of the interview; number of months the event occurred before the survey (according to DSS data)
Interviewer variables: age, years of schooling, marital status

In the univariate analysis, we used the Wald statistic to determine whether or not a variable would be included in the multivariate model; those with $p < 0.25$ were retained. In the multivariate model, variables that did not significantly ($p < 0.05$) contribute to the model were excluded, and a final model was fit.

Findings and Discussion

The analysis was based on 1925 MDHS respondents (930 women in the birth history sample; 995 women in the pregnancy history sample) who were matched with their records in the DSS and who had at least one birth or pregnancy during the 15-year period before the 1994 MDHS (i.e., June 1979 to May 1994; Fig. 1). The number

with a pregnancy history is slightly larger than the number with a birth history as women with only a non-live pregnancy termination would be included in the pregnancy history analysis sample but not in the birth history analysis sample.

As could be anticipated because of randomization, the birth and pregnancy history samples did not differ significantly in terms of major socio-demographic background factors such as marital status, number of years of schooling, religion, migration status during the study's reference period, or place of residence (data not shown). Thus, any observed differences in the validation study outcomes were likely due to the type of maternity history, not to those socio-demographic factors.

Possible contamination

The DSS women were older, had more years of schooling, and were of lower parity than the women in the adjacent, non-DSS villages. However, only the age difference was statistically significant (top panel of Table 1). [We note that the Family Planning and Health Services project was begun in half of the Matlab DSS area in 1977 and led to striking reductions in fertility starting that year [26]. This could explain the slightly older age distribution of women in the DSS area as the number of women aged 15–17 in 1994 would be lower there than elsewhere because of the fertility decline (i.e., 1994–1977 = 17).] The difference between age distributions of women in the DSS villages adjacent to non-DSS villages and women in all DSS

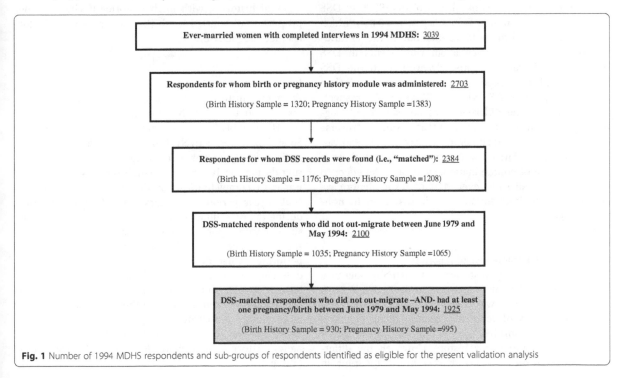

Fig. 1 Number of 1994 MDHS respondents and sub-groups of respondents identified as eligible for the present validation analysis

Table 1 Background characteristics and indicators of possible contamination for women interviewed in adjacent non-DSS and DSS villages and the women interviewed in all DSS villages, MDHS, 1994

Group of variables and indicator	Place of residence		
	Non-DSS villages	DSS villages	
		DSS villages adjacent to Non-DSS villages	All DSS villages
Number of women	225	292	2703
Background characteristics			
Percent with no schooling	56.4	51.7	54.7
Percent currently married	96.0	94.2	94.5
Percent with age <30 years	55.5	41.5*	48.4
Mean age	30.1	32.7*	31.2
Mean years of schooling	2.10	2.41	2.23
Mean parity	4.31	4.24	3.92
Indicators of possible contamination			
Maternal age heaping (percent of reported ages ending in 0 or 5)	16.9	20.5	19.6
Percent of women who reported complete dates for all births	90.7	97.9*	98.3
Heaping of birth intervals (percent of all intervals 12–48 months reported in multiples of 12)	14 ($n = 616$)	14 ($n = 764$)	15 ($n = 6498$)

*$p < 0.05$ for the test of equality of means (percentages) in non-DSS and adjacent DSS villages

villages is likely due to unique characteristics of the former group of villages.

Regarding the indicators of potential contamination, there was virtually no difference between areas in heaping of birth intervals (bottom panel of Table 1). On the other hand, women in the DSS were more likely to know the complete birth dates of all their births (98 % in DSS villages vs. 91 % in non-DSS villages; $p < 0.01$), which could be attributed to contamination due to the continuous questioning of women about vital events in DSS households. However, surprisingly, women in the DSS were more likely to report an age ending in 0 or 5 than women in the non-DSS villages (21 vs. 17 %, respectively), although the difference was not statistically significant. It is interesting to note that a similar "reverse contamination" was documented as part of the 1980 validation study in Matlab [3]. In summary, though there is some evidence of contamination, we expect the effect to be relatively small since over 90 % of respondents gave complete birth dates for all their births, even in non-DSS villages.

Results are now described for each hypothesis in turn.

Hypothesis 1: completeness of reporting

Birth and pregnancy histories had virtually identical completeness of live birth reporting at 99 % (Table 2). A child's survival status was a very important predictor of the completeness of reporting. Among living children, the percentages omitted were 0.2 in the birth history and 0.0 in the pregnancy history. However, the difference between the two histories is more apparent in

terms of reporting non-surviving children (Table 2). Among dead children, birth histories had a higher proportion omitted (7.0 % compared to 4.2 % in the pregnancy history sample, $p = 0.07$). Among mothers with no formal education and older mothers (30+ years), statistically significant differences exist between the two types of histories, with birth histories having a higher proportion of omitted live births than pregnancy histories (data not shown).

Infant deaths

Pregnancy histories performed slightly better than birth histories in terms of the completeness of infant death reporting (Table 2); infant death completeness rates were 86 and 82 %, respectively, though this difference was not statistically significant. For the 315 infant deaths occurring during the 10 years preceding the survey, reporting was more complete for infant deaths during the most recent 5-year period (0–4 years before the survey) than during the preceding 5-year period (5–9 years before the survey), with reporting completeness of 88 and 81 %, respectively. For both reference periods, birth histories performed worse than pregnancy histories, although the differences were not statistically significant. In the birth history sample, completeness was 86 % for infant deaths occurring 0–59 months before the survey and 78 % for infant deaths occurring during the 60–119 months before the survey. Corresponding percentages in the pregnancy history sample were 90 and 82 %, respectively (Table 2).

Table 2 Number of events and corresponding completeness rates (%) in the survey

Event type	Questionnaire type					
	Both		Birth history		Pregnancy history	
	Actual no. of events	Completeness (%)	Actual no. of events	Completeness (%)	Actual no. of events	Completeness (%)
Number of women[a]	1925	–	930	–	995	–
Live births	5425	99.2	2666	99.0	2759	99.4
All infant deaths 0–119 months before survey	315	84.1	138	81.9	177	85.9
Infants deaths 0–59 months before survey	151	88.1	69	85.5	82	90.2
Infant deaths 60–119 months before survey	164	80.5	69	78.3	95	82.1
Neonatal deaths	192	82.3	84	81.0	108	83.3
Early neonatal	135	80.7	58	79.3	77	81.8
Late neonatal	57	86.0	26	84.6	31	87.1
Post neonatal	123	87.0	54	83.3	69	89.9
Living children	4718	99.9	2339	99.8	2379	100.0
Dead children*	707	94.5	327	93.0	380	95.8

*Observed difference between birth histories and pregnancy histories were marginally significant ($p = 0.07$) among dead children
[a]Number of women who did not out-migrate between June 1979 and May 1994 and whose last pregnancy occurred during that period

Among infant deaths, the completeness of death reporting was lower for deaths that occurred earlier during the first year of life. For the 10 years preceding the survey, 83 and 81 % of neonatal deaths were captured by pregnancy and birth histories, respectively. Completeness rates were even lower for early neonatal deaths: 82 % of those deaths were captured by pregnancy histories compared with 79 % by birth histories (Table 2).

From the univariate analysis, the following variables were deemed appropriate ($p < 0.25$) for inclusion in the multiple logistic regression predicting omission: current survival status of the child, mother's age, parity, interviewer's years of schooling, and interviewer's marital status. These variables, along with a variable on questionnaire type (birth history versus pregnancy history) were included in the logistic regression model. Three covariates remained in the final model: child's survival status, maternal age, and parity (Table 3). After adjusting for these three variables, the odds of live birth omission were 2.0 times greater for birth histories than for pregnancy histories and this was borderline significant ($p = 0.050$).

Hypothesis 2: validity of fertility measures
Differences between actual (DSS) and reported (MDHS) "total fertility" for the 36-month period before the survey were small. Cumulative rates to age 39 were also similar for the periods 3–6 years and 6–9 years before the survey (Table 4). Birth histories and pregnancy histories did not differ significantly in the validity of those aggregate fertility measures. (Note that all of these fertility estimates are higher than those from the area-level analysis by definition because in the present analyses, we

excluded women who did not experience a pregnancy or birth between 1979 and 1994 [as noted in Fig. 1]).

Hypothesis 3: accuracy of time placement
Birth and pregnancy histories performed identically in terms of the correct placement of live births (44 % for each, Table 5). Backward displacement and forward displacement were symmetric in the MDHS (29 and 28 %, respectively), with virtually no difference. In addition, there was no statistically significant difference between birth histories and pregnancy histories in the mean absolute number of months displaced, hovering around 15 months.

Table 3 Logistic regression estimates (using generalized estimating equations) of the odds (and 95 % confidence interval) of a missed live birth using birth or pregnancy histories, adjusted for survival status of the live birth, maternal age, and parity

Parameter	Adjusted odds ratio	95 percent CI
Questionnaire type*		
Birth history (RC)	1.0	–
Pregnancy history	2.0	(1.0, 3.9)
Current survival status of live birth**		
Alive (RC)	1.0	–
Dead	22.5	(9.7, 52.4)
Maternal age at interview (in years)**	0.8	(0.8, 0.9)
Parity**	1.7	(1.4, 2.0)

Data sources: 1994 Matlab Demographic and Health Survey (MDHS); Matlab Demographic Surveillance System (DSS)
RC reference category
*$p < 0.10$ for the test of whether the adjusted odds ratio differs from 1.0
**$p < 0.05$ for the test of whether the adjusted odds ratio differs from 1.0

Table 4 DSS and MDHS estimates of "total fertility" (15–49 years) and "cumulative fertility" (15–39 years) among women sampled for the validation analysis, and the DSS-MDHS difference by the three most-recent 36-month intervals before the survey, according to type of questionnaire

Months before survey	Fertility measure	Questionnaire type					
		Birth history			Pregnancy history		
		DSS estimate	MDHS estimate	Difference	DSS estimate	MDHS estimate	Difference
0–35	Total fertility (15–49)	4.9	4.7	+0.2	5.7	5.3	+0.4
	Cum. fertility (15–39)	4.8	4.6	+0.2	5.5	5.1	+0.4
36–71	Cum. fertility (15–39)	4.7	4.8	−0.1	4.8	4.8	0.0
72–107	Cum. fertility (15–39)	5.3	5.1	+0.2	5.2	5.3	−0.1

Data sources: 1994 Matlab Demographic and Health Survey (MDHS); Matlab Demographic Surveillance System (DSS)
Note: "Total fertility" (15–49) is defined here as five multiplied by the sum of age-specific fertility rates, ages 15–49. "Cumulative fertility" (15–39) is defined as five multiplied by the sum of age-specific fertility rates, ages 15–39. "Total fertility" is in quotes because it was calculated only for the women who met the inclusion criterion for the present validation analysis, i.e., women who had given birth in the DSS within the 15 years before the survey

Differentials in displacement of births in time were explored according to the sex of the live birth, survival status at the time of the survey, and number of months before the survey. Birth and pregnancy histories performed similarly with respect to displacement according to each of those characteristics. Overall, female births were more likely to be displaced than male births;

Table 5 Percent of matched live births that are backward displaced, reported correctly, or forward displaced relative to the actual date, mean displacement (in months), and percent displaced according to two covariates, by questionnaire type

Variable and category	Questionnaire type		
	Both types	Birth history	Pregnancy history
Number of matched births (N)	5356	2636	2720
Percent displaced			
Backward displaced (i.e. reported too old)	28.5	27.9	29.2
Reported correctly	43.9	43.9	43.9
Forward displaced (i.e., reported too young)	27.6	28.2	26.9
Mean number of months displaced			
Backward displaced	−15.6	−15.2	−16.1
Forward displaced	+15.5	+15.5	+15.4
Percent displaced by characteristic of the event			
Survival status at time of interview			
Alive	53.9	54.0	53.8
Dead	71.7	72.3	71.2
Number of months before survey			
0–59	27.6	26.6	28.7
60–119	63.0	64.0	62.1
120–179	76.1	75.7	76.6

however, this differential was not statistically significant (not shown). There was, however, a striking observation in terms of displacement according to survival status (Table 5). The date of birth was displaced for 72 % of matched live births that later died, compared with 54 % of matched live births that were still alive at the time of the survey ($p < 0.05$). There was also a strong and significant relationship between displacement and the number of months since the child was born. Twenty-eight percent of live births that occurred 0–59 months before the survey were displaced, compared with 63 and 76 % of live births occurring 60–119 and 120–179 months before the survey, respectively ($p < 0.05$).

Pregnancy histories have a higher proportion of deaths correctly reported within the age ranges for early neonatal, neonatal, and infant mortality. However, the difference was only significant for infant deaths. Ninety-seven percent of 157 matched infant deaths in the pregnancy history sample were reported within the correct age range, compared with only 90 % of 126 matched infant deaths in the birth history sample ($p = 0.015$). Corresponding estimates for neonatal deaths were 94 and 90 % in the pregnancy history and birth history samples, respectively; for early neonatal deaths, the corresponding values were 93 and 89 %, respectively (Table 6).

Regarding heaping of age at death (on month 12 for infant deaths and month 1 for neonatal deaths), birth histories had a higher percentage of infant deaths heaped on month 12 than did pregnancy histories (4 and 1 %, respectively; $p = 0.07$). The two types of maternity history were virtually identical with respect to the percentage of matched neonatal deaths heaped on month 1 (3.6 vs. 3.7 %) (not shown).

Data quality is a concern in any data collection undertaking, and over the decades, demographers have examined quality of data from various population-based surveys. Most tests of data quality are either reliability

Table 6 Percent of matched death events reported within the correct age range in the MDHS

Age group of death (in DSS) and measure	Questionnaire type		
	Both types	Birth history	Pregnancy history
Infant deaths			
Number of matched events	283	126	157
Percent reported in correct age range*	93.6	89.7	96.8
Neonatal deaths			
Number of matched events	172	76	96
Percent reported in correct age range	91.9	89.5	93.8
Early neonatal deaths			
Number of matched events	120	52	68
Percent reported in correct age range	90.8	88.5	92.6

*$p < 0.05$ for the test of equality of proportions between birth and pregnancy histories

tests, tests against some known pattern, or comparisons with one or more other sources. One example is tests of age heaping (e.g., when ages ending in 0 or 5 are over-represented). Very few such tests can actually document the validity of the collected data. Thus, demographic surveillance systems offer a unique opportunity to assess the validity of birth and pregnancy history data collected in the manner of a typical DHS survey, the primary source of national fertility, and child mortality estimates in many less-developed countries.

Our three study hypotheses concerning comparable validity of birth and pregnancy histories were generally supported by the data. The "total fertility" measures calculated after matching cases on an individual level were accurate for both birth and pregnancy histories, and the small differences between the survey and gold standard estimates are fairly consistent with what was observed in a previous area-level validation [8] that also used the 1994 MDHS. Results for aggregate measures in the present analysis differed from the results presented in the earlier analysis by Bairagi et al. [8] because the present analysis includes data from a specific sample of women who met the inclusion criteria for this validation analysis, (i.e., they had a birth recorded in the DSS in the 15 years before the survey and did not out-migrate during that period) while the aggregate measures in the previous analyses were area-level measures with all women from the MDHS (and DSS) included.

When calculating woman years for the age-specific birth rates, the present analysis used the DSS maternal date of birth for women less than 28 years of age, not the reported (MDHS) date of birth. Only younger women born in the DSS area had known date of birth, so we could not assess the effect of misreporting of

women's ages for all women. Our analysis of a possible contamination effect was based on women's reported ages and dates of birth and suggests that there are some inaccuracies in age and date of birth reporting. However, we expect that inaccuracies of maternal age reporting would only have a minor effect on the results.

Both birth and pregnancy histories were close to perfect in terms of the completeness of live birth reports; completeness rates were 99 %. The regression analysis showed, however, that when adjusting for the survival status of the child, maternal age at the time of interview, and parity—three factors observed to have a strong, statistically significant association with live birth omission in this analysis—the odds of a missed live birth were two times higher if a birth history was used rather than a pregnancy history. Also for infant deaths, use of a birth history led to significantly more of these being reported at 12 months (and thus outside the interval for infant deaths) than was true for the pregnancy history. Therefore, for estimation of infant and child mortality, a pregnancy history is preferred.

Although a pregnancy history is a natural, chronological account of all pregnancies, it will take longer to administer than a birth history because of the additional level of information being asked and recorded. Also, a pregnancy history is more delicate to administer than a birth history since women may not want to discuss pregnancy losses. For example, in contexts where abortion is illegal and/or stigmatized, such pregnancy terminations may be difficult to disclose to an interviewer.

Because no previous individual-level validation studies have included both birth and pregnancy histories within the same study, there is no frame of reference against which our findings can be compared. The previous validation study conducted by Becker and Mahmud [3] in Matlab compared the validity of fertility information collected in backward and forward pregnancy histories. That study also documented completeness rates of about 98 % for live births in both backward and forward pregnancy histories.

There is no significant advantage of one type of maternity history over the other in terms of the time placement of live births. For births that were not correctly placed in time, displacement was symmetric; that is, equal proportions of live births were backward displaced and forward displaced. This finding is contrary to results of previous assessments in which there was a documented greater tendency for backward displacement of live births [3, 27, 28]. The present study does, however, corroborate findings from other assessments in terms of the significantly greater time displacement for births that later died, compared with current survivors [2, 29]. This latter observation might warrant further consideration in contexts with high rates of infant and under-five mortality.

Completeness was lower for deaths earlier during the first year of life. In addition, unlike the comparability of birth and pregnancy histories in terms of fertility estimation, when the priority is on measuring mortality within the first year of life, a pregnancy history is the better instrument to use. Deaths are more likely to be omitted in surveys than are surviving children, and this study shows this pattern with the lowest completeness rates for children who died in the early neonatal period. The poorer performance of both types of histories in capturing deaths that occurred during the first month of life is particularly salient given the increased global attention being paid to neonatal health and survival [30–32].

Regarding generalizability of this study's findings, a number of factors need to be considered. First, long-term exposure of DSS residents to demographic surveillance and public health interventions could render the DSS population quite different from other populations in terms of the recall and reporting of information in a survey. However, in our analyses, only one of three indicators of such potential "contamination" showed evidence of such an effect—98 % of births had complete date information in the DSS area versus 91 % in the adjacent non-DSS villages. Though significant, this is not a major difference that would render the DSS population unique relative to other populations. As a result, the study's findings are likely to be applicable to other contexts, at least within rural Bangladesh. It is important to note that validation studies like this can only be done where demographic surveillance has been in place for a number of years.

Migration is another consideration. This analysis excluded all out-migrants from the DSS including those who returned at a later time. This is not customary for standard analyses of fertility and mortality using population-based surveys. Although one may argue that this exclusion introduces a selection bias, 88 % of all MDHS respondents with any DSS records met the criterion of no out-migration from the DSS area during the 15-year reference period for the analysis. (Note that migration between villages within the DSS area did not pose a problem because of the unique identification numbers that are used.) Thus, migration probably does not pose a significant threat to the generalizability of our findings.

It is now possible to conduct validation studies like this one in other sites. In particular, any of the INDEPTH sites with complete and continuous registration of births and deaths for 15 or more years could undertake a similar study [33]. The Navrongo site in Ghana is such an example. We recommend that such studies be done soon after a national DHS survey so the same interviewers can be employed, thus controlling for interviewer effects, which can sometimes be substantial in magnitude. Further validation research conducted in different populations representing different demographic scenarios (e.g., different levels and patterns of fertility, mortality, and migration) can provide additional insights on the best way to collect demographic data in surveys.

The ideal data collection system for estimation of fertility and mortality is a vital registration system, but the cost of such a system is prohibitive for many developing countries. The alternative in many countries is a DHS, which includes a full birth history questionnaire that can produce data to estimate fertility and infant and child mortality. There has been a recent movement toward demographic data collection with faster turnaround than the typical DHS. In this vein, mobile phones are now being used by local enumerators to collect questionnaire data in some countries; this platform has been shown to provide results in a much more timely fashion than a DHS [34].

Conclusions

Birth and pregnancy histories are comparable in terms of their completeness of live-birth reports. However, because birth histories are associated with a higher degree of age of death heaping at 12 months, resulting in the exclusion of deaths that should be included in infant mortality calculations, a pregnancy history is the preferred tool for estimating infant mortality. The lower completeness of neonatal and early neonatal death reporting in both types of histories is salient given the importance of neonatal survival as a global priority. Our study's findings are likely to be applicable to other contexts, at least within rural Bangladesh, although validation studies of this nature can only be done where demographic surveillance has been in place for a number of years.

Competing interests

The authors declare that they have no competing interests.

Author Contributions

DE carried out the field research, conducted the analysis, and was the lead writer of the manuscript. SB supported methodological design, reviewed findings from the analysis, and contributed to preparation of the manuscript. All authors read and approved the final manuscript.
Donna Espeut is an independent researcher, New York, USA.

Acknowledgements

The authors would like to acknowledge Dr. Radheshyam Bairagi, Mr. Delowar Hussain, and the Demographic Surveillance System staff at the International Centre for Diarrhoeal Disease Research, Bangladesh (ICDDR,B), as well as Mr. Keith Purvis of ICF Macro at the time of the field work, for their data management assistance during the preliminary stages of the analysis.

The 1994 Matlab Demographic and Health Survey (MDHS) was conducted by Mitra and Associates, on behalf of the National Institute for Population Research and Training, Bangladesh. Mr. S.N. Mitra of Mitra and Associates provided the authors with additional information pertaining to data collection (e.g., background characteristics of MDHS interviewers) required for the analysis.

The matching process and certain portions of the analysis could only be accomplished in Bangladesh. Bangladesh-based work was funded through a Mellon Foundation grant to the Population Studies Center at the Johns Hopkins University School of Hygiene and Public Health.

Sources of support: Mellon Foundation, Population Center, Johns Hopkins University.

References

1. Cleland J. Demographic data collection in less developed countries 1946–1996. Pop Studies. 1996;50(3):433–50.
2. Demographic and Health Survey (DHS) Program. Information available at www.dhsprogram.com.
3. Becker S, Mahmud S. A validation study of backward and forward pregnancy histories in Matlab, Bangladesh. International Statistical Institute, 1984. (World Fertility Survey Scientific Reports 52).
4. Pullum T, Becker S. Evidence of omission and displacement in DHS birth histories. Rockville, MD: ICF International; 2014 (*Methodological Report 11*).
5. Johnson K, Grant M, Khan S, Moore Z, Armstrong A, Sa Z. Fieldwork-related factors and data quality in the Demographic and Health Surveys Program. Calverton, MD: ICF Macro; 2009. DHS Analytical Studies No. 19.
6. Hill K, Choi Y. Neonatal mortality in the developing world. Demogr Res. 2006;14(18):429–52.
7. Becker S, Diop-Sidibe N. Does use of the calendar in surveys reduce heaping? Stud Fam Plann. 2003;34(2):127–32.
8. Bairagi R, Becker S, Kantner A, Allen KB, Datta A, Purvis K. An evaluation of the 1993–94 Bangladesh Demographic and Health Survey within the Matlab area. Honolulu, HI: East–west Center, Program on Population; 1997. Asia-Pacific Population Research Reports No. 11.
9. Curtis SL. Assessment of the quality of data used for direct estimation of infant and child mortality in DHS-II surveys. Calverton, Maryland: Macro International Inc.; 1995 (Occasional Papers No. 3).
10. Macro International Inc. An assessment of the quality of health data in DHS I Surveys. Calverton, Maryland: Macro International Inc.; 1994.
11. Demographic and Health Surveys Program. An assessment of DHS-I data quality. Columbia, MD: IRD/Macro Systems; 1990. Methodological Report #1.
12. Stanton C. Perinatal mortality in the Philippines: an investigation into the use of demographic survey data for the study of perinatal mortality and its determinants. Baltimore: The Johns Hopkins University School of Hygiene and Public Health; 1995 (Dissertation).
13. Garenne M. Do women forget births? A study of maternity histories in a rural area of Senegal (Niakhar). Popul Bull UN. 1994;36:43–54.
14. Becker S, Sosa D. An experiment using a month-by-month calendar in a family planning survey in Costa Rica. Stud Fam Plann. 1992;23(6):386–291.
15. Chidambaram VC, Cleland JG, Goldman N, Rutstein S. An assessment of the quality of WFS demographic data. In: Hill AG, Brass W, editors. The analysis of maternity histories. Liege: Editions Derouaux-Ordina; 1992. p. 183–215.
16. Arnold F. Assessment of the quality of birth history data in the Demographic and Health Surveys. Columbia: IRC/Macro International Inc.; 1990 (Methodological Reports I: An Assessment of DHS-I Data Quality).
17. Westoff CF, Goldman N, Moreno L. Dominican Republic Experimental Study: an evaluation of fertility and child health information. Columbia, MD: Institute for Resource Development/Macro Systems Inc.; 1990.
18. Singh S. Evaluation of data quality. In: Cleland J, Scott C, editors. The World Fertility Survey: An Assessment. Oxford: Oxford University Press; 1987. p. 618–43. DHS Methodological Reports No. 5.
19. Pullum T. An assessment of age and date reporting in the DHS surveys, 1985–2003. Calverton, MD: Macro International Inc.; 2006.
20. Cleland J, Johnson-Acsadi G, Marckwardt A. Cleland J, Scott C, editors. The world fertility survey: an assessment. Oxford: Oxford University Press, 987:31–75.
21. Mostafa G, MA Kashem Shaikh, K Ahmed, and JK van Ginneken. Demographic surveillance system—Matlab, volume twenty-five: registration of demographic events—1994. Scientific Report No. 77, October 1996.
22. Mitra SN, Ali MN, Islam S, Cross AR, Saha T. Bangladesh Demographic and Health Survey 1993–1994. Calverton, MD: National Institute of Population Research and Training, Mitra and Associates, and Macro International Inc.; 1994.
23. ISSA. Integrated System for Survey Analysis: Version 2.28. Calverton, MD: Macro International; 1995.
24. SPSS Inc. Released 1999. SPSS for Windows, Version 9.0. Chicago, SPSS Inc.
25. StataCorp. Stata Statistical Software: Release 6.0. College Station, TX: StataCorp LP; 1999.
26. Phillips JF, Stinson WS, Bhatia S, Rahman M, Chakraborty J. The demographic impact of the Family Planning—Health Services Project in Matlab, Bangladesh. Stud Fam Plann. 1982;13(5):131–40.
27. Arnold F. An assessment of data quality in the Demographic and Health Surveys. Demographic and Health Surveys World Conference—Proceedings, Volume II. Columbia, MD: IRD/Macro International Inc.; 1991.
28. Bairagi R, Aziz KMA, Chowdhury MK, Edmonston B. Age misstatement for young children in rural Bangladesh. Demography. 1982;19(4):447–58.
29. Marckwardt AM, Rutstein SO. Accuracy of DHS-II demographic data: Gains and losses in comparison with earlier surveys. Calverton, MD: Macro International Inc.; 1996 (DHS Working Papers No. 19).
30. Rajaratnam JK, Marcus JR, Flaxman AD, Wang H, Levin-Rector A, Dwyer L, et al. Neonatal, postneonatal, childhood, and under-5 mortality for 187 countries, 1970–2010: a systematic analysis of progress towards Millennium Development Goal 4. Lancet. 2010;375:1988–2008.
31. Oza S, Cousens SN, Lawn JE. Estimation of daily risk of neonatal death, including the day of birth, in 186 countries in 2013: a vital-registration and modelling-based study. Lancet Glob Health. 2014;2:e635–44.
32. McKinnon B, Harper S, Kaufman JS, Bergevin Y. Socioeconomic inequality in neonatal mortality in countries of low and middle income: a multicountry analysis. Lancet Glob Health. 2014;2:e165–173.
33. Sankoh OA, Kahn K, Mwageni E, Ngom P, Nyarko P, editors. (INDEPTH Network). Population and health in developing countries. Volume 1: population, health and survival at INDEPTH sites. Ottawa, Canada: IDRC; 2002.
34. Zimmerman L, Olaolorun F, Radloff. S. Accelerating and improving survey implementation with mobile technology: lessons from PMA2020 implementation in Lagos, Nigeria. African Population Studies (forthcoming).

5

Groundwater arsenic and education attainment in Bangladesh

Michael P. Murray[1*] and Raisa Sharmin[2]

Abstract

Background: Thousands of groundwater tube wells serving millions of Bangladeshis are arsenic contaminated. This study investigates the effect of these wells on the education attainment and school attendance of youths who rely on those wells for drinking water.

Methods: The analysis combines data from the 2006 Bangladesh Multiple Indicator Cluster Survey (2006 MICS) and the National Hydrochemical Survey (NHS) of Bangladeshi tube wells' contamination conducted between 1998 and 2000. The study uses multiple regression analysis to estimate the differences in education attainment and school attendance among the following: (i) youths who live where tube wells are safe, (ii) youths who live where tube wells are unsafe but who report drinking from an arsenic-free source, and (iii) youths who live where tube wells are unsafe but who do not report drinking from an arsenic-free source.

Results: Controlling for other determinants of education attainment and school attendance, young Bangladeshi males who live where tube wells are unsafe (by Bangladeshis standards) but who report drinking from arsenic-free sources are found to have the same education attainment (among 19- to 21-year-olds) and school attendance (among 6- to 10-year-olds), on average, as corresponding young Bangladeshi males who live where wells are safe. But young Bangladeshi males who live where tube wells are unsafe and who do not report drinking from an arsenic-free source attain, on average, a half-year less education (among 19- to 21-year-olds) and attend school, on average, five to seven fewer days a year (among 6- to 10-year-olds) than do other Bagladeshi males of those ages. The estimated effects for females are of the same sign but much smaller in magnitude.

Conclusion: Bangladeshi public health measures to shift drinking from unsafe to safe wells not only advance good health but also increase males' education attainment.

Keywords: Arsenic, Education, Groundwater, Bangladesh

Background

While groundwater arsenic has plagued many countries, including Argentina, Mexico, India, Nepal, the USA, and Vietnam [1], in Bangladesh, the problem has been called "the largest poisoning of a population in history" [2–4].

Arsenic poisoning is calamitous. The World Health Organization (WHO) reports that drinking arsenic-contaminated water on a regular basis increases the risk of numerous cancers and can lead to skin pigmentation changes and hyperkeratosis [5]. Drinking from arsenic-contaminated tube wells has chronically poisoned millions of Bangladeshis; building on Sohel et al. [6] and

Flanagan et al. [7] estimated in 2012 that in Bangladesh over 40.000 deaths per year are due to arsenic poisoning. According to Chen et al. [8], arsenic-contaminated drinking water more than doubled Bangladeshi's lifetime mortality risk from cancers of the liver, bladder, and lung (229.6 vs 103.5 per 100,000 population).

Extensive reviews are available for studies of the physical, neurological, social, and psychological consequences of arsenicosis in Bangladesh (e.g., [1, 9, 10]). The literature, however, appears mute on arsenic's effects on education attainment. Education generally increases lifetime earnings, with primary school education having the largest return [11, 12]. Moreover, greater education attainment by a country's population has been found to spur economic growth [13–15]. Given the economic importance of

* Correspondence: mmurray@bates.edu
[1]Department of Economics, Bates College, Lewiston, ME 04240, USA
Full list of author information is available at the end of the article

education, it seems worth asking whether the physio-logical effects and social stigma associated with drinking arsenic-contaminated water reduce education attainment for those who grow up drinking such water. In this paper, we report our estimates of the effects of drinking arsenic-contaminated water on both primary school attendance by young Bangladeshi boys and total years of education completed by young Bangladeshi males.

Children are struck especially hard by arsenic poison-ing. Given this study's focus on school attendance and education attainment, neurological and social effects of arsenicosis are particularly pertinent as reduced cogni-tive capacity inhibits education attainment, and shun-ning by peers could discourage school attendance.

Studies have established adverse effects of arsenic on children's verbal comprehension, long-term memory [16], attention [16], cognitive development [17, 18], neurobehav-ioral development such as pattern memory and switching attention [19], and intelligence [20, 22]. Asadullah and Chaudhury [17] find significant effects of arsenic on math-ematics scores for Bangladeshi children. According to Chowdhury et al. [23] and Khandoker et al. [24], victims of lesions and blemishes frequently experience being ostra-cized and shunned within their families and local commu-nities, even to the extent of being excluded from marriage. Nasreen [25] provides several case studies of the adverse social effects of arsenicosis in Bangladesh.

Millions of groundwater wells were installed in Bangladesh from the 1970s onward [8], for the most part with funds from international agencies, with the goal of ending reliance on unsanitary surface water for drinking [26]. That a million or more of these wells were arsenic contaminated was long unknown [2–4, 27]. Esti-mates in the late 1990s [28, 29] revealed that some 35 mil-lion Bangladeshis were drinking their water from seriously contaminated wells. Subsequent efforts by the Bangladeshi government to alert households to the threat of arsenic-contaminated tube wells has reduced the proportion of the population drinking from such wells, but the number has remained high—the Bangladesh Bureau of Statistics and the United Nations Children's Fund [30] have esti-mated that 12.5 % of Bangladeshis, or 20 million people, still regularly drank arsenic-contaminated water in 2012–2013. An extensive literature assessing efforts to reduce arsenic poisoning has developed (e.g., [19] [31–34]).

The progress made by Bangladesh in reducing house-holds' reliance on arsenic-contaminated wells is evident in Table 1 which presents Bangladeshis' exposure to various levels of arsenic in their drinking water in 2000, 2009, and 2012–2013. In 2000, 42.1 % of wells had above the 10 parts per billion (ppb) arsenic that the World Health Organization deems the upper limit for safe drinking water [35]. Of wells, 24.9 % were above the Bangladesh safety limit of 50 ppb [17]. By 2012–2013, 24.8 % of

Table 1 Drinking water arsenic contamination exposure

Arsenic level (ppb)	Wells % above 2000[a]	Households % above level[b] 2009	Households % above level[c] 2012	Male youths % above level[d] 2006
10	48	32	24.8	62
50	25	13.4	12.5	34
100	16	6.2	–	18
200	9	3.4	2.8	8
300	5.1	1.8	–	2

ppb parts per billion
[a]Source: [27], Table 6.7
[b]Source: [7], Table 1
[c]Source: [29], Table WQ.2
[d]Authors' calculations from 2006 MICS and NHS data

households were found to be drinking water above the 10-ppb limit and 12.5 % above the 50-ppb limit.[1] Argos et al. [36] estimate that drinking groundwater containing more than 150 ppb of arsenic causes almost a doubling of mor-talities from all causes. Flanagan et al. [8] estimate that the percentage of households exposed to such a high level of arsenic was 8.9 % in 2000 and 4.8 % in 2009.

There is a regional variation in Bangladesh's ground-water arsenic levels. Contamination is greatest in the south and southeast of the country and least in the northwest and in north-central Bangladesh [28]. How-ever, highly contaminated groundwater has been found in some locales in the generally low-arsenic regions of northern Bangladesh [28]. In 2009 and 2012–2013, con-tamination rates in rural areas were about double than those in cities [30, 37].

Methods
Data and sampling
We relied on two publicly available data sets: (i) the 2006 Bangladesh Multiple Indicator Cluster Survey (2006 MICS) that was carried out by the Bangladesh Bureau of Statistics and UNICEF [37] and which has been cited as an example of "good practice" for inter-national data collection [38], and (ii) the oft-cited National Hydrochemical Survey (NHS) of wells con-ducted between 1998 and 2000 by the Department of Public Health Engineering of Bangladesh in consultation with the British Geological Survey [28].

The 2006 MICS is a nationally representative, ran-domly sampled, household survey with a response rate of 92.5 % [37]. The survey provides data on household socio-economic variables, including the head's and each individual's education attainment, local environment questions such as proximity of the household to indus-trial pollution sources, and questions specifically about local well-water arsenic contamination.

The NHS provided chemical test results for 3534 bore-holes from 61 of Bangladesh's 64 districts. The goal of the NHS was a random sample of tube wells, but logistical problems barred fully realizing this ideal [28]. The NHS reports surveyed well locations at the village level. We aggregated the arsenic levels to the sub-district level, the finest geographic detail available in the 2006 MICS data. Sub-districts in Bangladesh average about 150 km²., or 60 mi². Districts average 2300 km² or 890 mi². We designated as 'unsafe' sub-districts with average NHS well-water arsenic levels above Bangladesh's 50 ppb standard; we designated all other districts 'safe'.

Choosing a sub-sample of individuals to study for arsenic's effects on years of education required judgment. Tube wells were far from ubiquitous in Bangladesh in the late 1970s and early 1980s. Schoenfeld [33] found some urban areas in which under 40 % of households used tube wells in 1977, and clinical reports of physical effects did not begin until the early 1980s [2, 3, 27]. Thus, we did not know exactly which birth cohorts were fully exposed to the groundwater arsenic levels measured in the NHS. Estimates of arsenic's effects based upon individuals born before the general use of tube wells would underestimate those effects, but estimates based upon individuals too young would miss the full effect of arsenic on education. We estimated, by sex, well-water arsenic's effects on education attainment for youths who were aged 19 through 21 when sampled for the 2006 MICS, i.e., individuals born between 1985 and 1987. Of these ages, there were 7451 males and 9270 females in the 2006 MICS; one seventh of these youths were in sub-districts for which we had no tube well data and were therefore omitted from our analysis.

We chose individuals born between 1985 and 1987 for two reasons. First, the first clinical reports of arsenic poisoning occurred about this time [2, 27]; older individuals might have not felt the full impact of the growing number of arsenic-contaminated tube wells. Second, only 20 % of the sampled individuals between 19 and 21 years of age reported being in school and less than 7 % of the 22-year-olds reported being in school, so by age 19, most of arsenic's adverse effects on education had occurred.

Matching young men and women to the wells they drank from since childhood is not exact since where they lived in 2006 might not be where they lived for most of their childhoods. This source of measurement error looms largest for young adults who have moved from their parents' home because such individuals might well have moved away from their childhood sub-district. To reduce the attenuation bias from such measurement problems, we restricted attention to 19–21-year-olds who still lived with their parents. In the 2006 MICS, 80 % of the 19–21-year-olds still lived with their parents.

The Bangladeshi school system required school enrollment through grade V, which corresponds to ages 6 through 10. We examined, by sex, whether drinking arsenic-contaminated water affected school attendance of children aged 6 to 10 in 2006 when they were sampled for the 2006 MICS.

Key variables

This study focused attention on four variables: (i) an individual's years of education attained, (ii) the number of school days a child attended in the past week, (iii) whether the sub-district in which an individual lived in 2005 had safe or unsafe groundwater, and (iv) whether an individual was reported by the survey respondent to drink from an arsenic-free source (which we shall refer to as 'the individual drinks safely'). The NHS provided arsenic levels; the 2006 MICS provided the other three variables. The first two variables are integer valued; the second two are dummy variables.

Due to lack of extensive household-specific, year-by-year, data on the consumption of arsenic-contaminated water in Bangladesh, we of necessity measured exposure to arsenic-contaminated water by the average contamination level of local tube wells sampled in the 1998–2000 NHS. This 1998–2000 data was quite pertinent for several reasons. First, the natural hydrological traits of wells change little over time [39, 40]; we concluded from this that local tube well contamination was relatively stable from the mid- to late 1980s through 2006. Second, the 19–21-year-olds, whose total years of education by 2006 we studied, and the 6–10 year olds, whose school attendance we studied, grew up between 1985 and 2006, which were mostly years in which relatively few households were adjusting their behavior to avoid contaminated wells [33].

Control variables

Drinking arsenic-contaminated water is certainly not the only determinant of education attainment. Our multiple regression analysis controls for the well-known major determinants of education attainment. Mare [41] established that in the USA, the number of one's siblings, local-area economic conditions, and one's parents' financial resources and education are key determinants of a child's education attainment. More recently, Li et al. [42] and Huang [43] have confirmed these findings in a developing country context. Holmes [44] further established the importance of local wage and employment opportunities for decisions about continued schooling. We constructed six groups of control variables from the 2006 MICS data specific to our concern about arsenic contamination and other potential health threats:

1. Contamination awareness and avoidance: survey respondents reported whether they had heard of the well-water arsenic problem and whether they drank from arsenic-free sources.

2. Wealth/income indicators: (a) the household's z-score in the 2006 national distribution of wealth, (b) the square of the household's wealth z-score, (c) the household head's education level (seven categories), (d) the mean wealth z-score across sampled households in the sub-district in which the individual lives, and (e) the standard deviation of wealth z-scores for sampled households in the sub-district in which the individual lives. We view the mean and standard deviation of local wealth as indicating local income opportunities that compete with school for individuals' time.

3. Family circumstances, including the education of the household head and the number of other children competing for the households' resources.

4. Local environs indicators. Whether the sampled dwelling was as follows: (a) in a flood-prone area, (b) in a landslide-prone area, (c) located near industrial pollution, and (d) located near a garbage pile.

5. Housing security indicators: (a) did the respondent report security from eviction and (b) was the household squatting.

6. Indicator variables, one for each district, used to indicate where a household was located at the time of the survey.

We included in our regression models all the control variables in items 1–6, plus the individual's age reported in the 2006 MICS. Separate measures of mother's and father's education are available in too few cases to support regression analysis; we instead use the education of the household head to capture parental education. We also do not have a count of the number of siblings a child has. To proxy for the number of siblings, we use for youths 19–21 the number of other youths in the household, and for children 6–10 the number of other children in the household 0–16 years of age.

In our regression analyses, approximately 10 % of cases from the 2006 MICS were lost due to missing values on control variables.

Statistical analysis

We employed ordinary least squares (OLS) multiple regression analysis [45] to estimate the effects of tube wells' arsenic contamination on school attendance of 13,556 six- to ten-year-olds and on the education attainment of 4511 nineteen- to twenty-one-year-olds. To infer causal relationships from observational data, as opposed to experimental data, suitable controls were required for potentially confounding variables. Multiple regression allowed inclusion of such controls in our analysis.

Multiple regression has long been used for analyzing education attainment, dating back to at least 1980 [41] and has more recently been employed for such studies

in developing country contexts (e.g., [42–44]). For this paper, summary and regression statistics were all calculated using the regression routines of STATA 12™. The regression models all included dummy variables (binary zero-one variables) for the sub-district in which an individual lived in 2006. With many individuals in each sub-district, the regression disturbance terms were likely to be correlated within districts. The estimated standard errors we employed in the regressions accounted for this clustering of observations by sub-district [46].

Results

Bangladeshis in the 2006 MICS had generally completed their educations by age 21; only 6.8 % of the sampled Bangladeshi 22-year-olds reported still being in school. The average years of education of the sampled 22-year-olds was 7.4 years, with little difference between males and females. In 2005, on average, sampled primary school children attended school 5.3 out of 6 days per week, again with little difference between males and females.

Table 1 reveals that young Bangladeshis in the 2006 MICS tended to live in areas with somewhat greater than average arsenic exposure, although somewhat less often in the most affected areas. In 2006, almost two thirds of the sampled Bangladeshis aged 21 or less lived in communities in which the average well's arsenic level exceeded the WHO standard of 10 ppb or less [35]. Over a third of young Bangladeshis lived in communities in which the average well's arsenic level exceeded Bangladesh's own safe water standard of 50 ppb arsenic or less [20]; and 13 % lived in communities in which the average tube's well-water contained 150 ppb arsenic or more, which is the level Argos et al. [36] associate with a near doubling of all-causes mortality. The third of the sampled young Bangladeshis living in sub-districts with on-average unsafe well-water were, on average, exposed to arsenic levels of 145 ppb in their sub-district's well-water.

Authors' computations from the 2006 MICS and the NHS reveal that youths in households with a head who had completed primary schooling were 1.1 % more likely to live in communities with on-average unsafe drinking water than household heads with less education. (We designated as "unsafe" sub-districts with average NHS well-water arsenic levels above Bangladesh's 50 ppb standard; we designated all other districts "safe.") Perhaps surprisingly, youths in households with a head who had greater than median wealth were 4.8 % more likely to be exposed to arsenic-contaminated water than youths whose household heads had less than median wealth. Given the large sample size of the 2006 MICS, these computed differences are statistically significant at all conventional significance levels. Given these differences in education and wealth, simple comparisons of the mean education attainment between youths in safe and unsafe drinking water communities will reflect not only the effects of arsenic but also the effects of differences in parental wealth and, to a lesser degree, education.

Awareness of the arsenic problem was quite high among households sampled in the 2006 MICS, as evidenced by Table 2. In general, both awareness of the arsenic problem and reported reliance on arsenic-free sources rose with the local level of arsenic in wells. (Again, all of the differences in the table are statistically significant.) This pattern is unsurprising since the government focused its policy efforts on the most at-risk areas, and, the greater the risk, the more reason for people to "spread the word" about the problem.

Table 2 also reveals that decisions to drink safely in unsafe sub-districts differed sharply with both parental education and wealth. Among sampled children living in sub-districts with unsafe water, those whose household heads had completed primary school drank safely 16.4 % more often than the sampled children whose household heads had less education, and those whose households had above-median wealth drank safely 15.5 % more often than the sampled children from less wealthy households. Simple comparisons of the mean education attainment between those who drank safely in the unsafe districts and those who did not reflect not just differences in arsenic consumption but also differences in parental education and wealth. To reliably estimate the causal effects of arsenic using the 2006 MICS data, one must control for parental wealth and education.

Table 3 summarizes the education attainment of the sampled Bangladeshi youths aged 19 to 21 and the attendance patterns for sampled Bangladeshi children age 6–10 in this nationally representative sample. Our interest is in whether drinking from arsenic-contaminated wells results in a lower number of years of education attained and/or in fewer days of school attended in the

Table 2 Parental arsenic awareness and youths drinking safely

Percentage of youths with parents who in 2006 reported of having heard of arsenic problem	
Safe dub-districts[a]	72.7 %
Unsafe sub-districts[b]	92.9 %
Total	79.6 %
Percentage of youths in unsafe sub-districts who in 2006 were reported to drink safely	
Head did not complete primary school	50.2 %
Head completed primary school	66.6 %
Below-median wealth	47.0 %
Above-median wealth	65.5 %
Total	56.9 %

[a]Safe means tube well arsenic content in sub-district is ≤50 ppb
[b]Unsafe means tube well arsenic content in sub-district is >50 ppb

Table 3 Education attainment and school attendance in 2006 for young bangladeshis

Age	Males Avg. years ed.	Males % in school	Females Avg. years educ.	Females % in school
15	5.96	53.2	6.70	56.2
16	6.48	45.3	7.16	45.2
17	6.96	42.0	7.40	32.2
18	6.87	29.4	7.35	23.2
19	7.51	23.3	7.49	17.7
20	7.19	22.0	7.38	12.7
21	7.91	24.3	7.39	11.7

Age	Boys 6–10 Avg. days attended last week	Girls 6–10 Avg. days attended last week
6–10	5.26	5.32

Mean education attainment in 2006 for youths 19–21	
Safe sub-districts	7.92 years
Unsafe sub-districts	7.82 years

Mean education attainment in 2006 for youths 19–21 in unsafe sub-districts	
Reported to drink safely	8.25 years
Not reported to drink safely	7.18 years

Source: Authors' calculations from 2006 MICS

past week. We estimate the effect of drinking arsenic-contaminated water by comparing three groups of sampled individuals: (i) individuals who lived in sub-districts with safe groundwater, (ii) individuals who lived in sub-districts with unsafe groundwater who report drinking from arsenic-free sources, and (iii) individuals who lived in sub-districts with unsafe groundwater who did not report drinking from arsenic-free sources.

Education was compulsory for 6- to 10-year-olds; we focus on the school attendance of these children. For older youths, our concern is with their ultimate years of education attained. Since school participation rates were still nearly 30 % or higher for youths younger than 19, we choose to focus primarily on youths 19–21.

Table 3 summarizes the mean education attainment by the sampled 19–21-year-olds in sub-districts with safe water and in sub-districts with unsafe water. Table 3 also reports, for the sampled 19–21-year-olds who lived in the unsafe sub-districts, their mean education attainment was broken down by whether the youth drank safely or not. These data offer seemingly conflicting stories about how arsenic affects education attainment. Between safe and unsafe districts, the mean education attainment differed by 0.09 years. Since 40 % of the sampled youths in unsafe districts drank unsafely and 60 % drank safely, the 0.09 difference implies that those who drank unsafely averaged 0. 225 (i.e., 0.09/0.4) fewer years of education than others—groundwater arsenic seems to have mattered only modestly. But on average, the sampled youths in the unsafe sub-districts who drank safely attained 1.07 more years of education than their sampled neighbors who drank instead from contaminated sources—groundwater arsenic seems to have mattered quite a lot.

The seeming conundrum arises because differences in the mean education attainment reflect not only differing exposure to groundwater arsenic but also differing parental wealth and education (and differences in yet other determinants of education attainment, as well). To resolve the conundrum, we need to control for the multiple determinants of education attainment.

We report in Table 4 regressions of education outcomes on tube well contamination for the sampled males 19–21 years old. These regressions also included controls for parental wealth, parental education, and other likely determinants of education attainment. We do not report results for females because the estimated effects of living in an unsafe sub-district were much smaller in magnitude for females than for males. The smaller effects for females are consonant with the speculation of Asadullah [47] that observed lower levels of arsenic among Bangladeshi females [47, 48] are due to females drinking less per pound of body weight than do males (if this speculation is correct, a given level of a tube well's toxicity is less consequential for local females than for local males).[2]

Our first regression examined how groundwater arsenic affected expected years of education for males between 19 and 21 years of age. The dependent variable

was the years of education attained by 2006. Table 4, column 1 contains estimated coefficients for the dummy variable "unsafe" and for the interaction of "unsafe" with the "drinks safely" dummy (with their robust, clustered standard errors in parentheses). Males living in the unsafe sub-districts are estimated to suffer a loss of one-half of a year of education relative to males who live in the safe sub-districts; males in the unsafe-water sub-districts who drink safely are estimated to experience no such deficit.

Table 5 reports estimates of the covariates' coefficients from the regression reported in column 1 of Table 4. Parental education, parental wealth, and the presence of other youths in the household were all statistically significant with the expected signs. The local mean wealth variable had a statistically significant negative estimated coefficient.

Nearly two thirds of the sampled Bangladeshi youths faced wells with average arsenic exceeding the stricter WHO standard of 10 ppb. Table 4, column 2 reports coefficient estimates for a regression which added a dummy variable indicating an average local arsenic level between 10 and 50 ppb and an interaction between that dummy and the dummy for drinking safely.

Primary school boys' behavior exposed the roots of older boys' reduced schooling due to arsenic. Columns 3 and 4 of Table 4 report regressions with the explanatory variables used for columns 1 and 2, but with the dependent variable "days of school attended in the past week." In Bangladesh's 40-week school year, we estimated that boys who drank from unsafe water sources annually missed 4.8 to 6.9 more school days than did peers who drank safely. The estimated effect of arsenic levels between 10 and 50 ppb was imprecisely measured and statistically insignificant.

Table 5 reports estimates of the covariates' coefficients from the regression reported in column 3 of Table 4. Parental education and parental wealth were statistically significant with the expected signs. The estimated effect of other youths in the household was small and statistically insignificant. The mean and standard deviation of local wealth were jointly significant. The environmental and housing variables were jointly insignificant, though being in a flood-prone area did have a statistically significant negative effect.

Discussion

We employed data from Bangladesh's 1998–2000 National Hydrological Survey and 2006 Multiple Indicator Cluster Survey to estimate the effect of groundwater arsenic on males' education attainment and school attendance in Bangladesh. The former survey provided a large and geographically diverse sample of tube-wells whose arsenic contamination was known. The latter survey

Table 4 Unsafe water's effects on males' years of education (19–21-year-olds) and days of school attended (6–10-year-olds)

Variable	Years of education		Days of school attended	
Regression	1	2	3	4
Unsafe water	−.501[a] (0.134)	−.565[a] (0.167)	−.119[b] (0.053)	−.170[a] (0.067)
Unsafe*drink safe	0.494[a] (0.140)	0.497[a] (0.141)	0.107[c] (0.056)	0.105[c] (0.056)
10–50-ppb arsenic	–	−0.158 (0.150)	–	−0.057 (0.056)
10–50 ppb*drink safe	–	0.140 (0.150)	–	−0.027 (0.053)
R^2	0.3294	0.3296	0.0489	0.0491
# observations	4511	4511	13,556	13,556

Samples: youths in the 2006 MICS with well contaminations from the 1998/2000 NHS
[a]Statistically significant at 0.01 level
[b]Statistically significant at 0.05 level
[c]Statistically significant at 0.10 level

Table 5 Regression 1 and 3 covariates' estimated effects

Variable	Years of education (19–21-year-olds)			Days attended (6–10-year-olds)		
	Coef.	Robust std. err.	t	Coef.	Robust std. err.	t
Household wealth	1.366[a]	0.080	17.18	0.115[a]	0.026	4.41
Household wealth sqd.	−.194[a]	0.032	−6.12	−.031[a]	0.011	−2.75
Number of other youths in hours	−.130[a]	0.024	−5.39	0.001	0.011	0.11
Age	0.099[b]	0.052	1.91	0.055[a]	0.009	6.22
Head primary incomplete	0.247[b]	0.129	1.92	0.098[c]	0.043	2.29
Head primary complete	0.867[a]	0.121	7.17	0.160[a]	0.042	3.84
Head some secondary	1.486[a]	0.126	11.83	0.109[a]	0.042	2.60
Head secondary or more	2.425[a]	0.140	17.31	0.268[a]	0.046	5.87
Head non-std. schooling	−0.527	0.794	−0.66	0.376[a]	0.126	2.99
Head education missing	0.024	0.838	0.03	0.657[a]	0.126	5.23
Heard of arsenic prob.	0.557[a]	0.118	4.75	0.073[b]	0.038	1.92
Mean subdistrict wealth	−.812[a]	0.260	−3.12	−0.154	0.107	−1.44
Std. dev. sub-district wealth	0.202	0.333	0.61	0.018	0.139	0.13
Flood prone	0.224[b]	0.135	1.66	−.118[c]	0.055	−2.13
Garbage pile	−0.059	0.258	−0.23	0.125	0.211	0.60
Landslide prone	−0.570	0.679	−0.84	0.027	0.331	0.08
Industrial pollution	1.359[a]	0.324	4.20	−0.201	0.325	−0.62
Safe from eviction	0.443[c]	0.198	2.23	−0.001	0.055	−0.01
Squatter household	−1.062	0.666	−1.60	−0.092	0.153	−0.60

[a]Statistically significant at 0.01 level
[b]Statistically significant at 0.10 level
[c]Statistically significant at 0.05 level

provided measures of education attainment, school attendance, and myriad control variables, including households' responses to the question "Do you drink from arsenic free sources?" We concluded from our regression analyses of groundwater arsenic's effects on education that, on average, drinking water unsafe by Bangladesh's standards reduces by half a year, on average, a Bangladeshi boys' accumulation of schooling and reduces by 5 to 7 days a year a young Bangladeshi boy's school attendance. Hence, public health measures to shift drinking from unsafe to safe wells not only advance good health but also increase education attainment.

The estimated effect of drinking from Bangladesh-safe but WHO-unsafe wells is negative and of non-trivial magnitude but is quite imprecisely estimated. We are not alone in imprecisely estimating arsenic's effects at low levels. The National Research Council reports that the shape of arsenic's dose response curve for cancer remains unclear for low doses [49].

The regressions also offered a measure of our success in identifying the effects of arsenic: the estimates resolved the conundrum of Table 3 in which education attainment for the youths who reported drinking safely in the unsafe sub-districts was greater than the education

attainment of the youths who drank safely by dint of living in a safe sub-district. In our regressions, which controlled for other determinants of education, we estimated that the sampled individuals who lived where groundwater was safe attained the same levels of education as sampled individuals who drank safely despite living where groundwater was unsafe. Passing this test lends increased creditability to the estimates of how much less education was attained by the individuals who drank from locally unsafe wells.

The results in Table 5 indicate that parental wealth, education, and awareness of the arsenic problem positively influence youths' educational outcomes. Young males in wealthier sub-districts tend to attain less education than young males from other districts (when parental wealth is controlled for separately), but local wealth does not affect the school attendance by young boys. We interpret the local wealth variable as indicating the local income opportunities that compete with school for older youths' time. Such opportunities are less apt to matter for young boys because for them, attending school is mandatory.

In unreported regressions, we found that adding males as young as 15 to the sample hardly changed arsenic's estimated effects. Apparently, arsenic poisoning takes its education toll by age 15. Adding individuals as old as 25 cuts the estimated adverse effect to about three tenths of a year (but still confirms the finding of no adverse effect for those who drink safely). We attribute the lower estimate when including older individuals to older individuals having been less exposed to arsenic in the early 1980s than younger individuals were subsequently.

Limitations

Correlational models like ours do not offer the iron-clad protection from bias that well-designed experiments can: in correlational models, omitted relevant variables can bias the results of an analysis. Our analysis, like most regression analyses, requires attention to such biases because we do not have as rich an array of covariates available to us as we would wish. In particular, our data are a single cross-section, not a panel, of individuals. Consequently, we cannot track the dynamic determinants of education attainment. Our reliance on a cross-sectional correlational model is limited with respect to three classes of variables: economic, health, and policy variables. Here, we attend briefly to the nature of the biases we risk by not having better measures of such variables.

To fully understand why an individual attains the schooling he or she does, one would favor a detailed examination of the individual's economic circumstances over the course of the individual's childhood. With only a single cross-section, we miss the fluctuations in households' economic circumstances that affect education attainment. We observe a household's wealth at a single moment of time, which provides only a partial picture of a household's economic history. Because wealth fluctuates less over time than does income, observing a household's wealth at one moment of time is more informative about the household's economic circumstances over time than is observing the household's current income. But wealth does, nonetheless, vary over time, and to the extent that wealth varied differentially across sub-districts with high and low levels of groundwater arsenic, our measures of arsenic's effects on education attainment are biased. However, such biases are apt to be lessened by our model's inclusion of both local aggregate mean wealth and local aggregate variation in wealth.

A potentially more serious concern is our lack of data about the non-arsenic related health status of individuals both over time and in the period we observe. If high levels of arsenic in groundwater are correlated with other health threats, such as malaria-carrying mosquitos, for which we have no measures, then our estimate of groundwater arsenic's effect on education attainment will be biased. However, to the extent that individuals in a threatened area cannot avoid a specific health threat, both the estimated effect of arsenic contamination for those who drink arsenic-contaminated water and the

estimated effect for those in the same sub-district who drink from a safe source would be biased toward reduced education attainment. Thus, if such health threats are substantially correlated with groundwater arsenic contamination, we would expect to see an effect of groundwater arsenic on education attainment for those who live in arsenic-unsafe sub-districts yet drink safely. This was not the case. A remaining concern for our results are health threats that are avoidable, as we would expect that households which avoided unsafe water would also have taken measures like bed nets to avoid diseases such as malaria. The question, then, is, "How correlated was arsenic contamination with such avoidable health threats?" We employ as control indicators of industrial pollution and garbage dumps in the vicinity of an individual's home, but these are crude measures, so both avoidable environmental threats and avoidable ecological threats to health could cause biases in our results.

The third class of variables for which time series data would be valuable is policy-related variables. The effect of groundwater arsenic on residents of a sub-district is influenced by government policy. Moreover, government policy interventions are almost surely more intense in areas with the worst arsenic contamination. Both the extent of government policies in place during the childhoods of our observed individuals and the time path of those policies matter for the severity of groundwater arsenic's effects. By focusing on 19- to 21-year-olds born between 1984 and 1986, we capture the effects of groundwater arsenic averaged across the policy practices in place between 1984 and 2006. Our reading of the empirical literature about arsenic policies' efficacy suggests that policies shifted relatively few households from contaminated to safe supplies for two thirds of that time or more [33].

Our reliance on a single cross-section risks yet another bias. An arsenic level measured at one moment in time likely mismeasures individuals' long-run exposure to arsenic, which is the truly relevant exposure. Consequently, our estimates suffer some attenuation bias. Since arsenic levels in wells do not change much over time, attenuation bias arises chiefly from individuals not always having lived in the sub-district in which they were observed in 2005. The more individuals moved between childhood and 2005, the greater their contribution to such attenuation bias. To reduce this bias, we restricted the sample of 19–21-year-olds to individuals who still lived with their parent or grandparent when sampled; this shrank the 19–21-year-old sub-sample by 17 %.

The striking safety of drinking safely

Our multiple regression analysis controls for a large number of covariates that have been found by others to affect education attainment, including household wealth, parental education, number of other youths in the household, age, local environmental and economic indicators, and district of residence, as well as the household head's awareness of the arsenic problem. Those controls negate many potential sources of bias. Our results also offer a striking check on the validity of our results. We estimate that males who did not report drinking from an arsenic-free water source and lived where tube-wells were unsafe obtained half-a-year less education than males who lived where tube wells were safe, but we also estimate that individuals who lived in unsafe sub-districts but drank water from arsenic-free sources suffered essentially zero adverse education effect from the local tube wells' contamination. That the estimated effect of living in an unsafe sub-district disappears for those who did not drink the contaminated water strongly suggests that what we estimate as arsenic's effect on education attainment was, indeed, arsenic's effect and not a spurious result stemming from omitted variables.

Conclusions

In 2012–2013, 20 million Bangladeshis regularly drank water containing more than 50 ppb of arsenic, the Bangladesh standard for contamination, and 40 million regularly drank water containing more than the 10 ppb of arsenic deemed unsafe by the World Health Organization [29]. Given the horrific health consequences of regularly drinking arsenic-contaminated water [1, 9, 10], Bangladeshis' extensive reliance on arsenic-contaminated water, while much improved over levels of reliance in the past, still has severe adverse public health consequences. This paper's analysis finds further that young Bangladeshi males who live where tube wells are unsafe and who do not report drinking from an arsenic-free source attain, on average, a half-year less education (among 19- to 21-year-olds) and attend school, on average, five to seven fewer days a year (among 6- to 10-year-olds) compared to other Bangladeshi males of those ages. Hence, Bangladeshi public health measures to shift drinking from unsafe to safe wells not only advance good health but also increase education attainment for males.

Endnotes

[1]The figures in Table 1 for 2000 are the percentages of wells above specified thresholds [27], while those for 2009 and those for 2012–2013 are based on tests of households' drinking water [8, 30]. Since even in 2000 some households avoided sources known to be contaminated, the figures in Table 1 overstate how much households' exposure has changed since 2000, but there is widespread agreement that households substantially reduced their reliance on arsenic-contaminated sources over the decade.

[2]The regression results for females are available from the authors upon request. In our largest samples, girls

aged 11–25, the estimated effect of drinking from contaminated sources is a tenth of a year decrease in education attained; that estimate has a p value of 0.102.

Competing interests
The authors declare that they have no competing interests.

Authors' contributions
MPM and RS developed the conceptual framework of the research in conversations together. RS found and first downloaded the data and conducted and wrote up the preliminary analyses that focused on males and females together. RS also participated in the analysis plan for the empirical work reported here and advised on the form and content of the paper's several drafts. MPM replicated the downloaded data and preliminary analyses and advised on the form and content of the write-up of the preliminary analyses. MPM performed the regression analysis reported here, in consultation with RS. He also wrote the later drafts with the advice of RS. Both authors read and approved the final version of the manuscript.

Acknowledgements
This paper has benefitted from the very helpful suggestions of an anonymous reviewer. We are also grateful to Rosanne Ducey for editorial assistance. Only the authors are responsible for remaining errors or omissions.

Author details
[1]Department of Economics, Bates College, Lewiston, ME 04240, USA.
[2]University of Waterloo, Waterloo, Canada.

References
1. Brinkel J, Khan MH, Kraemer A. A systematic review of arsenic exposure and its social and mental health effects with special reference to Bangladesh. Int J Environ Res Public Health. 2009;6:1609–19.
2. Smith AH, Lingas EO, Rahman M. Contamination of drinking-water by arsenic in Bangladesh: a public health emergency. Bulletin of the World Health Organ. 2000;78(Jan):1093–103.
3. Ratan Kr Dhar, Bhajan Kr Biswas, Gautam Samanta, Badal Kr Mandal, D. Chakraborti, Shibtosh Roy, Abu Jafar et al. Groundwater arsenic calamity in Bangladesh. Current Science. 1997; 73, no. 1: 48–59.
4. Khan AW. Arsenic contamination in ground water and its effect on human health with particular reference to Bangladesh. J Prev Soc Med. 1997;16: 65–73.
5. IPCS. Arsenic and arsenic compounds. Geneva: World Health Organization; 2001. International Programme on Chemical Safety (Environmental Health Criteria 224).
6. Sohel N, Persson LA, Rahman M, Streatfield PK, Yunus M, Ekström EC, et al. Arsenic in drinking water and adult mortality: a population-based cohort study in rural Bangladesh. Epidemiology. 2009;20(6):824–30.
7. Flanagan SV, Johnston RB, Zheng Y. Arsenic in tube well water in Bangladesh: health and economic impacts and implications for arsenic mitigation. B World Health Organ. 2012;90(11):839–46.
8. Yu C, van Geen A, Graziano JH, Pfaff A, Madajewicz M, Faruque P, et al. Reduction in urinary arsenic levels in response to arsenic mitigation efforts in Araihazar, Bangladesh. Environ Health Perspect. 2007;115(June):917–23.
9. Safiuddin S, Shirazi M, Yusoff S. Arsenic contamination of groundwater in Bangladesh: a review. Int J Phys Sci. 2011;6(30):6791–800.
10. Rahman MM, Chowdhury UK, Mukherjee SC, Mondal BK, Paul K, Lodh D. Chronic arsenic toxicity in Bangladesh and West Bengal, India—a review and commentary. J Toxicol Clin Toxicol. 2001;39(7):683–700.
11. Psacharopoulos G. Returns to investment in education: a global update. World Dev. 1992;22(9):1325–43.
12. Psacharopoulos G, Patrinos HA. Returns to investment in education: a further update. Educ Econ. 2004;12(2):111–34.
13. Barro R. Economic growth in a cross-section of countries. Quart J Econ. 1991;106(2):407–43.
14. Lucas R. On the mechanics of economic development. J Monet Econ. 1988;22:3–42.

15. Gregory MN, David R, David W. A contribution to the empirics of economic growth. Quart J Econ. 1992;107(2):407–37.

16. Calderon J, Navarro ME, Jiminez-Capdeville ME, Santos-Diaz MA, Golden A, Rodriguez-Leyva I, et al. Exposure to arsenic and lead and neuropsychological development in Mexican children. Environ Res. 2001;85:69–76.

17. Asadullah MN, Chaudhury N. Poisoning the mind: arsenic contamination of drinking water wells and children's educational achievement in rural Bangladesh. Econ Educ Rev. 2011;30(5):873–88.

18. Rosado JL, Ronquillo D, Kordas K, Rojas O, Alatorre J, Lopez P, et al. Arsenic exposure and cognitive performance in Mexican schoolchildren. Environ Health Perspect. 2007;155:1371–5.

19. Tsai S-Y, Chou H-Y, The HW, Chen C-M, Chen C-J. The effects of chronic arsenic exposure on the neurobehavioral development in adolescence. NeuroToxicology. 2003;24:747–53.

20. Wasserman GA, Liu X, Parvez F, Ahsan H, Factor-Litvak P, Kline J, et al. Water arsenic exposure and children's intellectual function in Araihazar, Bangladesh. Environ Health Perspect. 2004;112:1329–33.

21. Wasserman GA, Liu X, Parvez F, Ahsan H, Factor-Litvak Kline PJ, et al. Water arsenic exposure and intellectual function in 6-year-old children In Araihazar, Bangladesh. Environ Health Perspect. 2007;115(2):285–9.

22. Von Ehrenstein OS, Poddar S, Yuan Y, Mazumder DG, Eskenazi B, Basu A, et al. Children's intellectual function in relation to arsenic exposure. Epidemiology. 2007;18:44–51.

23. Chowdhury MAI, Uddin MT, Ahmed MF, Ali MA, Rasul SMA, Hoque MA, et al. Collapse of socio-economic base of Bangladesh by arsenic contamination in groundwater. Pak J Biol Sci. 2006;9(9):1617–27.

24. Khandoker A, Khan M, Krämer A, Mori M. Social consequences of arsenicosis and mental health of arsenicosis patients: evidence from an arsenic-affected area of Bangladesh. Gesundheitswesen. 2010;72(8/9):72.

25. Nasreen, Mahbuba. Social impacts of arsenicosis. Arsenic contamination: Bangladesh perspective 2003: 340–353.

26. Maddison D, Catala-Luque R, Pearce D. Valuing the arsenic contamination of groundwater in Bangladesh. Environ and Resour Econ. 2005;31(4):459–76.

27. Saha KC. Chronic arsenical dermatoses from tube-well water in West Bengal during 1983–87. Indian J Dermatol. 1995;40:1–12.

28. Bangladesh Bureau of Statistics and Department of Public Health Engineering. Arsenic contamination of groundwater in Bangladesh. In: Kinniburgh DG, Smedley PL, editors. British Geological Survey Technical Report WC/00/19. Keyworth: British Geological Survey; 2001.

29. Frisbie S, Ortega R, Maynard D, Sarkar B. The concentrations of arsenic and other toxic elements in Bangladesh's drinking water. Environ Health Persp. 2002;110:1147–53.

30. Bangladesh Bureau of Statistics (BBS) and UNICEF. Bangladesh multiple indicator cluster survey 2012–2013, Progotir Pathey: final report, 2014, Dhaka, Bangladesh.

31. Bennear L, Tarozzi A, Pfaff A, Balasubramanya S, Ahmede KM, van Geen A. Impact of a randomized controlled trial in arsenic risk communication on household water-source choices in Bangladesh. J Environ Econ Manag. 2013;65:225–40.

32. Opar A, Pfaff A, Seddique AA, Ahmed KM, Graziano JH, van Geen A. Responses of 6500 households to arsenic mitigation in Araihazar, Bangladesh. Health Place. 2007;13(1):164–72.

33. Schoenfeld A. Area, village, and household response to arsenic testing and labeling of tubewells in Araihazar, Bangladesh. New York: Columbia University; 2005. Master Thesis, Earth and environmental science journalism.

34. Howard GM, Ahmed M F, Shamsuddin AJ, Mahmud SG, Deere D. Risk assessment of arsenic mitigation options in Bangladesh. J Health Popul Nutr. 2006;24(3):346–55.

35. World Health Organization. Exposure to arsenic: a major public health concern. Geneva: Public Health and Environment; 2010. p. 1–5.

36. Argos M, Kalra T, Rathouz PJ, Chen Y, Pierce B, Parvez F, et al. Arsenic exposure from drinking water, and all-cause and chronic-disease mortalities in Bangladesh (HEALS): a prospective cohort study. Lancet. 2010; 376:252–8.

37. Bangladesh Bureau of Statistics and United Nations Children's Fund. Multiple indicator cluster survey 2009: vol. 1, technical report. Dhaka: Bangladesh Bureau of Statistics/UNICEF 2010; 2010.

38. Chan M, Michel K, Julian L-L, Thoraya O, Julian S, Michel S, et al. Meeting the demand for results and accountability: a call for action on health data from eight global health agencies. PLoS Med. 2010;7(1):e1000223.

39. Cheng Z, van Geen A, Seddique A, Ahmed KM. Limited temporal variability of arsenic concentrations in 20 wells monitored for 3 years in Araihazar, Bangladesh. Environ Sci Technol. 2005;39(13):4759–66.

40. van Geen A, Versteeg R, Stute M, Horneman A, Dahr R, Gelman A, et al. Spatial variability of arsenic in 6000 tube wells in a 25 km^2 area of Bangladesh. Water Resours Res. 2003;39(5):1140.

41. Mare RD. Social background and school continuation decisions. J Am Stat Assoc. 1980;75(370):295–305.

42. Li Q, Zang W, An L. Peer effects and school dropout in rural China. China Econ Rev. 2013;27:238–48.

43. Huang J. Intergenerational transmission of educational attainment: the role of household assets. Econ Educ Rev. 2013;33:112–23.

44. Holmes J. Measuring the determinants of school completion in Pakistan: analysis of censoring and selection bias. Econ Educ Rev. 2003;22(3):249–64.

45. Murray Michael P. Econometrics: a modern introduction. Boston: Prentice Hall; 2006.

46. Wooldridge JM. Cluster-sample methods in applied econometrics. Am Econ Rev. 2003;93:133–8.

47. Asadullah MN. Poisoning the mind: arsenic contamination and cognitive achievement of children 2008; Vol. 4510. World Bank Publications.

48. Tondel M, Rahman M, Magnuson A, Chowdhury IA, Faruquee MH, Ahmad SA. The relationship of arsenic levels in drinking water and the prevalence rate of skin lesions in Bangladesh. Environ Health Perspect. 1999;107(9):727.

49. National Resource Council. Arsenic in drinking water. Washington, D.C.: Natl Acad Press 2001; (Update).

6

White rice consumption and risk of esophageal cancer in Xinjiang Uyghur Autonomous Region, northwest China: a case-control study

Li Tang[1], Fenglian Xu[2], Taotao Zhang[3], Jun Lei[4], Colin W. Binns[1] and Andy H. Lee[1*]

Abstract

This study investigated the association between white rice consumption and the risk of esophageal cancer in remote northwest China, where the cancer incidence is known to be high. A case-control study was conducted during 2008–2009 in Urumqi and Shihezi, Xinjiang Uyghur Autonomous Region of China. Participants were 359 incident esophageal cancer patients and 380 hospital-based controls. Information on habitual white rice consumption was obtained by personal interview using a validated semi-quantitative food frequency questionnaire. Logistic regression analyses were performed to assess the association between white rice consumption and the esophageal cancer risk. Confounding variables including socio-demographics, family history, dietary and lifestyle factors were adjusted in the multivariate model. The esophageal cancer patients reported lower consumption levels of white rice-based products, including cooked white rice and porridge, when compared to the control group. Overall, regular consumption of white rice foods was inversely associated with the esophageal cancer risk, the adjusted OR being 0.34 (95 % CI 0.23 to 0.52) for the highest (>250 g) versus the lowest (<92 g) tertile of daily intake. Similar reductions in risk were also apparent for high consumption levels of cooked white rice and porridge. In conclusion, habitual white rice consumption was associated with a reduced risk of esophageal cancer for adults residing in northwest China. Our findings provide evidence to support the continued consumption of white rice.

Keywords: Case-control study, White rice, Esophageal cancer, Xinjiang, China

Background

Globally, esophageal cancer is the eighth most common malignancy and the sixth leading cause of cancer-related deaths. In 2008, more than 480,000 new cases were diagnosed and approximately 407,000 deaths were attributable to this disease [1]. The incidence rates of esophageal cancer vary substantially between countries and regions, which suggest that dietary and lifestyle factors may play an important role in its aetiology [2].

Rice is a staple food for more than half of the world's population [3]. White rice, produced through a series of refining processes, is the predominant type of rice consumed in Asian countries [4]. A few studies have found

that the consumption of white rice may be linked to the development of type 2 diabetes [5, 6]. However, further substantive evidence is required to confirm its effect.

Xinjiang Uyghur Autonomous Region, located in the northwest of China, is one of the areas constituting the so-called 'Asian Esophageal Cancer Belt' [7]. Factors found to be consistently associated with an increased risk of esophageal cancer in this 'cancer belt' include a diet poor in fruit and vegetables intake, tobacco smoking and alcohol drinking [7]. According to a survey undertaken in Xinjiang between 2005 and 2008, the incidence of esophageal cancer was 30.2 per 100,000 adults, much higher than the national average of 19.3 per 100,000 [8]. White rice-based products, especially cooked white rice and porridge, are commonly consumed in China. In view of the lack of epidemiological data, the present study investigated the association

* Correspondence: Andy.Lee@curtin.edu.au
[1]School of Public Health, Curtin University, GPO Box U 1987, Perth, WA 6845, Australia
Full list of author information is available at the end of the article

between white rice consumption and the risk of esophageal cancer in this remote area of China.

Methods

Study design and participants

A hospital-based case-control study of esophageal cancer was conducted in Urumqi and Shihezi, Xinjiang Uyghur Autonomous Region of China, between January 2008 and December 2009. Subjects were recruited from Xinjiang Tumour Hospital, Shihezi People's Hospital, Kuitong Hospital and No. 1 Affiliated Hospital of Shihezi University.

Medical records and pathology reports were searched to identify incident patients diagnosed within the past 12 months. Pathological diagnoses were based on the International Classification of Disease for Oncology (ICD-O-3 codes: C150-C155, C158, C159) [9]. Patients without histopathological confirmation and those reported memory problems were excluded. Of the total 364 incident patients identified, 359 consented to participate in the study.

Controls were recruited from inpatient wards at the same hospitals from the Departments of Ophthalmology, Orthopedic, Respiratory Disease and Physiotherapy. Exclusion criteria for controls were previous diagnosis of any malignant disease, on long-term medical diet, and self-reported memory problems. Whenever more controls were available than could be interviewed, the final selection was made using random numbers. Of the 400 eligible controls recruited to frequency matched with cases by gender and age (within 5 years), 380 eventually gave their consent to be interviewed. No significant differences in age, gender and demographics were found between participants and non-participants.

The study protocol was approved by the participating hospitals and the Human Research Ethics Committee of Curtin University (approval number HR 56/2006), and conformed to the provisions of the Declaration of Helsinki. Written informed consent was obtained from all participants, who were assured of confidentiality of the information provided and their right to withdraw at any time without prejudice.

Data collection

All participants were interviewed personally by trained hospital staff, usually in the presence of their next-of-kin to help the recall of past events. The structured questionnaire used composed sections on demographic characteristics, anthropometry, past and family medical history, diet, and lifestyle such as cigarette smoking and alcohol drinking. Information on dietary habits was collected using a 137-item semi-quantitative food frequency questionnaire which had been validated in both Han and ethnic minority groups [10]. The questionnaire included fruits, vegetables, meat and white rice products

commonly consumed in northwest China. Frequency and amount of intake were recorded in detail. The reference recall period for dietary variables was set at 5 years before diagnosis for cases and 5 years before interview for controls. The energy content of each food or beverage item was obtained from the Chinese Food Composition Tables to calculate total energy intake (kcal/day) [11].

Statistical analysis

Chi-square and t tests were used to compare the sample characteristics between case and control groups. Total white rice intake (g/day) was defined as the sum of daily consumption of cooked white rice, porridge and glutinous rice. For each exposure variable of interest, the tertiles corresponding to the distribution of controls were used to derive the cutoff points, resulting in three increasing levels of exposure, with the lowest level of intake being the reference category. However, glutinous rice intake was categorised as a binary variable due to its low and infrequent consumption by the Xinjiang adults.

Both crude and adjusted odds ratio (OR) and corresponding 95 % confidence interval (CI) were computed using unconditional logistic regression analyses. Confounding variables included in the separate models were age (years), gender, education level (none/primary, secondary, tertiary), annual income (<5000 yuan, 5000–20,000 yuan, > 20,000 yuan), body mass index (5 years ago, kg/m^2), vegetable consumption (g/day), fruit consumption (g/day), meat consumption (g/day), total energy intake (kcal/day), smoking status (never, ever), alcohol drinking (never/seldom, often) and family history of cancer in first-degree relatives (no, yes). These variables were either established or plausible risk factors from the literature. All statistical analyses were performed in the SPSS package version 20.

Results

Table 1 summarises characteristics of the sample by case-control status. The participants were on average 61 (SD 11.4) years old with mean body mass index 24.1 (SD 3.7) kg/m^2. Most (about 72 %) of them were male. About half the participants were smokers and regularly drank alcoholic beverages. Compared to the controls, patients with esophageal cancer tended to belong to the ethnic minority group, have lower education level but a family history of esophageal cancer, have a marginally lower daily energy intake, and consume significantly less vegetables and fruits in daily life. With respect to white rice-based products, the cases reported lower levels of cooked rice and porridge intake than the controls, whereas less than half the participants ate glutinous rice on a daily basis for both groups.

Table 2 presents the results of logistic regression analyses. Overall, regular consumption of white rice foods

Table 1 Comparison of demographic factors and white rice consumption between case and control groups in northwest China

Variable	Cases n (%)	Controls n (%)	p^a
Gender			0.623
Male	260 (72.4 %)	269 (70.8 %)	
Female	99 (27.6 %)	111 (29.2 %)	
Ethnic group			0.001
Han	270 (75.2 %)	322 (84.7 %)	
Minority	89 (24.8 %)	58 (15.3 %)	
Education level			<0.001
None/primary	183 (51.0 %)	136 (35.8 %)	
Secondary	140 (39.0 %)	191 (50.3 %)	
Tertiary	36 (10.0 %)	53 (13.9 %)	
Annual income (yuan^b)			0.112
<5000	130 (36.2 %)	132 (34.7 %)	
5000–20,000	177 (49.3 %)	171 (45.0 %)	
>20,000	52 (14.5 %)	77 (20.3 %)	
Smoking status			0.188
Never	164 (45.7 %)	192 (50.5 %)	
Ever	195 (54.3 %)	188 (49.5 %)	
Alcohol drinking			0.216
Never/seldom	193 (53.8 %)	187 (49.2 %)	
Often	166 (46.2 %)	193 (50.8 %)	
Family history of cancer in first-degree relatives			<0.001
No	306 (85.2 %)	356 (93.7 %)	
Yes	53 (14.8 %)	24 (6.3 %)	
Age at interview (years): mean (SD)	61.4 (11.0)	60.6 (11.8)	0.338
BMI (5 years ago, kg/m^2): mean (SD)	24.3 (3.8)	24.0 (3.6)	0.181
Vegetable consumption (g/day): mean (SD)	677.8 (542.6)	874.3 (621.8)	<0.001
Fruit consumption (g/day): mean (SD)	342.0 (410.6)	463.1 (480.6)	<0.001
Meat consumption (g/day): mean (SD)	232.1 (263.1)	242.3 (264.1)	0.601
Energy intake (kcal/day): mean (SD)	4310 (2681)	4709 (2716)	0.047
Total white rice (g/day): mean (SD)	137.8 (188.0)	208.7 (208.9)	<0.001
Cooked white rice (g/day): mean (SD)	79.5 (133.1)	111.2 (132.9)	0.001
Porridge (g/day): mean (SD)	53.0 (83.9)	95.2 (148.3)	<0.001
Glutinous rice	157 (43.7 %)	183 (48.2 %)	0.228

^{a}Chi-square or t-test for difference between cases and controls
^{b}1 yuan ≅ 0.16 USD

was inversely associated with the esophageal cancer risk, and the dose-response relationship was significant (p for trend < 0.001). The adjusted OR was 0.34 (95 % CI 0.23 to 0.52) for adults consuming over 250 g relative to those less than 92 g per day. Similar reductions in cancer risk were also apparent for high consumption levels of cooked white rice and porridge, but not from eating glutinous rice. Further subgroup analysis by ethnicity (Han versus Uyghur minority people) produced similar results which were omitted for brevity.

Discussion

The present study provided the first report on the inverse association between habitual white rice consumption and esophageal cancer risk. Our results were somewhat different from a previous study undertaken in India which observed similar frequency of rice consumption between esophageal cancer patients and controls [12]. Despite the lack of a comprehensive biological mechanism underlying the relationship between white rice and esophageal cancer development, an experimental study has demonstrated the

Table 2 Crude and adjusted odds ratio (95 % confidence interval) of esophageal cancer risk for white rice consumption in northwest China

Daily intake (g)	Cases n (%)	Controls n (%)	Crude OR (95 % CI)	Adjusted OR[a] (95 % CI)
Total white rice				
<92	195 (54.3 %)	125 (32.9 %)	1.00	1.00
92–250	101 (28.1 %)	130 (34.2 %)	0.50 (0.35, 0.70)	0.51 (0.36, 0.74)
>250	63 (17.5 %)	125 (32.9 %)	0.32 (0.22, 0.47)	0.34 (0.23, 0.52)
Cooked white rice				
<30	187 (52.1 %)	128 (33.7 %)	1.00	1.00
30–140	95 (26.5 %)	120 (31.6 %)	0.54 (0.38, 0.77)	0.64 (0.44, 0.92)
>140	77 (21.4 %)	132 (34.7 %)	0.40 (0.28, 0.57)	0.48 (0.33, 0.71)
Porridge				
<28	194 (54.0 %)	124 (32.6 %)	1.00	1.00
28–100	106 (29.5 %)	136 (35.8 %)	0.50 (0.36, 0.70)	0.52 (0.36, 0.75)
>100	59 (16.4 %)	120 (31.6 %)	0.31 (0.21, 0.46)	0.34 (0.22, 0.50)
Glutinous rice				
no	202 (56.3 %)	197 (51.8 %)	1.00	1.00
yes	157 (43.7 %)	183 (48.2 %)	0.84 (0.63, 1.12)	0.93 (0.68, 1.28)

[a]From separate logistic regression models adjusting for age (years), gender, education level (none/primary, secondary, tertiary), annual income (<5000 yuan, 5000–20,000 yuan, > 20,000 yuan), body mass index (5 years ago, kg/m^2), vegetable consumption (g/day), fruit consumption (g/day), meat consumption (g/day), total energy intake (kcal/day), smoking status (never, ever), alcohol drinking (never/seldom, often) and family history of cancer in first-degree relatives (no, yes)

anti-carcinogenic property of white rice through its growth-inhibiting and immunopotentiating effects on leukemic cells [13]. Even after the refining process, white rice still contains antioxidant nutrients and essential amino acids which are required for a good health [14].

In this study, a standardised identification procedure had been implemented that ensured the ascertainment of cases was maximised and complete. To avoid misclassification of the case-control status, we recruited only incident patients who had been diagnosed with esophageal cancer within the past 12 months and subsequently confirmed with pathology. All controls were carefully screened. It was possible that some esophageal cancer patients might have modified their dietary behaviours since the onset of the disease. Therefore, the reference period for the dietary recall was set at 5 years before diagnosis to minimise reverse causation.

Several other issues should be considered when interpreting the findings. The use of hospital-based controls may lead to Berksonian bias if their characteristics are different from those of the general population. Four hospitals serving the entire catchment region were used for recruitment to reduce the selection bias. Although the recall of habitual white rice consumption should not be affected by the case-control status, dietary assessment was made based on self-report, which probably introduced some recall error in the response of participants, especially since the recall period of dietary intakes was set at 5 years ago. Face-to-face interviews were thus arranged in the presence of next-of-kin to help improve the accuracy of their responses. Information bias and recall bias were unlikely because all participants remained blind to the study hypothesis, while the protective role of white rice has not yet been established. It may be argued that white rice consumption is a marker of an (unidentified) healthy lifestyle against esophagus disease development. Therefore, plausible demographic and lifestyle confounding factors, including fruit and vegetables consumption, were adjusted for in the logistic regression analyses. Nevertheless, the possibility of residual confounding effects could not be ruled out. Finally, future studies with information on the pathologic severity of esophageal cancer at the time of diagnosis are recommended to enable a more comprehensive profile of the patients.

Conclusions

In conclusion, inverse associations were observed between white rice products and the esophageal cancer incidence among Xinjiang adults. Further prospective cohort studies in this high risk area of China and elsewhere are required to confirm the effects of long term consumption.

Competing interests
The authors declare that they have no competing interests.

Authors' contributions
All authors read and approved the final manuscript.

Acknowledgements
Thanks are due to the esophageal cancer patents and control participants who agreed to be interviewed, and to the medical and nursing staff of the participating hospitals for their assistance in recruitment. No funding was received.

Author details
[1]School of Public Health, Curtin University, GPO Box U 1987, Perth, WA 6845, Australia. [2]National Drug and Alcohol Research Centre, University of New South Wales, Sydney, NSW, Australia. [3]School of Medicine, Shihezi University, Shihezi, Xinjiang, China. [4]Xinjiang Tumour Hospital, Urumqi, Xinjiang, China.

References
1. Ferlay J, Shin H, Bray F, Forman D, Mathers C, Parkin D. Cancer incidence and mortality worldwide. Lyon: International Agency for Research on Cancer; 2010 (http://globocan.iarc.fr, accessed on 2 October 2013).
2. Carr JS, Zafar SF, Saba N, Khuri FR, El-Rayes BF. Risk factors for rising incidence of esophageal and gastric cardia adenocarcinoma. J Gastrointest Cancer. 2013;44:143–51.
3. Economic Research Service, United States Department of Agriculture. Rice: Overview. 2012. (http://www.ers.usda.gov/topics/crops/rice.aspx#.UcmOWPmnrzx, accessed on 5 October 2013).
4. Hu EA, Pan A, Malik V, Sun Q. White rice consumption and risk of type 2 diabetes: meta-analysis and systematic review. BMJ. 2012. doi:10.1001/archinternmed.2010.109.
5. Nanri A, Mizoue T, Noda M, Takahashi Y, Kato M, Inoue M, et al. Rice intake and type 2 diabetes in Japanese men and women: the Japan Public Health Center-based Prospective Study. Am J Clin Nutr. 2010;92:1468–77.
6. Sun Q, Spiegelman D, van Dam RM, Holmes MD, Malik VS, Willett WC, et al. White rice, brown rice, and risk of type 2 diabetes in US men and women. Arch Intern Med. 2010;170:961–9.
7. Zheng S, Vuitton L, Sheyhidin I, Vuitton DA, Zhang Y, Lu X. Northwestern China: a place to learn more on esophageal cancer. Part one: behavioural and environmental risk factors. Eur J Gastroenterol Hepatol. 2010;22:917–25.
8. Ainiwaer J, Li D, Zhang L, Xiaheding Y, Tuerxunnayi, Liu Y. A survey of esophageal cancer incidence in Yili, Xinjiang between 2005 and 2008. Xinjiang Med J. 2011;41:112–4 [in Chinese].
9. Garbbert HE, Shimoda T, Hainaut P, Nakamura Y, Field JK, Inoue H. Tumours of the Oesophagus. In: Hamilton SR, Aaltonen LA, editors. World Health Organization classification of tumours pathology and genetics of tumours of the digestive system. Lyon: IARC Press; 2000. p. 9–30.
10. Zhang T. [Investigation on dietary factors and lifestyles of esophageal cancer patients in Xinjiang]. Master Thesis, Shihezi University, 2010. [in Chinese].
11. Chinese Center for Disease Control and Prevention. China Food Composition Table. 2d ed. Beijing: Peking University Medical Press, 2009:78–183.
12. Sehgal S, Kaul S, Gupta BB, Dhar MK. Risk factors and survival analysis of the esophageal cancer in the population of Jammu, India. Indian J Cancer. 2012;49:245–50.
13. Liao HF, Chen YY, Yang YC, Wang CS, Chen YJ. Rice (Oryza sativa L.) inhibits growth and induces differentiation of human leukemic U937 cells through activation of peripheral blood mononuclear cells. Food Chem Toxicol. 2006;44:1724–9.
14. Patil SB, Khan MK. Germinated brown rice as a value added rice product: A review. J Food Sci Technol. 2011;48:661–7.

7

The opioid effects of gluten exorphins: asymptomatic celiac disease

Leo Pruimboom[1,2*] and Karin de Punder[1,3]

Abstract

Gluten-containing cereals are a main food staple present in the daily human diet, including wheat, barley, and rye. Gluten intake is associated with the development of celiac disease (CD) and related disorders such as diabetes mellitus type I, depression, and schizophrenia. However, until now, there is no consent about the possible deleterious effects of gluten intake because of often failing symptoms even in persons with proven CD. Asymptomatic CD (ACD) is present in the majority of affected patients and is characterized by the absence of classical gluten-intolerance signs, such as diarrhea, bloating, and abdominal pain. Nevertheless, these individuals very often develop diseases that can be related with gluten intake. Gluten can be degraded into several morphine-like substances, named gluten exorphins. These compounds have proven opioid effects and could mask the deleterious effects of gluten protein on gastrointestinal lining and function. Here we describe a putative mechanism, explaining how gluten could "mask" its own toxicity by exorphins that are produced through gluten protein digestion.

Keywords: Asymptomatic celiac disease, Celiac disease, Gliadin, Gluten, Exorphins

Background

Gluten is the main structural protein complex of wheat consisting of glutenins and gliadins. Glutenins are polymers of individual proteins and are the fraction of wheat proteins that are soluble in dilute acids. Prolamins are the alcohol-soluble proteins of cereal grains that are specifically named gliadins in wheat [1], which can be further degraded to a collection of opioid-like polypeptides called *exorphins* in the gastrointestinal tract [2]. Gliadin epitopes from wheat gluten and related prolamins from other gluten-containing cereal grains, including rye and barley, can trigger celiac disease (CD) in genetically susceptible people [3], and accumulating data provide evidence for the deleterious effects of gluten intake on general human health. Nevertheless, until now, there is no consent about the possible detrimental health effects of gluten intake because of often failing gastrointestinal symptoms even in individuals with proven CD. By describing our "silent opioid hypothesis," we hope to shine light on this highly conflictive scientific item. Our review process and literature search was based on the use of the following key words: gluten, gliadin, celiac disease, asymptomatic celiac disease, gluten and transglutaminase, gluten and exorphins, gluten and intolerance, gluten and DPP IV, gluten and substance P, DPP IV, gluten and neoantigens, celiac disease and epidemiology, and gluten-free diet. Literature inclusion criteria included in vitro, in vivo, and human trial studies; indexed publications; full-text papers; and research methodology. Papers were excluded when not indexed and when methodology did not reach minimal criteria, and papers older than 2005 were excluded when more actual publications were available.

Asymptomatic celiac disease

CD normally presents itself with a number of typical signs and symptoms of malabsorption: diarrhea, muscle wasting, and weight loss. Other gastrointestinal (GI) symptoms like abdominal pain, bloating, and flatulence are also common. Curiously, a large group of patients that have been diagnosed with CD through screening for CD-specific antibodies and duodenal biopsy [3, 4] lack these classical symptoms, a condition that is also referred to as "asymptomatic CD" (ACD). Many disorders are present in patients with ACD, including diabetes

* Correspondence: cpni.pruimboom@icloud.com
[1]Natura Foundation, Edisonstraat 66, 3281 NC Numansdorp, Netherlands
[2]Department of Laboratory Medicine, University Medical Center Groningen (UMCG), University of Groningen, P.O. Box 30.001, 9700 RB Groningen, Netherlands
Full list of author information is available at the end of the article

mellitus type I [5, 6], severe hypoglycemia in diabetes mellitus type I [7], psoriasis [8], sleep apnea in children [9], neoplasia [10], atopic dermatitis [11], depression [8], subclinical synovitis in children [12], autism [13], schizophrenia [14], and irritable bowel syndrome (IBS) [8], suggesting that gluten intake is related to the development of these conditions.

ACD is present in a large group of diagnosed celiac patients [15, 16]. A study based on the data of the National Health and Nutrition Examination Survey showed that only 17 % of patients with serologically diagnosed CD suffer from the classical celiac symptoms [17]. A human study in 2089 elderly individuals looking for possible persistence of anti-gliadin antibody (AGA) positivity showed that 54 % of the AGA-positive patients suffered from intestinal inflammation, but only a small number of them complained about gastrointestinal symptoms [18]. The rate of elderly people suffering from mild inflammation in the gut mucosa and being AGA-negative is, according to a recent Swedish-population-based study, only 3.8 % [19], again showing that gluten can cause inflammatory injury in the gut, without suffering any gastrointestinal symptoms. The presence of possible ACD is further recognized by the National Institute for Health and Care Excellence (UK) [20]. According to the guidance for CD screening issued in 2009, it is recommended to screen for CD when patients suffer from diabetes mellitus type I, IBS, thyroid hormone disturbances, Addison's disease, epilepsy, lymphoma, rickets, repetitive miscarriage, Sjögren's disease, and Turner disease. The following question arises: why do patients with ACD, with proven inflammatory signs, not suffer from pain, bloating, and other typical symptoms? Could it be that substances present in gluten with opioid effects mask the deleterious effects, functioning as masking compounds of gastrointestinal symptoms, converting the causal factor of CD, gluten, into a silent killer?

CD is characterized by the presence of serum antibodies against tissue transglutaminase

The most reliable way to diagnose CD is through small intestinal biopsy and measurement of the presence of serum antibodies against tissue transglutaminase (tTG), the main endomysial auto-antigen in CD [21–23]. Tissue TG deamidates glutamine residues from the gliadin peptide into glutamic acid, leading to enhanced immunogenicity of the resulting modified peptides. In addition, tTG can, in the absence of any other protein substrate, crosslink with gliadin, producing a tTG-gliadin complex, which can be considered a neo-antigen with possible immune toxicity [24, 25]. Both symptomatic and asymptomatic CD are associated with certain immune system-related genetic polymorphisms, of which the HLA-DQ2

and HLA-DQ8 polymorphisms are expressed in the majority of CD patients [3]. However, many more genes, all related to a more pro-inflammatory activity of the immune system, are also linked with increased CD susceptibility [26]. A recent study by Sironi et al. [27] showed that several interleukin/interleukin receptor genes, involved in the pathogenesis of CD, have been subjected to pathogen-driven selective pressure. Particularly, CD alleles of IL18-RAP, IL18R1, IL23, IL18R1, and the intergenic region between IL2 and IL21 display higher frequencies in populations exposed to high microbial/viral loads, suggesting that these variants protected humans against pathogens. Since CD occurred after the increase of hygiene management and the incorporation of cereals into the human diet, it can be assumed that individuals bearing these genotypes are better protected against pathogens but at the same time are more susceptible for autoimmune diseases in general and CD specifically [28]. Although the above-described events explain the development of the typical inflammatory symptoms of CD and even the flattening of the gut lining through this immune response, they do not explain the phenomenon that many patients suffer from ACD at the level of the intestine and often, in parallel, suffer from extra-gastrointestinal disorders [8].

Gliadin is degraded to a collection of polypeptides called exorphins in the gastrointestinal tract

Breakdown of gliadin from wheat is achieved through hydrolysation by intestinal pepsin, leucine aminopeptidase, and elastase, resulting in the release of immune-reactive and opioid-like peptides, including gliadinomorphin-7 (Tyr-Pro-Gln-Pro-Gln-Pro-Phe) from α-gliadin [2]. Further breakdown of these peptides, which are rich in proline, depends on the enzyme dipeptidyl peptidase IV (DPP IV), capable of cleaving N-terminal dipeptides with proline at the second (penultimate) position [29–31]. The remaining tripeptide (in the case of gliadinomorphin-7) with proline in the center is slowly hydrolyzed and acts as a selective competitive inhibitor for DPP IV [32–34].

Whereas total breakdown of gliadin into isolated amino acids prevents the presence of the gluten epitopes which are known to provoke a pro-inflammatory response of the immune system in genetically susceptible people [35, 36], a possible DPP IV deficiency/inactivity could result in the incomplete breakdown of gluten, and thereby increase the presence of immune-reactive and opioid-like peptides, also known as gluten exorphins [36–39]. Gluten is not the only source of exorphins. Dairy products and certain vegetables such as soy and spinach also contain proteins, which can be converted in bioactive exorphins [40].

Gliadin from gluten and casein from dairy products show surprisingly high substrate specificity for DPP IV when compared with other endogenous DPP IV substrates. For example, DPP IV shows higher affinity for gliadin and casein than for substance P (SP) [41] and glucagon-like peptide (GLP) [42]. Gliadin is highly specific for DPP IV [36], which is further evidenced by its binding affinity with human DPP IV. By using an enzyme-linked immunosorbent assay, it was shown that binding of gliadin and casein to DPP IV inhibited DPP IV binding to anti-DPP IV by 52 and 44 %, respectively [43]. The fact that gliadin has a high affinity for DPP IV might explain why so many patients with proven CD are asymptomatic. Inhibition of DPP IV by gliadin can result in increased levels of non-metabolized gliadin molecules with opioid activity that can inhibit the typical abdominal pain associated with classical CD (Fig. 1).

Opioid pathways could be responsible for the development of ACD

It is surprising that a large group of patients, positive for the presence of CD antibodies and with proven histological CD, do not suffer from any gastrointestinal symptoms. If it is the opioid effects of gluten itself masking the classical symptoms of CD, then symptoms should be provoked when patients are given naloxone, a natural antagonist of morphine.

Opioid effects on intestinal transit time

Gastric emptying and intestinal transit are influenced by endogenous and exogenous opioid substances. It is known for long that morphine increases gastrointestinal transit time in humans and that this can be reversed by naloxone [44]. Early research showed that gluten exorphins induced a significant increase in transit time, and this effect was abolished when naloxone was administered [45]. A more recent study supports these early findings. In a single-center study, Urgesi et al. [46] observed that patients suffering from CD show a significantly longer small bowel transit time. In the discussion, the authors mention different pathways explaining their findings but do not mention the possible effect of opioids on intestinal transit time.

Gluten-derived exorphins mimic endogenous opioid activity

Stimulation of insulin production after meal intake is considered an endogenous opioid activity. Early research in rodents showed that oral administration of gluten exorphin A5 stimulated insulin production after food intake. The postprandial increase of insulin release by gluten exorphin was completely abolished by the opioid antagonist naloxone, implying that gluten exorphins maintain bioavailability for the peripheral nervous system within the gastrointestinal tract and pancreatic tissues [47]. Elevated circulating prolactin levels were

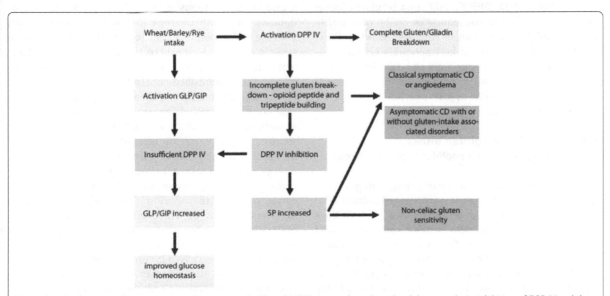

Fig. 1 The development of symptomatic and asymptomatic CD and NCGS. Incomplete gluten breakdown results in inhibition of DPP IV and the possible increase of SP, leading to intestinal and extra-intestinal gluten-induced disorders. Gluten-derived DPP IV inhibition also increases the presence of GIP and GLP in the gut, leading to improved glucose homeostasis

observed in individuals diagnosed with CD [48]. A short gluten-free diet period lowered prolactin levels in these patients, suggesting that gluten (or gluten-derived substances), similar to endogenous opioids, directly affects prolactin secretion. This was further evidenced by Fanciulli et al. [49]. In rats, by using an opioid antagonist unable to cross the blood-brain barrier (naloxone methobromide), intraccrebroventricular (ICV)-injected gluten exorphins stimulated prolactin release through activation of opioid receptors probably also outside the brain.

Gluten exorphins influence behavior and pain perception
A recent review of the literature concluded that food-derived exorphins are bioactive and affect behavioral traits such as spontaneous behavior, memory, and pain perception in rodents. The highest behavioral influence was measured for casein and spinach-derived exorphins (respectively, B-casomorphin and rubiscolin) [50]. Only one of the reviewed studies described the effects of gliadin exorphins in this context. Takahashi et al. [51] showed that ICV-administered gliadin exorphin A5 induced antinociceptive effects and orally delivered gliadin exorphin A5 modified learning and anxiety behavior during several laboratory stressors in mice, thus indicating that orally delivered exorphins can influence both the peripheral and central nervous system and suggesting that gluten exorphins possess opioid activity that could potentially mask symptoms in ACD patients.

Besides explaining the lack of intestinal symptoms through gluten exorphin opioid activity in individuals suffering from ACD, DPP IV inhibition by gluten intake can have many other consequences on human health. DPP IV inhibition is known to have anti-diabetic effects but at the same time could be responsible for the presence of extra-intestinal symptoms and disorders in ACD and the occurrence of intestinal and extra-intestinal symptoms and disorders in CD and non-celiac gluten sensitivity (NCGS) patients (described below).

DPP IV inhibition by gluten intake
DPP IV blockage by gliadin peptides improves glucose homeostasis
Casein is not the only protein competing with gluten as a substrate for DPP IV (a nice overview of natural DPP IV substrates is provided by Gorrel et al. [52]). Other N-terminal dipeptides with proline at the second position, like the incretins, GLP and glucose-dependent insulinotropic polypeptide (GIP), both important regulators of glucose metabolism and essential to gut function, compete with gluten as substrates for DPP IV [52–57]. Carbohydrate intake increases the secretion of both incretins, which are normally rapidly broken down by DPP IV [58]. In a recent review [58], it is described how the

inhibiting effect of gliadin on DPP IV increases the presence of GLP and GIP, by using whole wheat as a natural DPP IV inhibitor. DPP IV inhibition by gliadin could explain the "health promoting" effects of whole wheat intake, as the suppression of GLP and GIP breakdown has anti-diabetic effects [58] (Fig. 1). Contrasting data were found in a randomized, controlled, and open-labeled study [59]. Two days of DPP IV inhibition increased GLP and GIP levels but did not affect glucose values, transit time, or gastric emptying in healthy subjects, suggesting that short exposure to DPP IV inhibition does not affect any function related with DPP IV. The latter makes sense when observing the toxic effects of gluten as a natural DPP IV inhibitor. When patients suffering from NCGS followed a gluten-free diet and were re-challenged with gluten intake, it took approximately 7 days before new symptoms were provoked [60]. Longer use of gluten and synthetic DPP IV inhibitors have been shown to influence gastric emptying and transit time significantly. It is even so that deceleration and slowing of transit time are considered the most important mechanisms by which DPP IV inhibitors influence glucose homeostasis [56, 61, 62].

DPP IV blockage by gliadin peptides induces intestinal and extra-intestinal disorders
Breakdown of SP is also dependent on DPP IV activity. SP has neurological, immunological, and endocrinological functions and influences pain sensitivity, gut peristaltic, inflammation, and social interaction [63]. Increased concentrations of SP in the gut can produce abdominal pain with diarrhea [64] and angioedema with swelling and abdominal pain [65]. High SP levels in the gut can even produce pancreatitis together with abdominal pain, diarrhea, and vomiting [66]. A recent double-blind placebo-controlled human trial showed that the intake of a small amount of gluten (4.375 g/day for 1 week) significantly increased intestinal and extra-intestinal symptoms in individuals with self-reported gluten sensitivity [67]. Typical intestinal symptoms such as bloating and abdominal pain were increased after 1 week of gluten intake, as were extra-intestinal symptoms, such as depression and apthous stomatitis. Because in patients suffering from NCGS no known intestinal lesions or other biomarkers such as antibodies against gluten/gliadin/self-antigens seem to be present [68], their symptoms have to be explained by different pathways. NCGS presents itself with intestinal symptoms like diarrhea, abdominal discomfort, and flatulence, while headache, lethargy, attention-deficit/hyperactivity disorder, ataxia, or oral ulceration appears as an extra-intestinal symptom [3, 67]. Most, if not all, of these symptoms can be explained by

increased levels of SP [64, 69, 70], suggesting that, in NCGS patients, gliadin blocks DPP IV activity and thereby inhibits SP breakdown. Thus, interventions targeting SP release in this group of patients could be a possible strategy to alleviate their intestinal and extra-intestinal symptoms [67] (Fig. 1).

DPP IV inhibition increases the development of angioedema

DPP IV inhibition by synthetic inhibitors, such as sitagliptin, is known to increase the possibility of developing angioedema [71]. CD produces the same symptoms as angioedema, and both disorders are so similar that, in general, it is advised to screen people with hereditary angioedema for CD [72]. Skin disorders, CD, and angioedema seem to be associated as seen in patients suffering from gluten-induced chronic urticaria [73] of which approximately 40 % also experience angioedema [74]. Even guidelines for the management of urticaria are similar as for angioedema [74, 75], suggesting that both disorders have the same etiology, which could be CD and/or increased levels of SP through DPP IV inhibition. A study by Ramsay et al. [76] indicated that patients with gastrointestinal disorders (CD, morbus Crohn, colitis) suffer from mast-cell-induced inflammation. Interestingly enough, mast-cell inflammation can be induced by SP [77]. DPP IV inhibition by gluten would also explain the relationship between gluten intake and skin disorders [78, 79]. Many skin diseases, including acne vulgaris, are associated with higher serum levels of SP [69], which can be induced by blockage of DPP IV [65]. Another gluten intake-related disorder, major depression, is also related with DPP IV inhibition; low serum DPP IV is an important marker for depression [80], and gluten could function as an inhibitor of DPP IV.

Gliadin peptides can cause anatomical changes at the level of the brain

Recent research in humans has shown that gluten intake can even cause anatomical changes at brain level, although neurological symptoms are absent. Anatomical MRI shows silent neurological changes, including bilateral decrease in cortical gray matter and caudate nuclei volumes in celiac patients compared to controls [81]. Negative correlations were found between the duration of the disease and the volumes of the affected regions. Similar neurological changes were observed in a retrospective examination of the brain by MRI of patients suffering from biopsy-proven CD who were referred for a neurological opinion by their gastroenterologist [82]. Patients were divided into subgroups based on their primary neurological complaint (balance disturbance, headache, and sensory loss). The outcome was that CD

patients suffer from a significant loss of cerebellar volume compared with healthy controls. Affected area were brain regions below and above the tentorium cerebelli. These changes were the highest in the headache subgroup and unexpected for the patient's age. The headache group had an average loss of white matter in these regions two times more than the subgroup with balance disturbance and six times more than the subgroup suffering from sensory loss. One possible explanation for the loss of white matter in people suffering from CD is the presence of gluten-induced autoimmune vasculitis [83]. Another more recent hypothesis explaining the loss of white matter caused by reactions against gluten is related with the complementary immune system. The complement protein C1Q is known to bind and help eliminate complexes of immune globulins bound to antigens [84]. C1Q further is considered a "punishment factor" of the central neurological system, produced by strong synapsis and marking weak synapsis for possible phagocytosis by neighboring glia cells [85]. The process of synapsis breakdown should be considered normal in early life with the purpose of remodeling the central nervous system during neurological development [86]. Increased expression of C1Q has been observed in patients suffering from Alzheimer [87], autism [88], and schizophrenia [89]. Severance et al. [84] showed that C1Q binds preferentially to immune globulins coupled with casein and gluten antigens. Their results suggest that the increased expression of C1Q increased synaptic breakdown and could be responsible for schizophrenia onset. We speculate that the increased presence of gliadin peptides, induced by DPP IV inhibition, could be responsible for stimulating C1Q expression and, thereby increases disease susceptibility for these neurodevelopmental and neurodegenerative disorders.

Conclusions

The precise pathway leading to the development of ACD still needs to be discovered. However, the putative mechanism presented in this review could explain this intruding phenomenon. The incomplete breakdown of the gluten protein, resulting in the presence of gliadin peptides with opioid effects, makes it plausible to suggest that the opioid effects of gluten exorphins could be responsible for the absence of classical gastrointestinal symptoms of individuals suffering from gluten-intake-associated diseases. Moreover, the partial digestion of gluten, leading to DPP IV inhibition, could also account for the presence of extraintestinal symptoms and disorders in ACD and the occurrence of intestinal and extra-intestinal symptoms and disorders in CD and NCGS patients. If so, then individuals suffering from any of these conditions should be recognized in time and engage in a gluten-free lifestyle to prevent gluten-induced symptoms and disorders.

Competing interests

The authors declare no conflict of interest.

Authors' contributions

LP wrote the first manuscript based on an extensive literature review. KP revised the manuscript and added several sections to the manuscript, including the figure. The final manuscript was revised and accepted by both authors. Both authors read and approved the final manuscript.

Author details

[1]Natura Foundation, Edisonstraat 66, 3281 NC Numansdorp, Netherlands. [2]Department of Laboratory Medicine, University Medical Center Groningen (UMCG), University of Groningen, P.O. Box 30.001, 9700 RB Groningen, Netherlands. [3]Institute of Medical Psychology, Charité University Medicine Berlin, Hufelandweg 14, 10117 Berlin, Germany.

References

1. Tatham AS, Shewry PR. Allergens to wheat and related cereals. Clin Exp Allergy. 2008;38(11):1712–26. doi:10.1111/j.1365-2222.2008.03101.x.
2. Trivedi MS, Shah JS, Al-Mughairy S, Hodgson NW, Simms B, Trooskens GA, et al. Food-derived opioid peptides inhibit cysteine uptake with redox and epigenetic consequences. J Nutr Biochem. 2014;25(10):1011–8. doi:10.1016/j.jnutbio.2014.05.004.
3. Troncone R, Jabri B. Coeliac disease and gluten sensitivity. J Intern Med. 2011;269(6):582–90. doi:10.1111/j.1365-2796.2011.02385.x.
4. Strohle A, Wolters M, Hahn A. Celiac disease–the chameleon among the food intolerances. Med Monatsschr Pharm. 2013;36(10):369–80. quiz 81–2.
5. Bybrant MC, Ortqvist E, Lantz S, Grahnquist L. High prevalence of celiac disease in Swedish children and adolescents with type 1 diabetes and the relation to the Swedish epidemic of celiac disease: a cohort study. Scand J Gastroenterol. 2014;49(1):52–8. doi:10.3109/00365521.2013.846403.
6. Hansson T, Dahlbom I, Tuvemo T, Frisk G. Silent coeliac disease is over-represented in children with type 1 diabetes and their siblings. Acta Paediatr. 2015;104(2):185–91. doi:10.1111/apa.12823.
7. Khoury N, Semenkovich K, Arbelaez AM. Coeliac disease presenting as severe hypoglycaemia in youth with type 1 diabetes. Diabet Med. 2014; 31(12):e33–6. doi:10.1111/dme.12488.
8. Pinto-Sanchez MI, Bercik P, Verdu EF, Bai JC. Extraintestinal manifestations of celiac disease. Dig Dis. 2015;33(2):147–54. doi:10.1159/000369541.
9. Parisi P, Pietropaoli N, Ferretti A, Nenna R, Mastrogiorgio G, Del Pozzo M, et al. Role of the gluten-free diet on neurological-EEG findings and sleep disordered breathing in children with celiac disease. Seizure. 2015;25:181–3. doi:10.1016/j.seizure.2014.09.016.
10. Brito MD, Martins A, Henrique R, Mariz J. Enteropathy-associated T cell lymphoma as a complication of silent celiac disease. Hematol Rep. 2014; 6(4):5612. doi:10.4081/hr.2014.5612.
11. Ress K, Annus T, Putnik U, Luts K, Uibo R, Uibo O. Celiac disease in children with atopic dermatitis. Pediatr Dermatol. 2014;31(4):483–8. doi:10.1111/pde.12372.
12. Iagnocco A, Ceccarelli F, Mennini M, Rutigliano IM, Perricone C, Nenna R, et al. Subclinical synovitis detected by ultrasound in children affected by coeliac disease: a frequent manifestation improved by a gluten-free diet. Clin Exp Rheumatol. 2014;32(1):137–42.
13. Knivsberg AM, Reichelt KL, Hoien T, Nodland M. A randomised, controlled study of dietary intervention in autistic syndromes. Nutr Neurosci. 2002;5(4): 251–61. doi:10.1080/10284150290028945.
14. Jackson J, Eaton W, Cascella N, Fasano A, Warfel D, Feldman S, et al. A gluten-free diet in people with schizophrenia and anti-tissue transglutaminase or anti-gliadin antibodies. Schizophr Res. 2012;140(1–3): 262–3. doi:10.1016/j.schres.2012.06.011.
15. Anderson RP, Henry MJ, Taylor R, Duncan EL, Danoy P, Costa MJ, et al. A novel serogenetic approach determines the community prevalence of celiac disease and informs improved diagnostic pathways. BMC Med. 2013; 11:188. doi:10.1186/1741-7015-11-188.
16. Bizzaro N, Tozzoli R, Villalta D, Fabris M, Tonutti E. Cutting-edge issues in celiac disease and in gluten intolerance. Clin Rev Allergy Immunol. 2012; 42(3):279–87. doi:10.1007/s12016-010-8223-1.
17. Rubio-Tapia A, Ludvigsson JF, Brantner TL, Murray JA, Everhart JE. The prevalence of celiac disease in the United States. Am J Gastroenterol. 2012; 107(10):1538–44. doi:10.1038/ajg.2012.219. quiz 7, 45.
18. Ruuskanen A, Kaukinen K, Collin P, Krekela I, Patrikainen H, Tillonen J, et al. Gliadin antibodies in older population and neurological and psychiatric disorders. Acta Neurol Scand. 2013;127(1):19–25. doi:10.1111/j.1600-0404. 2012.01668.x.
19. Walker MM, Murray JA, Ronkainen J, Aro P, Storskrubb T, D'Amato M, et al. Detection of celiac disease and lymphocytic enteropathy by parallel serology and histopathology in a population-based study. Gastroenterology. 2010;139(1):112–9. doi:10.1053/j.gastro.2010.04.007.
20. National Institute for Health and Care Excellence. http://www.nice.org.uk/guidance/CG86/informationforpublic. Accessed May 2015.
21. Dieterich W, Ehnis T, Bauer M, Donner P, Volta U, Riecken EO, et al. Identification of tissue transglutaminase as the autoantigen of celiac disease. Nat Med. 1997;3(7):797–801.
22. Frulio G, Polimeno A, Palmieri D, Fumi M, Auricchio R, Piccolo E, et al. Evaluating diagnostic accuracy of anti-tissue Transglutaminase IgA antibodies as first screening for Celiac Disease in very young children. Clin Chim Acta. 2015;446:237–40. doi:10.1016/j.cca.2015.04.035.
23. Fasano A, Catassi C. Clinical practice. Celiac disease. N Engl J Med. 2012; 367(25):2419–26. doi:10.1056/NEJMcp1113994.
24. Colomba MS, Gregorini A. Are ancient durum wheats less toxic to celiac patients? A study of alpha-gliadin from Graziella Ra and Kamut. ScientificWorldJournal. 2012;2012:837416. doi:10.1100/2012/837416.
25. Di Pisa M, Pascarella S, Scrima M, Sabatino G, Real-Fernandez F, Chelli M, et al. Synthetic peptides reproducing tissue transglutaminase-gliadin complex neo-epitopes as probes for antibody detection in celiac disease patients' sera. J Med Chem. 2015;58(3):1390–9. doi:10.1021/jm5017126.
26. Qiao SW, Iversen R, Raki M, Sollid LM. The adaptive immune response in celiac disease. Semin Immunopathol. 2012;34(4):523–40. doi:10.1007/s00281-012-0314-z.
27. Sironi M, Clerici M. The hygiene hypothesis: an evolutionary perspective. Microbes Infect. 2010;12(6):421–7. doi:10.1016/j.micinf.2010.02.002.
28. Pruimboom L, Fox T, Muskiet FA. Lactase persistence and augmented salivary alpha-amylase gene copy numbers might have been selected by the combined toxic effects of gluten and (food born) pathogens. Med Hypotheses. 2014;82(3):326–34. doi:10.1016/j.mehy.2013.12.020.
29. Augustyns K, Van der Veken P, Senten K, Haemers A. The therapeutic potential of inhibitors of dipeptidyl peptidase IV (DPP IV) and related proline-specific dipeptidyl aminopeptidases. Curr Med Chem. 2005;12(8):971–98.
30. De Meester I, Durinx C, Bal G, Proost P, Struyf S, Goossens F, et al. Natural substrates of dipeptidyl peptidase IV. Adv Exp Med Biol. 2000;477:67–87. doi:10.1007/0-306-46826-3_7.
31. Vanhoof G, Goossens F, De Meester I, Hendriks D, Scharpe S. Proline motifs in peptides and their biological processing. FASEB J. 1995;9(9):736–44.
32. Augustyns K, Bal G, Thonus G, Belyaev A, Zhang XM, Bollaert W, et al. The unique properties of dipeptidyl-peptidase IV (DPP IV / CD26) and the therapeutic potential of DPP IV inhibitors. Curr Med Chem. 1999;6(4):311–27.
33. Mentlein R. Dipeptidyl-peptidase IV, (CD26)-role in the inactivation of regulatory peptides. Regul Pept. 1999;85(1):9–24.
34. Rahfeld J, Schierhorn M, Hartrodt B, Neubert K, Heins J. Are diprotin A (Ile-Pro-Ile) and diprotin B (Val-Pro-Leu) inhibitors or substrates of dipeptidyl peptidase IV? Biochim Biophys Acta. 1991;1076(2):314–6.
35. Bethune MT, Khosla C. Oral enzyme therapy for celiac sprue. Methods Enzymol. 2012;502:241–71. doi:10.1016/B978-0-12-416039-2.00013-6.
36. Hausch F, Shan L, Santiago NA, Gray GM, Khosla C. Intestinal digestive resistance of immunodominant gliadin peptides. Am J Physiol Gastrointest Liver Physiol. 2002;283(4):G996–G1003. doi:10.1152/ajpgi.00136.2002.
37. Detel D, Persic M, Varljen J. Serum and intestinal dipeptidyl peptidase IV (DPP IV/CD26) activity in children with celiac disease. J Pediatr Gastroenterol Nutr. 2007;45(1):65–70. doi:10.1097/MPG.0b013e318054b085.
38. Ozuna CV, Iehisa JC, Gimenez MJ, Alvarez JB, Sousa C, Barro F. Diversification of the celiac disease alpha-gliadin complex in wheat: a 33-mer peptide with six overlapping epitopes, evolved following polyploidization. Plant J. 2015. doi:10.1111/tpj.12851.
39. Shan L, Molberg O, Parrot I, Hausch F, Filiz F, Gray GM, et al. Structural basis for gluten intolerance in celiac sprue. Science. 2002;297(5590):2275–9. doi:10.1126/science.1074129.

40. Teschemacher H. Opioid receptor ligands derived from food proteins. Curr Pharm Des. 2003;9(16):1331–44.

41. Kikuchi M, Fukuyama K, Epstein WL. Soluble dipeptidyl peptidase IV from terminal differentiated rat epidermal cells: purification and its activity on synthetic and natural peptides. Arch Biochem Biophys. 1988;266(2):369–76.

42. Castillo GM, Reichstetter S, Bolotin EM. Extending residence time and stability of peptides by protected graft copolymer (PGC) excipient: GLP-1 example. Pharm Res. 2012;29(1):306–18. doi:10.1007/s11095-011-0542-2.

43. Vojdani A. Identification of etiology of autism. 2005. Google Patents.

44. Yuan CS. Gastric effects of mu-, delta- and kappa-opioid receptor agonists on brainstem unitary responses in the neonatal rat. Eur J Pharmacol. 1996; 314(1–2):27–32.

45. Tovoli F, Masi C, Guidetti E, Negrini G, Paterini P, Bolondi L. Clinical and diagnostic aspects of gluten related disorders. World J Clin Cases. 2015;3(3):275–84. doi:10.12998/wjcc.v3.i3.275.

46. Urgesi R, Cianci R, Bizzotto A, Costamagna G, Riccioni ME. Evaluation of gastric and small bowel transit times in coeliac disease with the small bowel PillCam(R): a single centre study in a non gluten-free diet adult Italian population with coeliac disease. Eur Rev Med Pharmacol Sci. 2013; 17(9):1167–73.

47. Fukudome S, Shimatsu A, Suganuma H, Yoshikawa M. Effect of gluten exorphins A5 and B5 on the postprandial plasma insulin level in conscious rats. Life Sci. 1995;57(7):729–34.

48. Delvecchio M, Faienza MF, Lonero A, Rutigliano V, Francavilla R, Cavallo L. Prolactin may be increased in newly diagnosed celiac children and adolescents and decreases after 6 months of gluten-free diet. Horm Res Paediatr. 2014;81(5):309–13. doi:10.1159/000357064.

49. Fanciulli G, Dettori A, Tomasi PA, Demontis MP, Gianorso S, Anania V, et al. Prolactin and growth hormone response to intracerebroventricular administration of the food opioid peptide gluten exorphin B5 in rats. Life Sci. 2002;71(20):2383–90.

50. Lister J, Fletcher PJ, Nobrega JN, Remington G. Behavioral effects of food-derived opioid-like peptides in rodents: Implications for schizophrenia? Pharmacol Biochem Behav. 2015. doi:10.1016/j.pbb.2015.01.020.

51. Takahashi M, Fukunaga H, Kaneto H, Fukudome S, Yoshikawa M. Behavioral and pharmacological studies on gluten exorphin A5, a newly isolated bioactive food protein fragment, in mice. Jpn J Pharmacol. 2000;84(3):259–65.

52. Gorrell MD. Dipeptidyl peptidase IV and related enzymes in cell biology and liver disorders. Clin Sci (Lond). 2005;108(4):277–92. doi:10.1042/CS20040302.

53. Aertgeerts K, Ye S, Shi L, Prasad SG, Witmer D, Chi E, et al. N-linked glycosylation of dipeptidyl peptidase IV (CD26): effects on enzyme activity, homodimer formation, and adenosine deaminase binding. Protein Sci. 2004; 13(1):145–54. doi:10.1110/ps.03352504.

54. Blom WA, Lluch A, Stafleu A, Vinoy S, Holst JJ, Schaafsma G, et al. Effect of a high-protein breakfast on the postprandial ghrelin response. Am J Clin Nutr. 2006;83(2):211–20.

55. Kim NH, Yu T, Lee DH. The nonglycemic actions of dipeptidyl peptidase-4 inhibitors. Biomed Res Int. 2014;2014:368703. doi:10.1155/2014/368703.

56. Tambascia MA, Malerbi DA, Eliaschewitz FG. Influence of gastric emptying on the control of postprandial glycemia: physiology and therapeutic implications. Einstein (Sao Paulo). 2014;12(2):251–3.

57. Tolle S. GLP-1 analogues in treatment of type 1 diabetes mellitus. Dtsch Med Wochenschr. 2014;139(42):2123–6. doi:10.1055/s-0034-1387304.

58. Cavazos A. Mejia EGd. Identification of bioactive peptides from cereal storage proteins and their potential role in prevention of chronic diseases. Comprehensive Reviews in Food Science and Food Safety. 2013;12(4):364–80.

59. Rhee NA, Ostoft SH, Holst JJ, Deacon CF, Vilsboll T, Knop FK. The impact of dipeptidyl peptidase 4 inhibition on incretin effect, glucose tolerance, and gastrointestinal-mediated glucose disposal in healthy subjects. Eur J Endocrinol. 2014;171(3):353–62. doi:10.1530/EJE-14-0314.

60. Biesiekierski JR, Newnham ED, Irving PM, Barrett JS, Haines M, Doecke JD, et al. Gluten causes gastrointestinal symptoms in subjects without celiac disease: a double-blind randomized placebo-controlled trial. Am J Gastroenterol. 2011;106(3):508–14. doi:10.1038/ajg.2010.487. quiz 15.

61. Edholm T, Degerblad M, Gryback P, Hilsted L, Holst JJ, Jacobsson H, et al. Differential incretin effects of GIP and GLP-1 on gastric emptying, appetite, and insulin-glucose homeostasis. Neurogastroenterol Motil. 2010;22(11):1191–200. doi:10.1111/j.1365-2982.2010.01554.x. e315.

62. Tasyurek HM, Altunbas HA, Balci MK, Sanlioglu S. Incretins: their physiology and application in the treatment of diabetes mellitus. Diabetes Metab Res Rev. 2014;30(5):354–71. doi:10.1002/dmrr.2501.

63. Karl T, Hoffmann T, Pabst R, von Horsten S. Extreme reduction of dipeptidyl peptidase IV activity in F344 rat substrains is associated with various behavioral differences. Physiol Behav. 2003;80(1):123–34.

64. Sohn W, Lee OY, Lee SP, Lee KN, Jun DW, Lee HL, et al. Mast cell number, substance P and vasoactive intestinal peptide in irritable bowel syndrome with diarrhea. Scand J Gastroenterol. 2014;49(1):43–51. doi:10.3109/00365521.2013.857712.

65. Grouzmann E, Livio F, Buclin T. Angiotensin-converting enzyme and dipeptidyl peptidase IV inhibitors: an increased risk of angioedema. Hypertension. 2009;54(3):468–70. doi:10.1161/HYPERTENSIONAHA.109.135244.

66. Waeber B, Buclin T, Grouzmann E. Angioedema during ACE and DPP-4 inhibition. Rev Med Suisse. 2010;6(231):28–31.

67. Di Sabatino A, Volta U, Salvatore C, Biancheri P, Caio G, De Giorgio R, et al. Small amounts of gluten in subjects with suspected nonceliac gluten sensitivity: a randomized, double-blind, placebo-controlled, cross-over trial. Clin Gastroenterol Hepatol. 2015. doi:10.1016/j.cgh.2015.01.029.

68. Di Sabatino A, Corazza GR. Nonceliac gluten sensitivity: sense or sensibility? Ann Intern Med. 2012;156(4):309–11. doi:10.7326/0003-4819-156-4-201202210-00010.

69. Bowe WP, Logan AC. Acne vulgaris, probiotics and the gut-brain-skin axis - back to the future? Gut Pathog. 2011;3(1):1. doi:10.1186/1757-4749-3-1.

70. Herpfer I, Katzev M, Felge B, Fiebich BL, Voderholzer U, Lieb K. Effects of substance P on memory and mood in healthy male subjects. Hum Psychopharmacol. 2007;22(8):567–73. doi:10.1002/hup.876.

71. Gosmanov AR, Fontenot EC. Sitagliptin-associated angioedema. Diabetes Care. 2012;35(8), e60. doi:10.2337/dc12-0574.

72. Csuka D, Kelemen Z, Czaller I, Molnar K, Fust G, Varga L, et al. Association of celiac disease and hereditary angioedema due to C1-inhibitor deficiency. Screening patients with hereditary angioedema for celiac disease: is it worth the effort? Eur J Gastroenterol Hepatol. 2011;23(3):238–44. doi:10.1097/MEG.0b013e328343d3b2.

73. Caproni M, Bonciolini V, D'Errico A, Antiga E, Fabbri P. Celiac disease and dermatologic manifestations: many skin clue to unfold gluten-sensitive enteropathy. Gastroenterol Res Pract. 2012;2012:952753. doi:10.1155/2012/952753.

74. Powell RJ, Du Toit GL, Siddique N, Leech SC, Dixon TA, Clark AT, et al. BSACI guidelines for the management of chronic urticaria and angio-oedema. Clin Exp Allergy. 2007;37(5):631–50. doi:10.1111/j.1365-2222.2007.02678.x.

75. Curto-Barredo L, Silvestre JF, Gimenez-Arnau AM. Update on the treatment of chronic urticaria. Actas Dermosifiliogr. 2014;105(5):469–82. doi:10.1016/j.ad.2012.12.019.

76. Ramsay DB, Stephen S, Borum M, Voltaggio L, Doman DB. Mast cells in gastrointestinal disease. Gastroenterol Hepatol (N Y). 2010;6(12):772–7.

77. Hide M, Yanase Y, Greaves MW. Cutaneous mast cell receptors. Dermatol Clin. 2007;25(4):563–75. doi:10.1016/j.det.2007.06.013. ix.

78. Abenavoli L, Proietti I, Leggio L, Ferrulli A, Vonghia L, Capizzi R, et al. Cutaneous manifestations in celiac disease. World J Gastroenterol. 2006; 12(6):843–52.

79. Kotze LM. Dermatitis herpetiformis, the celiac disease of the skin! Arq Gastroenterol. 2013;50(3):231–5. doi:10.1590/S0004-28032013000200041.

80. Maes M, De Meester I, Verkerk R, De Medts P, Wauters A, Vanhoof G, et al. Lower serum dipeptidyl peptidase IV activity in treatment resistant major depression: relationships with immune-inflammatory markers. Psychoneuroendocrinology. 1997;22(2):65–78.

81. Bilgic B, Aygun D, Arslan AB, Bayram A, Akyuz F, Sencer S, et al. Silent neurological involvement in biopsy-defined coeliac patients. Neurol Sci. 2013;34(12):2199–204. doi:10.1007/s10072-013-1448-z.

82. Currie S, Hadjivassiliou M, Clark MJ, Sanders DS, Wilkinson ID, Griffiths PD, et al. Should we be 'nervous' about coeliac disease? Brain abnormalities in patients with coeliac disease referred for neurological opinion. J Neurol Neurosurg Psychiatry. 2012;83(12):1216–21. doi:10.1136/jnnp-2012-303281.

83. Pratesi R, Gandolfi L, Friedman H, Farage L, de Castro CA, Catassi C. Serum IgA antibodies from patients with coeliac disease react strongly with human brain blood-vessel structures. Scand J Gastroenterol. 1998;33(8):817–21.

84. Severance EG, Gressitt KL, Halling M, Stallings CR, Origoni AE, Vaughan C, et al. Complement C1q formation of immune complexes with milk caseins and wheat glutens in schizophrenia. Neurobiol Dis. 2012;48(3):447–53. doi:10.1016/j.nbd.2012.07.005.

85. Fourgeaud L, Boulanger LM. Synapse remodeling, compliments of the complement system. Cell. 2007;131(6):1034–6. doi:10.1016/j.cell.2007.11.031.

86. Stevens B, Allen NJ, Vazquez LE, Howell GR, Christopherson KS, Nouri N, et al. The classical complement cascade mediates CNS synapse elimination. Cell. 2007;131(6):1164–78. doi:10.1016/j.cell.2007.10.036.

87. Benoit ME, Tenner AJ. Complement protein C1q-mediated neuroprotection is correlated with regulation of neuronal gene and microRNA expression. The Journal of neuroscience : the official journal of the Society for Neuroscience. 2011;31(9):3459–69. doi:10.1523/JNEUROSCI.3932-10.2011.

88. Ashwood P, Wills S, Van de Water J. The immune response in autism: a new frontier for autism research. J Leukoc Biol. 2006;80(1):1–15. doi:10.1189/jlb. 1205707.

89. Zakharyan R, Khoyetsyan A, Arakelyan A, Boyajyan A, Gevorgyan A, Stahelova A, et al. Association of C1QB gene polymorphism with schizophrenia in Armenian population. BMC medical genetics. 2011;12:126. doi:10.1186/1471-2350-12-126.

"Girl Power!": The Relationship between Women's Autonomy and Children's Immunization Coverage in Ethiopia

Jane O. Ebot

Abstract

Background: Although immunizations are efficient and cost effective methods of reducing child mortality, worldwide, approximately 2 million children die yearly of vaccine-preventable diseases. Researchers and health organizations have detailed information on the positive relationship between women's autonomy and children's health outcomes in developing countries.

Methods: This study investigates the links between women's household autonomy and children's immunization status using data from a nationally representative sample of children aged 12–30 months ($N = 2941$) from the 2011 Ethiopia Demographic and Health Survey.

Results: The results showed that women's socioeconomic status and household autonomy were significantly associated with children's immunization status.

Conclusion: Overall, the implications of this study align with those of the Millennium Development Goal #3: improvements in women's household autonomy are linked to more positive child health outcomes.

Keywords: Immunization, Household autonomy and health, Ethiopia, Children

Background

Reducing child mortality rates in Sub-Saharan Africa (SSA) has been one of the leading focuses of the Millennium Development Goals (MDG). The target of MDG 4 focuses on reducing child mortality rates by two thirds by 2015 [1]. As a way to achieve country-specific MDG 4 targets, SSA countries have created national immunization programs as efficient and cost effective ways to reduce child mortality and the number of children with life-threatening infectious diseases. The World Health Organization (WHO) recommends children be fully immunized by age 1 to prevent most of the common childhood diseases. Fully immunized children receive one dose of tuberculosis (BCG); three doses of diphtheria, pertussis, and tetanus (DPT) and polio; and one dose of measles [2]. In 2012, an estimated 2,000,000–3,000,000 deaths were averted by vaccinations, yet approximately 19,000,000 children were not fully immunized, 16,000,000 of whom resided in eight SSA countries [2].

Health organizations have stressed the importance of maternal decision-making in improving children's health outcomes in developing countries. During the 1994 Cairo International Conference on Population and Development, policymakers from around the world called for greater focus on improving women's autonomy to address health needs in developing countries [1]. MDG 3 promotes gender equality and women's autonomy as important means of improving women's and children's health outcomes [3]. Yet limited and uneven progress from the MDG 3 has necessitated more precise research detailing the importance of women's autonomy. Therefore, the aim of this analysis is to investigate the association between Ethiopian women's household autonomy and children's immunization status, which is important for both theoretical and policy reasons.

Ethiopia is the setting for this analysis because it is characterized by both low levels of full immunization coverage and women's autonomy. Ethiopia, SSA's second poorest

Correspondence: jebot@usaid.gov
Service Delivery Improvement Division, Office of Population and Reproductive Health, Bureau for Global Health, United States Agency for International Development (USAID), 2100 Crystal Drive, Arlington, VA 22202, USA

country based on gross domestic product [4], is one of the few African countries that is expected to reach its country-specific MDG 4: between 1990 and 2010, under-five mortality rates declined from 167 to 88 deaths per 1000 children, an average annual decline of 6.3 % [5]. Among the many government-sponsored health sector initiatives, the increase of immunization coverage has been a key method toward successfully meeting MDG 4. As of 2010, progress in immunization coverage against diphtheria, pertussis, tetanus, and measles increased, though more than 75 % of Ethiopian children were still not fully vaccinated [6]. Given these low levels of immunizations, it is critical to research ways to increase their coverage.

Many studies have linked greater women's household autonomy and reductions in infant mortality [7] and better child nutritional outcomes [8, 9]. Decision-making, or autonomy, is the capacity to manipulate and have control over one's personal environment, in order to make decisions about one's own livelihood or those of family members [10]. More autonomous women have increased decision-making abilities concerning marriage candidates [11], contraception [12], sexual activity [13], and access to health care and resources [14]. More autonomous women can also improve their children's health compared to less autonomous women. As children's primary caregivers, women are typically the first to recognize symptoms in sick children and invest time and income to improve their children's health and nutrition [15]. Even before children are born, more autonomous women would have more access to safe delivery services and antenatal care, which would influence the knowledge and access they have in relation to vaccine campaigns and information [10]. Yet male heads of household most often make health care and household financial decisions in traditional societies [15]. Women's limited household autonomy may draw limited benefits for their children from available access to child health care. For example, Woldemicael and Tenkorang analyzed the association between women's autonomy and health-seeking behavior in Ethiopia and the results showed that more autonomous Ethiopian women were more likely to access health care compared to Ethiopian women with little household autonomy [14]. Woldemicael [16] used Demographic Health Surveys (DHS) data from Ethiopia and Eritrea to show that net of socioeconomic status, sole decision-making about visits to family/relatives increased the use of antenatal care in both countries, though sole decision-making about household purchases increased antenatal care only in Eritrea. Therefore, women's household autonomy becomes a means through which women can use health services to reduce their young children's risks of mortality and morbidity.

Early marriages, high fertility rates, and low levels of educational attainment, coupled with deep-rooted patriarchal beliefs regarding the role and status of women, have negatively affected Ethiopian women's autonomy. By age 16, most Ethiopian women leave their families and communities for their new husband's village or home [6]. Women who marry early typically have less mobility and autonomy than unmarried women or women who did not marry early and are at greater risk of intimate partner violence [17–19]. Additionally, Ethiopian women have high adolescent birth and total fertility rates which are negatively associated with children's health and care: the 2010 adolescent birth rate was 109 births per 1000 women, the 15th highest in the world, and the current total fertility rate is 5.39 births per woman [19, 20, 21].

Although researchers have found clear relationships between women's autonomy and health outcomes, certain limitations necessitate further study. First, few studies have focused on the relationship between women's household autonomy and children's immunization status, despite its recognized importance improving children's health and odds of survival [22]. Second, prior to the inclusion of questions on women's household status in the DHS and the Multiple Indicator Cluster Surveys (MICS), many scholars used women's education as a proxy measure of women's autonomy. Educational attainment is a pathway through which women can improve their livelihoods and children's health outcomes [23], yet it does not take into account other means through which women can gain autonomy, especially for those who have not received any formal education: approximately 50 % of Ethiopian women aged 15–49 years of age had not received any formal education as of 2011 [6].

This study builds on work by Singh et al. [22] and Singh et al. [24] by including both a household decision-making index and individual-level measure of women's household autonomy from the 2011 Ethiopia Demographic and Health Survey (EDHS) empowerment and gender modules [22, 24]. This method allows for an overall understanding of women's household autonomy and also highlights the importance of each separate measure of decision-making within the composite household measure. For example, increased decision-making abilities concerning visits to family/relatives may improve children's immunization status compared to decisions regarding daily food preparation because the former symbolizes a lack of physical mobility for women, a factor that policymakers must consider when implementing micro-level initiatives to improve women's autonomy and children's health [25]. In addition, including dimensions of women's autonomy may tap into socioeconomic and demographic characteristics that are specific to a culture or social context. Without including additional analyses of specific elements of women's household autonomy, explanations for its effects on health outcomes are limited.

Methods

Data

Data come from the 2011 EDHS. The 2011 EDHS has complete interviews from 16,702 households; 16,515 women aged 15–49 years; and 14,110 men aged 15–59 years. This study's sample was limited to the 2941 children aged 12–30 months of married women aged 15–49 years in the survey. The child age limits were based on WHO recommendations that children be fully immunized by 12 months of age. There is a 30-month upper limit to cover the cases where children were somewhat late in getting all the vaccines.

Dependent variable

This analysis focuses on children's immunization status, an important health indicator because it is one of the earliest ways parents can prevent common childhood diseases/infections. The EDHS collected information on children's immunizations from vaccination cards and mothers' verbal responses. The vaccination cards represent routine vaccines whereas maternal recall encompasses both routine vaccines and those done through immunization campaigns. Immunization status was coded as a multi-response categorical variable based on WHO standards: a value of "0" was assigned to children who had received no vaccines, a value of "1" was assigned to children who were partially vaccinated (had received one to seven WHO-recommended vaccines), and a value of "2" was assigned to children who were fully vaccinated (received all eight vaccines).

Independent variables

The primary independent variable, women's household autonomy, was gauged through EDHS questions asking women about their household decision-making abilities: "Who usually makes the final decision on the purchase of major household goods; visits to family/relatives; women's earnings; and women's own health care?" Responses to each of these questions were coded into three categories: the woman made the sole decision, the woman made the decision jointly with her husband/partner, or the husband/partner made the sole decision. The household autonomy index reflects the number of decisions in which a woman participated alone or jointly with her husband. Specifically, it was created by summing up the total number of decisions in which a woman participated alone or jointly with her husband and ranged in all four scenarios. It ranged from 0 to 4: a low score on the household autonomy index indicates a lower level of household autonomy whereas a high score on the autonomy index indicates a higher level of household autonomy.

I included two dichotomous measures of women's health access: women who delivered their last child in a hospital/clinic/health care facility versus women who delivered at home and women who received some form of antenatal care for their latest pregnancy versus women who received no antenatal care.

The analysis also included measures of mothers' and fathers' socioeconomic status. Mothers' educational attainment was measured in three categories due to small cell counts at the higher levels of education: no education, primary school education, and secondary school and higher. Fathers' educational attainment was measured in four categories: no education, primary school education, secondary school education, and higher. Women's occupation was coded into four categories: no occupation, manual, agriculture, and professional sector. Women's household wealth status was measured as an index constructed by the EDHS: poorest, poorer, middle, richer, richest. Other control variables included women's religion, age in years, polygamous marriage, age at first marriage, child's age, child sex, number of children under 5 years of age in the household, region, and urban/rural residential location.

Methods

I employed ordinal logistic regressions for the multivariate analyses. "Partially immunized" and "fully immunized" statuses were contrasted against the reference category of "not vaccinated" children. Sample weights were used to make the results nationally representative.

Ethical clearance

This study is based on an analysis of survey data with all identifying information removed. The 2011 EDHS was approved by the Ethiopia Health and Nutrition Research Institute (EHNRI) Review Board, the National Research Ethics Review Committee (NRERC) at the Ministry of Science and Technology, the Institutional Review Board of ICF, and the CDC. All study participants gave informed consent before participation, and all information was collected confidentially. Use of this data was granted by ICF International.

Results

Descriptive statistics

Table 1 presents weighted descriptive statistics. About 15 % of Ethiopian children did not receive any vaccine, though most children were partially vaccinated. Only 24 % of children were fully immunized, meaning that they received all eight doses of vaccines specified by the WHO. The household autonomy index mean of 3.1 means that on average, most women made about three out of four decisions alone or jointly. More specifically, individual decision-making showed that across all scenarios, most women made decisions jointly with their husband/partner rather than solely. Approximately 89 %

Table 1 Women's reports of autonomy, socioeconomic status, and their children's immunization status in Ethiopia (weighted data)

	N (percent %)	CI
Immunization status		
No vaccinations (reference category)	521 (14.9)	(11.9, 18.5)
Partially vaccinated	1588 (61.0)	(57.4, 64.5)
Fully vaccinated	832 (24.1)	(21.3, 27.1)
Mean number of vaccinations	4.7 (mean)	(4.4, 5.0)
Autonomy index (0–4)	3.1 (mean)	(3.0, 3.2)
Household decision-making		
Person who makes final decision on household purchases		
Mother	185 (4.3)	(3.3, 5.6)
Joint	1647 (61.3)	(58.0, 64.5)
Husband/partner (reference category)	1109 (34.4)	(31.3, 37.7)
Person who makes final decision on visits to family/friends		
Mother	594 (14.4)	(12.5, 16.5)
Joint	1550 (62.0)	(58.8, 65.1)
Husband/partner (reference category)	797 (23.6)	(21.2, 26.2)
Person who makes final decisions regarding respondent's earnings		
Mother	294 (9.2)	(7.6, 11.2)
Joint	2555 (87.4)	(85.3, 89.3)
Husband/partner (reference category)	92 (3.3)	(2.3, 4.7)
Person who makes final decisions on respondent's health care		
Mother	453 (12.0)	(10.3, 13.9)
Joint	1633 (59.8)	(56.5, 63.0)
Husband/partner (reference category)	855 (28.2)	(25.3, 31.3)
Health care		
Home delivery	2495 (89.8)	(87.8, 91.4)
Antenatal care	1139 (36.0)	(33.0, 39.1)
Socioeconomic status		
Mothers' individual level of educational attainment		
No education (reference category)	2040 (68.8)	(65.5, 71.9)
Primary school	740 (26.9)	(22.1, 27.9)
Secondary school and higher	161 (4.4)	(5.1, 7.9)
Fathers' individual level of educational attainment		
No education (reference category)	1508 (51.0)	(47.4–54.6)
Primary school	1071 (39.6)	(36.3–43.1)
Secondary school	189 (4.9)	(3.7–6.4)
Higher	173 (4.5)	(3.3–6.0)

Table 1 Women's reports of autonomy, socioeconomic status, and their children's immunization status in Ethiopia (weighted data) *(Continued)*

	N (percent %)	CI
Women's occupation		
No occupation (reference category)	1645 (47.2)	(43.7, 50.7)
Manual	215 (7.2)	(5.6, 9.2)
Agriculture	586 (26.9)	(23.8, 30.3)
Professional	495 (18.7)	(16.0, 21.8)
Household wealth		
Poorest (reference category)	904 (23.0)	(19.8, 26.5)
Poorer	513 (22.1)	(19.7, 24.7)
Middle	474 (20.9)	(18.6, 23.4)
Richer	482 (19.3)	(16.5, 22.5)
Richest	568 (14.7)	(12.7, 16.8)

Source: 2011 EDHS; N = 2941

of women delivered their last child at home, and only 36 % of women received some form of antenatal care. Finally, about 68 % of mothers did not receive a formal education, 47 % of mothers were not in the labor force, and households were evenly spread across the wealth index.

Table 2 presents ordinal logistic regression results testing the association between women's household autonomy and Ethiopian children's immunization status. Results from this table confirm the importance of women's household autonomy for child health: net of socioeconomic status, women's household autonomy was a significant predictor of children's immunization status. Beginning with the baseline model that only included the household autonomy index, every one unit increase in women's household autonomy was associated with an expected 16 % increase in the odds of a child being partially immunized compared to the reference category of a child having no vaccines. In model 2, I included health access measures, which slightly diminished the household autonomy effect. Relative to women who did not receive antenatal care, women who received antenatal care had increased odds of children being partially immunized compared to having no vaccines. The inclusion of the socioeconomic variables in model 3 did not dampen the household autonomy effect: net of health care access, education, occupation, and household wealth, increases in women's household autonomy continued to have significant and positive effect on the odds of children being partially immunized versus not vaccinated at all.

The second half of the table displays results predicting full immunization status versus no vaccines. Model 1 shows that a one-unit increase in women's household autonomy is related to a 36 % increase in the odds of a child being fully immunized versus not having any vaccines. In model 2, the household

Table 2 Odds ratios from ordinal logistic regressions predicting Ethiopian children's immunization status[ae]

	Partially immunized (vs. no vaccines)			Fully immunized (vs. no vaccines)		
	Model 1	Model 2	Model 3	Model 1	Model 2	Model 3
Autonomy index	1.16*	1.13****	1.16**	1.36**	1.29**	1.32**
	(1.00, 1.35)	(0.98, 1.31)	(1.00, 1.33)	(1.13, 1.63)	(1.07, 1.56)	(1.10, 1.590)
Delivered at home		0.91	1.04		0.61	0.80
		(0.33, 2.53)	(0.39, 2.81)		(0.20, 1.88)	(0.27, 2.35)
Antenatal care		2.62***	2.45***		5.68***	4.95***
		(1.57, 4.38)	(1.46, 4.11)		(3.30, 9.79)	(2.89, 8.50)
Mothers' education[b]						
Primary school			1.76*			2.32**
			(1.09, 2.86)			(1.64, 4.01)
Secondary school and higher			2.31			3.72
			(0.44, 12.17)			(0.76, 18.20)
Fathers' education[b]						
Primary school			1.17			0.96
			(0.75, 1.82)			(0.58, 1.58)
Secondary school			0.98			0.73
			(0.34, 2.77)			(0.22, 2.36)
Higher			1.08			0.89
			(0.34, 3.39)			(0.25, 3.13)
Occupation[c]						
Manual			0.43*			0.43****
			(0.20, 0.95)			(0.16, 1.13)
Agriculture			1.28			1.57
			(0.82, 2.01)			(0.91, 2.73)
Professional			1.09			1.04
			(0.67, 1.76)			(0.61, 1.80)
Wealth index[d]						
Poorer			0.69			1.00
			(0.42, 1.13)			(0.53, 1.88)
Middle			0.65****			0.75
			(0.40–1.04)			(0.41, 1.36)
Richer			0.5*			0.99
			(0.32, 0.95)			(0.50, 1.94)
Richest			1.09			2.95****
			(0.341, 2.90)			(0.98, 8.81)
Constant	3.18	1.97	0.92	3.36	1.48	0.37
	(0.51, 19.72)	(0.32, 12.06)	(0.172, 4.92)	(0.46, 24.85)	(0.21, 10.63)	(0.06, 2.28)
Observations	2941	2941	2941	2941	2941	2941

*$p < 0.05$; **$p < 0.01$; ***$p < 0.001$; ****$p < 0.10$
[a]Each model controls for women's religion, mother's age in years, polygamous marriage, age at first marriage, child's age, child sex, number of children under 5 years of age in the household, region, and urban/rural residential location
[b]Reference category is no education
[c]Reference category is no occupation
[d]Reference category is poorest
[e]Confidence interval in parentheses
Source: 2011 Ethiopia Demographic and Health Surveys

autonomy index odds ratio is reduced in size yet remained highly statistically significant, net of health access. It should be noted that compared to women who received no antenatal care, women who received antenatal care had higher odds of children being fully immunized versus having no vaccines. The full array of socioeconomic-status variables in model 3 did nothing to diminish the statistical strength of women's household autonomy.

Table 3 shows the multinomial logistic regression results modeling the relationships between individual measures of women's household autonomy and immunization status. Looking across all the models, only decisions related to finances had a significant effect on partial immunization status. In the first full model, for example, compared to women who said their husband made the final decision on their earnings, women who said they made joint decisions about their earnings had 4.3 times higher odds of their children being partially immunized versus having no vaccines, net of all control variables. In the second full model, joint decisions on earnings (compared to husbands making the sole earnings decision) increased the odds of children being fully immunized by 8.1 times versus not being vaccinated.

Additional models analyzing the relationship between women's household autonomy and children's number of vaccines using negative binomial models (results not presented) showed a positive relationship: net of socioeconomic status and health access, 1-unit increases in women's household autonomy were related to 0.06-unit increases in the number of vaccines.

Discussion

Several studies have showed how women's autonomy is positively related to children's health outcomes [9, 14, 26], yet few have looked at how household autonomy is related to children's immunization status [22]. This study is built upon these prior analyses and tested the relationship between women's household autonomy and Ethiopian children's immunization status. The first key finding from this study was the importance of women's household autonomy for children's immunization status. This pattern is similar to results observed by Singh et al. [22] in Nigeria, where women's autonomy was also positively correlated with children's immunization status. Including mothers' and fathers' individual-level educational attainment, household wealth, and occupation did not dampen the robust and significant relationship between women's overall participation in decisions related to their movement, household purchases, earnings, use of antenatal care, and their children's immunization status. Women's socioeconomic status has been identified as a key means of improving household autonomy and gender equity:

more educated women are more likely to work outside the home in better paying occupations and have better access to health services and health-related knowledge than less educated women [27]. The results of this study show that for Ethiopian women, education was not a substitute for autonomy. That is, Ethiopian women's household autonomy is not solely created through access to education but through greater freedom to make decisions concerning their livelihoods. Therefore, policymakers should not only continue to provide Ethiopian women with safe and accessible schools but should also implement gender-related initiatives that specifically target women's autonomy within the home. Yet it should be noted that women's household autonomy was not as important to children's immunization as women's use of antenatal care. As suggested by Jennings et al. [28], women's household autonomy and antenatal care use might not be individually exclusive pathways for improving children's health. That is, women who make sole or joint decisions with their spouse or partner might be more likely to interpret antenatal care as either a "shared domain" or more likely to solicit antenatal care compared to women with low household autonomy [28–30].

A second key finding was the significance of individual measures of women's household autonomy. More specifically, women who had decision-making abilities related to financial allotments were more likely to have their child partially or fully immunized, compared to women who had no part in these decisions. Women with the freedom to make financial decisions means that they can decide to use their resources to pay for preventative health services for their children. More interesting is the result that women who made financial decisions jointly with their husband were even more likely to get their children vaccinated compared with women who made financial decisions independently. This finding may mean that joint decision-making represents cohesiveness between wives and husbands and an active way that men can improve children's health outcomes that is not necessarily related to socioeconomic status. Though many gender initiatives are typically female-focused, this result suggests that policymakers consider how initiatives that focus on improving marital communication and equity can both improve a sense of spousal togetherness and improvement in children's health outcomes.

There are some limitations to this study. First, the cross-sectional nature of the EDHS means that causal relationships between individual measures of women's household autonomy and children's immunization status cannot be established with certainty. Second, the EDHS does not ask questions about women's role within society as a whole, which might be related to children's immunization status. It is important for future research on women's autonomy to capture both household and

Table 3 Odds ratios from ordinal logistic regressions predicting Ethiopian children's immunization status using individual measures of women's autonomy[ae]

	Partially immunized (vs. no vaccines)			Fully immunized (vs. no vaccines)		
	Model 1	Model 2	Model 3	Model 1	Model 2	Model 3
Individual measures of women's autonomy[f]						
Person who makes final decision on household purchases						
Mother	2.11	1.92	1.86	2.12	1.68	1.67
	(0.84, 5.31)	(0.74, 4.99)	(0.74, 4.71)	(0.70, 6.44)	(0.52, 5.39)	(0.452, 5.32)
Joint	1.18	1.07	1.10	1.30	1.07	1.09
	(0.78, 1.78)	(0.70, 1.63)	(0.72, 1.66)	(0.80, 2.11)	(0.65, 1.75)	(0.66, 1.77)
Person who makes final decision on visits to family/friends						
Mother	1.15	1.01	1.00	1.55	1.28	1.26
	(0.66, 2.03)	(0.56, 1.82)	(0.55, 1.81)	(0.73, 3.28)	(0.60, 2.72)	(0.58, 2.72)
Joint	0.97	0.94	0.97	1.19	1.19	1.23
	(0.61, 1.53)	(0.59, 1.50)	(0.60, 1.55)	(0.70, 2.05)	(0.69, 2.05)	(0.71, 2.13)
Person who makes final decisions regarding respondent's earnings						
Mother	2.78****	2.78	3.38****	4.63*	4.96*	6.53**
	(0.87, 8.89)	(0.82, 9.40)	(1.00, 1.42)	(1.34, 15.98)	(1.22, 20.18)	(1.68, 25.54)
Joint	3.16**	3.57**	4.29**	4.71**	6.30***	8.13***
	(1.34, 7.49)	(1.53, 8.35)	(1.69, 10.89)	(1.86, 11.89)	(2.27, 17.54)	(2.59, 25.34)
Person who makes final decisions on respondent's health care						
Mother	1.40	1.47	1.42	1.91	2.00****	1.79
	(0.70, 2.81)	(0.73, 2.98)	(0.68, 2.93)	(0.87, 4.17)	(0.90, 4.41)	(0.79, 4.10)
Joint	1.08	1.10	1.06	1.22	1.28	1.19
	(0.71, 1.64)	(0.72, 1.70)	(0.67, 1.67)	(0.71, 2.09)	(0.74, 2.22)	(0.67, 2.12)
Health care						
Delivered at home		0.87	0.96		0.58	0.74
		(0.31, 2.45)	(0.37, 2.50)		(0.19, 1.81)	(0.26, 2.13)
Antenatal care		2.75***	2.54***		6.04***	5.08***
		(1.64, 4.60)	(1.54, 4.18)		(3.51, 10.39)	(2.98, 8.65)
Mothers education[b]						
Primary school			1.78*			2.30**
			(1.08, 2.94)			(1.31, 4.04)
Complete secondary school and higher			2.28			3.66****
			(0.47, 11.11)			(0.83, 16.27)
Fathers' education[b]						
Primary school			1.10			0.91
			(0.72, 1.68)			(0.55, 1.46)
Secondary school			1.05			0.80
			(0.35, 3.10)			(0.24, 2.67)
Higher			1.07			0.87
			(0.35, 3.31)			(0.25, 2.98)

Table 3 Odds ratios from ordinal logistic regressions predicting Ethiopian children's immunization status using individual measures of women's autonomy[a][e] *(Continued)*

Occupation[c]						
Manual occupation			0.56			0.57
			(0.26, 1.20)			(0.22, 1.50)
Agriculture occupation			1.34			1.64****
			(0.85, 2.11)			(0.93, 2.89)
Professional occupation			1.37			1.31
			(0.77, 2.40)			(0.69, 2.50)
Wealth index[d]						
Poorer			0.74			1.06
			(0.43, 1.27)			(0.55, 2.06)
Middle			0.66****			0.74
			(0.41, 1.06)			(0.40, 1.37)
Richer			0.52*			0.91
			(0.31, 0.87)			(0.47, 1.78)
Richest			1.09			2.87****
			(0.42, 2.85)			(0.97, 8.46)
Constant	1.40	0.78	0.27	1.08	0.37	0.69
	(0.21, 9.18)	(0.12, 5.15)	(0.04, 1.69)	(0.14, 8.33)	(0.05, 2.92)	(0.01, 0.45)
Observations	2941	2941	2941	2941	2941	2941

$*p < 0.05$; $**p < 0.01$; $***p < 0.001$; $****p < 0.10$
[a]Each model controls for women's religion, mother's age in years, polygamous marriage, age at first marriage, child's age, child sex, number of children under 5 years of age in the household, region, and urban/rural residential location
[b]Reference category is no education
[c]Reference category is no occupation
[d]Reference category is poorest
[e]Confidence interval in parentheses
[f]Reference group is husband makes final decision
Source: 2011 Ethiopia Demographic and Health Surveys

social measures of women's autonomy and to use longitudinal data to understand its long-term impact on children's health across the life course.

Conclusion

Research on immunization coverage is not only an important indicator of health care utilization but also a measureable indicator of the progress toward the 2015 MDG. Understanding factors that could assist women in seeking health care for their children is also important in advancing the MDG's gender-related initiatives. This study provides important insight into one of the many ways that empowering women shapes the lives of those around them.

Abbreviations
DHS: Demographic Health Surveys.

Competing interests
The author declares that he/she has no competing interests.

Acknowledgements
This research was supported by grant, 5 R24 HD042849, Population Research Center, awarded to the Population Research Center at The University of Texas at Austin by the Eunice Kennedy Shriver National Institute of Health and Child Development. Thank you to Dr. Robert Hummer, Sarah Blanchard, and Molly Dondero for their editorial assistance with this research.

References
1. Food and Agriculture Organization. Millennium Development Goals. Access September 4, 2012, from http://www.fao.org/mdg/en/.
2. World Health Organization. 2012a. Immunization, vaccines, and biologicals: World Immunization Week 2012. Access January 13, 2012, from http://www.who.int/immunization/newsroom/events/immunization_week/en/index.html.
3. United Nations Children's Fund. Millennium Development Goals: promote gender equality and empower women. Retrieved August 15, 2012, from http://www.unicef.org/mdg/index_genderequality.htm.
4. Central Intelligence Association. The world factbook: Ethiopia. Retrieved February 11, 2013.
5. The World Factbook 2013-14: Ethiopia. Washington, DC: Central Intelligence Agency; 2013
6. Central Statistical Agency [Ethiopia] and ICF International. Ethiopia Demographic and Health Survey 2011. Addis Ababa, Ethiopia and Calverton, Maryland, USA: Central Statistical Agency and ICF International; 2012
7. Ghuman SJ. Women's autonomy and child survival: a comparison of Muslims and non-Muslims in four Asian countries. Demography. 2003;40(3):419–36.

8. Brunson EK, Shell-Duncan B, Steele M. Women's autonomy and its relationship to children's nutrition among the Rendille of northern Kenya. Am J Hum Biol. 2009;21:55–64.

9. Doan R, Bisharat L. Female autonomy and child nutritional status: the extended-family residential unit in Amman, Jordan. Soc Sci Med. 1990;31:783–9.

10. Bloom SS, Wypij D, Das GM. Dimensions of women's autonomy and the influence on maternal health care utilization in a North Indian city. Demog. 2001;38:67–78.

11. Hindin MJ. For better or for worse? Women's autonomy and marital status in Zimbabwe. Soc Sci Res. 2002;31:151–72.

12. Hogan DP, Berhanu B, Hailemariam A. Household organization, women's autonomy, and contraceptive behavior in southern Ethiopia. Stud Fam Plann. 1999;30:302–14.

13. Hindin MJ, Muntifering CJ. Women's autonomy and timing of most recent sexual intercourse in Sub-Saharan Africa: a multi-country analysis. J Sex Res. 2011;48:511–9.

14. Woldemicael G, Tenkorang EY. Women's autonomy and maternal health-seeking behavior in Ethiopia. Matern Child Health J. 2010;14:988–98.

15. Ngom P, Debpuur C, Akweongo P, Adongo P, Binka FN. Gate-keeping and women's health seeking behavior in Navrongo, Northern Ghana. Afr J Reprod Health. 2003;7:17–26.

16. Woldemicael G. Do women with higher autonomy seek more maternal health care? Evidence from Eritrea and Ethiopia. Health Care Women Int. 2010;31:599–620.

17. Mahmud S, Amin S. Girls' schooling and marriage in rural Bangladesh. Res Soc Educ. 2006;15:71–99.

18. Gómez AM, Speizer IS. Community-level intimate partner violence and the circumstances of first sex among young women from five African countries. Reprod Health. 2010;7:8.

19. Gupta N, Mahy M. Adolescent childbearing in Sub-Saharan Africa: can increased schooling alone raise ages at first birth. Demogr Res. 2003;8:93–106.

20. United Nations Children's Fund. Ethiopia, statistics. Retrieved November 21, 2012.

21. Prakash R, Singh A, Pathak PK, Parasuraman S. Early marriage, poor reproductive health status of mother and child well-being in India. J Fam Plann Reprod Health Care. 2011;37:136–45.

22. Singh K, Haney E, Olorunsaiye C. Maternal autonomy and attitudes towards gender norms: associations with childhood immunization in Nigeria. Matern Child Health J. 2012;8(17):837-841.

23. Mirowsky J, Ross CE. Life course trajectories of perceived control and their relationship to education. Am J Sociol. 2007;112(5):1339–82.

24. Singh K, Bloom S, Brodish P. Gender equality as a means to improve maternal and child health in Africa. Health Care Women Int. 2013;1(36):57-69

25. Moursund A, Kravdal Ø. Individual and community effects of women's education and autonomy on contraceptive use in India. Popul Stud. 2003;57:285–301.

26. Boehmer U, Williamson JB. The impact of women's status on infant mortality rate: a cross-national analysis. Soc Indic Res. 1996;37(3):333–60.

27. Burchi F. Child nutrition in Mozambique in 2003: the role of mother's schooling and nutrition knowledge. Econ Human Biol. 2010;8(3):331–45.

28. Jennings L, Na M, Cherewick M, Hindin M, Mullany B, Ahmed S. Women's empowerment and male involvment in antenatal care: analyses of Demographic and Health Surveys (DHS) in selected African countries. BMC Pregnancy Childbirth. 2014;14:297–308.

29. Choi JY, Lee S-H. Does prenatal care increase access to child immunization? Gender bias among children in India. Soc Sci Med. 2006;63(1):107–17.

30. Mistry R, Galal O, Mistry R, Galal O, Lu M. Women's autonomy and pregnancy care in rural India: a contextual analysis. Soc Sci Med. 2009;69(6):926–33.

Perception and attitudes towards preventives of malaria infection during pregnancy in Enugu State, Nigeria

Nkechi G. Onyeneho[1*], Ngozi Idemili-Aronu[1], Ijeoma Igwe[1] and Felicia U. Iremeka[2]

Abstract

Background: The objective of this study is to explore and document perceptions and attitude associated with uptake of interventions to prevent malaria in pregnancy infection during pregnancy in Enugu State, Nigeria.

Methods: This is a cross-sectional study in three local government areas in Enugu State to identify the people's perceptions and attitudes towards sleeping under insecticide-treated bednets and uptake of recommended doses of intermittent presumptive treatment during pregnancy. In-depth interview guides were employed to collect data from health workers and mothers who delivered within 6 months preceding the study, while focus group discussion guides were employed in collecting data from grandmothers and fathers of children born within 6 months preceding the study.

Results: The people expressed fairly good knowledge of malaria, having lived in the malaria-endemic communities. However, some were ignorant on what should be done to prevent malaria in pregnancy. Those who were aware of the use of insecticide-treated bednets and intermittent presumptive treatment during pregnancy however lamented the attitude of the health workers, who make access to these interventions difficult.

Conclusions: Efforts to prevent malaria in pregnancy should focus on providing health education to pregnant women and their partners, who reinforce what the women are told during antenatal care. The attitude of health workers towards patients, who need these interventions, should be targeted for change.

Keywords: Perception, Attitude, Malaria-in-pregnancy, Insecticide treated bednets, Intermittent presumptive treatment, Nigeria

Background

Malaria remains a major challenge to attaining the health-related Millennium Development Goals and of public health in Nigeria, where half of the population suffers at least one episode of malaria in a year. Nigeria, where the disease accounts for 11 % of maternal mortality and 12–30 % of mortality in children under 5 years of age [1], is one of the hardest hit countries in Africa south of the Sahara. Malaria is endemic throughout Nigeria. Fifty percent of the adult population experience at least one malaria episode annually. Prevalence rate of malaria among children under 5 years of age in Nigeria was put at 51.5 % by rapid diagnostic test positive results [2]. Children under 5 years of age may suffer malaria attacks two to four times each year [3]. A study in Abeokuta, in the South-west of Nigeria, found a very high malaria prevalence rate of 62.4 % among women attending traditional birth homes [4]. Health facility prevalence of malaria in pregnancy in Nigeria is estimated at 48 % [5, 6]. The disease currently accounts for nearly 110 million clinically diagnosed cases per year, 60 % of outpatient visits, and 30 % hospitalizations [7]. Mortality range associated with malaria in pregnancy can vary 100-fold across the spectrum of birth weight and rises continuously with decreasing weight [8].

Malaria in pregnancy is also reported to have links with inter-uterine growth retardation [9]. It is estimated to cause up to 15 % of maternal anemia and about 35 %

* Correspondence: nkechi.onyeneho@unn.edu.ng
[1]Department of Sociology/Anthropology, University of Nigeria Nsukka, Nsukka 410001, Nigeria
Full list of author information is available at the end of the article

of preventable low birth weight as well as neonatal mortality [10]. Malaria-induced low birth weight is responsible for between 62,000 and 363,000 infant deaths every year in Africa, which translates to 3–17 deaths per 1000 live births [11]. Guyatt and Snow (2004) estimated that malaria in pregnancy caused 11.4 % of neonatal deaths and 5.7 % of infant deaths in malaria-endemic areas of Africa, resulting in approximately 100,000 infant deaths per year [12]. In a study of effects of the use of insecticide-treated bednets on birth outcomes in Southeast Nigeria, Igwe, Ebuchi, Imem, and Afolabi (2007) noted that malaria during pregnancy is also a significant drain on its economy and a major financial burden to the poor [13]. With these indices, achieving the Millennium Development Goals of reducing child and maternal deaths by two thirds and three quarters, respectively, by 2015 in Nigeria will require a more pragmatic approach to address malaria-related morbidity and mortality in Nigeria.

Current efforts to address malaria illnesses and deaths in Nigeria include the adoption of artemisinin-based combination therapy (artemether-lumefantrine and artesunate-amodiaquine) for the treatment of uncomplicated malaria. Furthermore, Nigeria is currently promoting home management of malaria using artemisinin combination therapy in line with the World Health Organization's recommendation in order to ensure prompt and appropriate access to management of malaria [14]. Sulphadoxine-pyrimethamine is exclusively reserved for preventing malaria during pregnancy. The use of insecticide treated bednets is also highly recommended for protection against contact with *Plasmodium falciparium* parasite. These are contained in the national antimalarial drugs updated 2012 [15].

The use of insecticide-treated bednets has not only remained one of the most important of all measures of protection against malaria; it has become the single most dependable intervention when used properly and efficacious in reducing maternal anemia, placental infection, and low birth weight [16]. Fegan, et al. also reported 44 % reduction in mortality due to insecticide-treated bednet use [17]. In realization of the effectiveness of insecticide treated bednets against malaria, improvements were made in the production of insecticide treated bednets. Between 2008 and 2010, a cumulative total of 289 million insecticide-treated bednets were delivered to sub-Saharan Africa, enough to cover 76 % of the 765 million persons at risk [18].

Despite the tragedy and economic loss caused by malaria, the majority of pregnant women in Nigeria do not have access to these insecticide-treated bednets. In Enugu State, for instance, the NPC and ICF Macro (2009) reports that only 9.7 % of the households surveyed had at least one net while only 3.9 % of the pregnant women slept under a treated net [7]. Reasons for the

low utilization may be attributable to a number of socio-cultural factors, including ignorance, poverty, beliefs, and gender issues as well as low utilization of antenatal clinic services among Nigeria women compared to women in other African countries and also the lack of malaria in pregnancy services existing in antenatal clinic's program [19].

The most promising preventive approach to using antimalarial drugs for pregnant women is intermittent presumptive treatment. Garner et al. estimated that effective prevention of malaria with chloroquine prophylaxis or intermittent presumptive treatment reduces the risk of low birth weight by as much as 43 % [20]. Intermittent presumptive treatment is based on the use of antimalarial drugs given in treatment doses at predefined intervals after quickening [21]. For many years, WHO recommended that pregnant women in malaria-endemic areas should receive an initial antimalarial treatment dose on their first contact with antenatal services, followed by weekly chemoprophylaxis with an effective and safe antimalarial drug [22].

The critical factors responsible for the current levels of utilization of intermittent presumptive treatment and insecticide-treated bednets in preventing malaria in pregnancy in Enugu remain unclear. This paper explored and documented the perceptions and attitude associated with uptake of interventions to prevent malaria in pregnancy infection during pregnancy in Enugu State, Nigeria.

Methods
Ethical statement
Ethical approval was received through the health research ethics committee of the University of Nigeria Teaching Hospital. The community leaders and members of the community involved in the study gave their verbal approval for the study. The verbal approval was considered sufficient to avoid a situation where the people will be uncooperative and less outspoken for fear of repercussions.

Study design
The study was exploratory and adopted a cross-sectional approach using qualitative methods of inquiry, based on in-depth interviews and focus group discussion designs. The study was designed to allow a description and analysis of community perceptions/attitudes towards insecticide-treated bednets and intermittent presumptive treatment in pregnancy sulphadoxine-pyrimethamine for preventing malaria in pregnancy employing qualitative inquiry in Enugu state, Nigeria. Community perception of the interventions is viewed from a perspective that recognizes an interaction among a number of variables, including the socio-demographic realities of the people as well as their

past experiences with the health system, health problems, and relevant interventions.

Study area

The locale for this study was the capital of Enugu State, Enugu Urban. The people of Enugu Urban belong largely to the Igbo ethnic group, which is one of the three largest ethnic groups in Nigeria. The name "Enugu" comes from two Igbo words "enu ugwu" or "top of the hill." The city's slogan is "perpetual apex pride." Nicknamed the "coal city" in the early 1900s, Enugu was a major center for the mining of coal but since the Biafra war, coal production has declined almost to a halt. Thus in recent years, the city's economy has diversified and is largely dominated by trading, commerce, and small-scale industry as well. A significant proportion of the population is also engaged in the civil service sector.

The major health care facility in Enugu urban is the Enugu State University Teaching Hospital and College of Medicine. There are also numerous private, missionary, and government-owned hospitals and clinics. The people of Enugu also have access to the University of Nigeria Teaching Hospital, located in Ituku Ozalla community of Nkanu West, a neighboring local government area (LGA) to Enugu South LGA.

Enugu urban has three LGA, namely Enugu South, Enugu East, and Enugu North (which is the major business district). Over the years, Enugu urban has grown enormously especially in areas of commerce, estate, and health facilities.

Study population and sampling

The target population for this study was women within the child bearing age of 15–49 years who gave birth within 6 months before the survey. Their mothers and husbands were also covered in the study. Health care providers were also interviewed. The distribution of data collected in each local government area is contained in Table 1 below.

A total of nine communities were randomly selected from each LGA. The focus group discussions were equally distributed across local government area. This gave a total of 24 focus group discussions (FGDs) with husbands and mothers of women (15–49 years), who delivered within 6 months before the survey and 30 in-depth interviews (IDI) with health workers and women (15–49 years), who delivered within 6 months before the survey, in the entire study (Table 1). Each focus group discussion session consisted of 8 to 10 participants, selected with the convenience sampling technique, after receiving community consent following social mobilization.

Groups were selected according to participants' availability. Women who delivered in less than 6 months to

Table 1 Distribution of Sample by LGA and Groups of Study Participants

Groups	Local government area						Total	
	Enugu/E peri urban		Enugu/ N urban		Enugu/S rural			
	FGD	IDI	FGD	IDI	FGD	IDI	FGD	IDI
Mothers of women who delivered within 6 months before the survey	4	–	4	–	4	–	12	–
Husbands of women who delivered within 6 months before the survey	4	–	4	–	4	–	12	–
Health workers	–	4	4	–	4			12
Women who delivered within 6 months before the survey	–	6		6		6		18
Total	8	10	8	10	8	10	24	30

the study were equally included in the study based on their availability and willingness to participate in the study. The health workers on the other hand were selected through a two stage sampling. First, 12 health facilities were randomly selected from the list of health facilities in the study LGAs. The officer in charge of the selected health facility was purposively selected for the study.

Before the commencement of the study, the state malaria control officer took the researcher to the community leaders and introduced the mission. The community leaders in turn mobilized the community members and informed them that the officials from the state capital have come to discuss issues relating to their health in the community. They were also informed that some of them will be needed for focus group discussions and another special group for in-depth interviews with the researcher.

Instrument and method of data collection

The instruments for data collection were focus group discussion and in-depth interview guides, which explored such themes as the common health problems in the communities, knowledge of malaria, practices in preventing malaria in pregnancy, perception of insecticide treated bednets and intermittent presumptive treatment in pregnancy, as well as antenatal care practices for protection against malaria infection during pregnancy. The discussions were tape recorded, where permission was granted. The discussion sessions were made informal with light refreshment served to the participants during discussion, in the case of the focus group discussions. The instruments were pre-tested in one urban and two rural communities in Nsukka local government area, for the sensitivity of the instrument. The pre-testing also provided opportunity for giving targeted orientation on the methods and objectives of the study to the data collectors. FGD and IDI sessions took an average of 45 min and 30 min, respectively.

The team spent approximately 1 week in each local government area for activities which included mobilization of the groups, actual discussion, interviews, and data cleaning. The focus group discussion and interviews were facilitated by social scientists from the Faculty of Social Sciences in the University of Nigeria, which is located within Enugu State. However, the facilitators were also from the same cultural background with the participants in the study.

Data analysis

Analysis of the data placed emphasis on the interpretation, description, and recording/writing of what was actually said. In going through the transcriptions, phrases with contextual or special connotations were noted and pulled out as illustrative quotes in developing the ethnographic summaries. To do this, relevant themes were developed for the coding and sorting of the qualitative data and Atlas.ti version 5.0 software was used in managing the qualitative data. The transcripts were first done in the local language and translated into English. In going through the transcriptions, phrases with contextual or special connotations were noted and pulled out as illustrative quotes.

The analysis commenced in the field while the data were reviewed and corrected for accuracy and clarity. All interviews and discussions were transcribed and the transcripts typed with MSWord processing package and converted into American standard code for information interchange rich text format (RTF) files. These were coded and sorted using the Atlas.ti version 6 program.

The next level of analysis began with the review of the interview and discussion experiences with the field assistants who facilitated and recorded interviews and discussions, this time to obtain their views on the factors that inhibited or animated discussions. A more detailed analysis began with the researchers reading the transcript. During the first reading, notes were made of major concepts. A second reading utilized a system of open coding. A rereading of the texts was done to discern patterns in the ordering and clustering of themes, which provided guide on the systematic development of themes and codes used in Atlas.ti software. This process ensured inter-coder reliability and facilitated triangulation of data from discussions and interviews.

Results

Social demographic characteristics of the respondents

A total of 246 persons ($N = 246$) were enlisted in the study and participated in the discussions ($n = 216$) and in-depth interviews ($n = 30$). Approximately one third of this was drawn from each of the participating LGA.

Respondents for the in-depth interviews were mainly 12 health workers and 18 women who delivered in less than 6 months prior to the study, 4 and 6, respectively from each LGA (Table 1). The health workers were mainly females with ages between 28 and 45 years. The women who delivered in less than 6 months before the study were aged between 20 and 31 years and were into civil service and trading.

Approximately half of the FGD participants fell into the two categories of focus group discussion participants, namely mothers and husbands of women who delivered less than 6 months before the study (see Table 2). The participants were aged between 25 to 61 years with a mean age of 39.7 years (39.7 ± 8.8 SD). A total of 112 participants were females. One hundred and fifty-one of the respondents were married, and 5 were widows while

Table 2 Distribution of FGD Participants by Socio-Demographic Characteristics

Socio-demographic characteristics	Frequency ($N = 216$)	Percentage
States		
Enugu east	68	32
Enugu north	81	37
Enugu south	67	31
Groups		
Mothers of women who delivered	112	52
Husband of women who delivered	104	48
Marital status		
Married	151	60
Widow	5	2
Never married	60	28
Educational level		
No formal education/Arabic	27	12
Primary	45	21.0
Secondary	111	52
Post-secondary	33	15
Occupation		
Unemployed	61	28
Civil servant	66	31
Trader	24	11
Artisan	65	30
Age group		
25–29	29	1311
30–34	24	1516
35–39	33	17
40–44	34	27
45–49	37	
50+	59	

60 were single. One hundred and thirty-four of the respondents had at least secondary education.

The FGD participants were drawn from various occupational categories and were fairly evenly distributed, with the exception of the group of traders (11.1 %). Twenty-eight percent (28.2 %) was unemployed while 30.6 percent and 30.1 percent were civil servants and artisans, respectively.

Common health problems
The discussions opened with a review of the common health problems in the communities. A number of health problems were mentioned, though with some variations between the urban/peri urban and rural LGAs. Non communicable health problems like hypertension and cardiac problems featured more in the urban/peri urban communities. On the other hand, infectious diseases featured more in the typical rural communities. Malaria featured very prominently all the communities irrespective of the level of status of the LGA (urban, peri urban, and rural). Below are samples of the quotes to illustrate the findings.

Malaria is a common thing in this community that when we see the symptoms, the people come complaining of high fever, they will complain of cold .... Malaria is the prevalent disease condition in this community because it is a tropical area. It is an endemic area for malaria and when the people come, they will complain of high fever, cough, and loss of appetite and more so malaria will be there. So there are signs and symptoms. We treat the people for malaria. [IDI, female health worker; Enugu South]

We have different diseases like cholera, malaria and eye problems, which are very common in our community.... [Participant: FGD, husbands; Enugu South LGA]

Malaria is more because it can come in different ways until that person goes for test and they confirm it to be malaria while that person must have been taking treatment for another sickness. So there are different malaria [Participant, FGD, grandmothers, Enugu North]

Knowledge of malaria in pregnancy
Virtually all the respondents, irrespective of community, indicated awareness of malaria. Participants in the focus group discussion sessions with grandmothers and husbands of the women who delivered recently gave graphic description of the problems of malaria in the community. The common problems faced by pregnant women included malaria, nausea, body pains, bleeding, among others. The following quote from the husband of a woman who just delivered a baby, less than

6 months preceding the survey, in a focus group discussion session in Enugu East, typifies the perception of health problems of pregnant women in the communities. According to him,

Their sickness during pregnancy includes malaria. It causes death of so many women in this community after and during the delivery. It causes the placenta to go out of its tracings. Unfortunately after delivery the person dies and leaves the baby. So many women when taken to the hospital during pregnancy their legs are swollen if the delivery is coming out. The other sickness is bleeding. The women will bleed to the extent no one can stop the blood she will now die. In some of the hospitals that would have given the person treatment and equality but what they demand is unreasonable... before the husband is able to comply she will die

Malaria was one of the common problems associated with pregnancy in the study area. According to a grandmother in a focus group discussion session in Enugu East LGA, "what I know is that pregnant women like having malaria; it is almost part of their experiences and they must go through it". Another grandmother in Enugu North local government area enumerated how the malaria in pregnant women affects their babies. According to her,

The problem it carries is that even a baby in the womb if delivered immediately is affected. In the hospital you will hear the nurse mention different type of malaria that the baby is born with. Some of these malaria types come with death.

These quotations pointed out the preponderance of malaria among the people. The pregnant women held the belief that exposure to sun, eating oily food, and drinking bad water cause malaria. In Enugu South focus group discussion session for older mothers, different perceptions on malaria causation were put forward.

...malaria is very rampant due to dirty environment and too much staying under the sun [Participant: FGD, grandmother; Enugu South]

...most women are very dirty, their lifestyle is very dirty. They don't cook their food well and they don't boil their water before drinking, so when you eat food that is not well cooked and drink water that is not boiled you can have malaria. [Participant: FGD, grandmother; Enugu East]
...

In Enugu North,

...everybody says malaria is caused by mosquitoes, I agree but it is not only mosquitoes that cause malaria. There are tiny insects that come out of the dirty stream near us, when these insects bite you, you can come down with malaria. These insects are worst than mosquitoes because net cannot prevent it. [Participant: FGD, husband; Enugu North]

...malaria is rampant here because of our bad weather. At times in the morning when the weather is supposed to be cool, the sun will be so hot and if you stay outside under that sun for a long time, you will fall sick. [Participant: FGD, husband; Enugu North]

The following quote from the husband of one of the participants in Enugu South threw more light on the knowledge of how people got malaria. According to him,

Malaria is a serious ailment to all living beings. Again malaria episodes are of different types. But that of pregnant women are always as a result of lack of blood.... Groundnut is not good for a pregnant woman. Similarly, too much of fresh fish in stew is bad. Mango and orange develop malaria

There seemed to be some effects of the health education given to the women in the health centers

...we have taught them that it is only mosquitoes that can cause malaria but previously they did not know that it is only mosquito. Some of them say sun, when they eat too much oil and all those stuff. [IDI, female health worker, Enugu South]

Prevention and treatment of malaria in pregnancy
Some of the participants held the view that malaria could not be prevented. This is reflected in a sample of quotation taken from the focus group discussion session.

Malaria is a continuous process and is everywhere as you can ask anybody. There is no protective means except bringing the hospital into this community.... Nothing can be done to stop malaria as it is a continuous process as we are looking for something to cure the malaria... a lot of malaria is man-made. [FGD: husband in Enugu South].

...there is nothing like prevention of malaria, I don't believe malaria can be prevented when everything around you gives you malaria, will you wear net and be working around? You cannot do that, so I don't think malaria can be prevented. [Respondent: IDI, mother; Enugu South]

Others who had used insecticide-treated bednets mentioned that they are used for preventing mosquito bites and of course malaria infections. According to a grandmother in an FGD session in Enugu North, the bednets are, "to prevent mosquito from biting them and stop malaria...". For a number of reasons, including ignorance, lack of access, poverty, and even perceived discomfort, it is not used fully. According to the same grandmother in Enugu North,

Some of them complain that it is too hot. My daughter in law complains that it is hot and does not like staying inside it.... I have it, I tie it on the window but at night I remove it because it is hot.... (General laughter).

She further demonstrated that the lack of use is due to ignorance and poverty. In her words, "some of the pregnant women do not know about insecticide treated bednets or its benefits, if there is any and they do not have money to buy it". In a focus group discussion session with the husbands in Enugu North, a man queried, "can one sleep under insecticide treated bednets she does not have?"

Similarly, participants in the different focus group discussion sessions indicated awareness of sulphadoxine-pyrimethamine/fansidar. However, they argued that it is not used in pregnancy because it was never prescribed by doctors. The commonly prescribed drugs for the prevention of malaria were Daraprim, which they called "Sunday-Sunday medicine" and chloroquine. In a focus group discussion session with mothers in Enugu, it was agreed that "they (health workers) gave Sunday-Sunday medicine.... They gave us chloroquine...." Chloroquine is good because doctor gave it....Doctors prescribed it...."

When asked if they know fansidar, one of the grandmothers in the focus group discussion session in Enugu East said,

I know it, but I take Sunday-Sunday. When I was pregnant I was given Sunday-Sunday.... If you are pregnant, Doctors do not prescribe Fansidar because it is strong. ... it is not good for pregnant women but could be useful if you are not pregnant [Respondent: IDI, mother, Enugu East].

A grandmother in Enugu North noted that it was beyond their capacity to say how a pregnant woman with malaria should be managed. According to her,

...when I used to deliver, mosquito was not as much as they are now; malaria is too common so I don't know the type of treatment because we are not doctors. Well, when I used to give birth, I used to go to the clinic and if I feel the symptoms of malaria and they used to give me Sunday - Sunday medicine and fruit....

A husband of one of the newly delivered women surveyed, in Enugu South, noted that,

Some of the others will go to Native Doctors, Hospital, clinic for treatment and even the people in the hospital don't know any wrong from right. Whereas, some of the herbalists know the type of herbs to be administered, in the hospital the nurses that are there will not want to treat the pregnant women for safe deliver.

Another husband from Enugu East emphasized that,

There are traditional birth attendants that can give drugs and herbs that will subside for the temporarily, since they are not real doctor who learn about drugs proper.

A grandmother in Enugu East noted that,

Most times, for stubborn malaria, they use mix alba, essom salt, and are advised to take anaema like boiled leaves and drink.

Another grandmother from Enugu North wondered why they should bother with knowing the ways of managing malaria in pregnancy when the doctors normally dispense "Sunday-Sunday" medicine to them. According to her, "it is like that question is higher than us because we are not doctors...."

In a focus group discussion session in Enugu North with husbands, participants threw more light on how their wives sought treatment when they were ill with malaria. According to one of the participants,

...whenever she is sick, we go the chemist first and buy some drugs. If there is any dealer there we asked him what drug to buy, if not we buy the one we know. If that does not work, we shall now go to nurse (auxiliary nurse) to give her injection, when we have tried all these ones and it doesn't work, we will now go to hospital. [Participant: FGD, husband; Enugu North]

Barriers for ITN and IPT use
Discussions from focus group discussion sessions in Enugu South and North with the women and husbands of pregnant women stressed the point that if the services in antenatal clinic were good, the cost and distance would not be a hindrance. They emphasized the fact that,

... pregnant women like to go for ante-natal but the problem is the quality of care. Most of the nurses are not qualified for the job. When you come for

ante-natal, they just stay there and be shouting at the pregnant women. When you complain of sickness, they do not give you anything; they just tell you that government did not give them drugs. This is very common with government hospitals, the private ones are better. [Respondent: IDI, woman; Enugu South]

...the roads are very bad, the pregnant women find it difficult to come out to the hospital because the transport people say that the road will spoil their buses. But if they hear that the government brought drugs, they will enter 'okada' (commercial motorcycle transportation) or trek to the hospital so that they can get these drugs. [Respondent: IDI, woman; Enugu South]
...my wife goes for ante-natal in a private clinic because she is more comfortable there. The environment of the clinic is clean, the nurses attend to her well, they give her ante-natal drugs and the doctor checks her every time she goes there. It is more expensive and far from our house but she will rather go there than go to government hospital and collect insults. [Participant: FGD, husband; Enugu South]

The people experienced a lot of problems with the orthodox health system, some of which included the attitude of the health workers, distance, and cost. In the alternative therefore, they sought traditional treatment. According to the husband of a recently delivered woman in Enugu South, they do not go to doctors "since the hospital is far. Traditional birth attendants, living in the village attended to them". Another husband from Enugu North argued,

.... Even if the drugs are sent to primary health centre the Nigerian Nurses will not give you the drugs. I witnessed, from the last bednet that was given, that the Nigerian Nurses deprived the people by saying how can they sleep under the Bed Net. I don't know how the Nigerian profess to humanitarian service as to enable them have one for mankind. We know that Nurses are the worst set of people, arrogant.

One could also trace the non-use to unavailability of these commodities across Enugu. The focus group discussions and in-depth interviews carried out during the course of this study revealed how the various participants (both men and women) and medical practitioners strongly indicated the unavailability of insecticide treated bednets, for instance.

In Enugu North focus group discussion session with husbands of pregnant women, a participant mocked:

What nets? There are no nets, they tell us that mosquito nets are available free of charge but when we ask for it they always tell us that government did not provide any net. [Participant: FGD, husband; Enugu North]

It is all a '419' scam, we always hear that WHO has provided mosquito nets for the hospital and for distribution but we have never seen it. We only see it in the market and it is very expensive. I am sure the government people sell it to those traders in the market. [Participant: FGD, adult male; Enugu North]
In-depth interviews in Enugu North and Enugu East.

...those who are in charge of insecticide treated bednets distribution should increase their efforts. They are not doing enough; they need to go from house to house to give out these nets. They should also make these nets available to hospitals and health centers so that it can be given to pregnant women when they visit. [Respondent: IDI, health worker; Enugu East]

...most women that come here say that they buy insecticide treated bednets from the market. Nobody has given me any net to give to the women that come here, so I advise the women to go and buy. [Respondent: IDI, health worker; Enugu North]

Health workers interviewed noted difference in the effectiveness of the urban and rural local government areas in the distribution of intermittent presumptive treatment in pregnancy and insecticide-treated bednets than others. According to one of the health workers interviewed,

In this local government, the ministry of health gives us our drugs; in fact they distribute it to all the local governments. At a certain time, I even heard that they were giving out insecticide treated bednets to people. [Respondent: IDI, health worker; Enugu North]

I understand that the ministry of health gives drugs freely to all the local government areas and it is left for the local government to know how to distribute it to the hospitals and health centers. Even the insecticide treated bednets, I heard that the local government people were going house to house to give people nets. [Respondent: IDI, health worker; Enugu North]

For reasons of unavailability of health commodities, as captured in the preceding quotes, pregnant women prefer to go to private hospitals for antenatal care and other healthcare needs; this is largely as a result of poor conditions of government owned health facilities, lack of drugs, and hospital equipments. Focus group discussion sessions held across Enugu local government areas threw more light on how serious this problem is,

... most of these government hospitals don't have anything; when my wife went there they could not even give her panadol. They always say that government did not give them any drug, so I decided that she should register in a private clinic even though they are expensive at least they would give her quality care [Participant: FGD, adult male; Enugu South]

If you go to our government hospitals, they are very dirty, the nurses are very rude. I even heard that they used to slap these pregnant women when they are in labor, so I did not even allow her to go there. We just went to a private hospital and registered. [Participant: FGD, adult male; Enugu North]
In these government hospitals, they give fake drugs. They give you chalk when you take it, what is happening will still be happening... [Participant: FGD, older mothers; Enugu South]
If a woman wants a safe delivery, she should just go to a private clinic. People say that government hospitals have equipment and drugs but it is a lie. When you go there they will still write drugs for you to go and buy and the equipments are not even working and you can never see doctor only rude nurses. Like now the doctors are on strike, so there is no need. [Participant: FGD, older mothers; Enugu North]

The attitude of health workers discouraged the women from going to hospital for antenatal care and even when they did, it was not done early in the pregnancy. For instance, the husband of a newly delivered woman in Enugu South mentioned that, "the normal month for this is four (4) months. But my wives treated them with herbs as they do not register in any of the hospital. I treat them with herbs."
Women who indicated that they took sulphadoxine-pyrimethamine reported that they got it from health facility/during antenatal care visit. Others indicated that they got it from the pharmacy. The qualitative data showed that women often receive a variety of services. According to a grandmother in Enugu South,

When we were pregnant in our days, they used to cut leaves, squeeze it and give to us to drink, if the child was disturbing you she will lie still until you deliver.
.... But now it is not easy, power keeps attacking them.
... Women have really died on the way. Labour can be prolonged with the cord twisting around the neck of the baby.

Some doctors considered administration of intermittent presumptive treatment in pregnancy as unnecessary. They preferred to wait for the pregnant woman to come down with malaria before they treat. This fact was deduced from an in-depth interview carried out with a health worker in Enugu North local government area,

> ...we use paludrine as a prophylactic dose in early pregnancy. We do not really administer intermittent presumptive treatment because from my own perspective and experience, we have a lot of fake drugs. So I rather treat malaria than give prophylactic drug that would harm the baby. [Respondent: IDI, health worker; Enugu South]

Discussion and conclusions

This study revealed different levels of awareness of malaria and how it should be managed during pregnancy. These levels of awareness were also found to reflect on actions taken to prevent malaria during pregnancy. Those who were aware used insecticide-treated bednets and intermittent presumptive treatment during pregnancy. These findings confirm findings from other studies. Studies on disease control and utilization of health promotion interventions have identified community perception as a major driver of the people's attitude towards the interventions. Those who hold this view argue that utilization of such health interventions is only partially explained by availability, while the major decider lies in the people's perception, which forms basis of their decision on whether or not to use the interventions [23–25]. The results of this study confirm these positions. Some scholars had also argued that assessment of the people's perceptions is germane to the development and delivery of appropriate health interventions [26]. This study investigated people's perceptions and attitudes towards use of health commodities designed for preventing malaria in pregnancy and showed results that corroborate earlier studies. The study indicated that pregnant women perceived high fever and general weakness as a normal sign of pregnancy. However, their perceptions of the preventive technologies affect the use of the same technologies considered safe, low cost, and effective in protecting women against malaria infection during pregnancy. This is not peculiar to Nigeria. A study by Njama, Dorsey, Guwatudde, Kigonya, Greenhouse, Musisi, and Kamya (2003) in Kampala city also indicated that 90 % of the care givers knew that mosquitoes cause malaria although they equally indicated other perceived causes such as drinking unboiled water and respiratory illnesses [27].

Despite awareness of the causes and implication of malaria in pregnancy, insecticide-treated nets (ITN) and intermittent preventive treatment (IPT) as preventive or treatment measure, and the health facilities to be the first place to go at the onset of illness, misconceptions and poor attitude of health workers towards patients affected the uptake of interventions related to malaria in pregnancy. Antenatal care at health facilities is key in the delivery of malaria in pregnancy prevention interventions [28–31]. However, the women seemed discouraged with the health system and rather go for alternative health care. Some studies have highlighted the social, cultural, and health system constraints to the use of health facilities [30]. Health workers' attitudes and behavior towards pregnant women and attitudes towards specific services offered can also potentially deter women from accessing ANC at health facilities [32].

The limitation of this study is the inability to generalize the results to larger populations. It is a qualitative study in which the inclusion of participants was not based on any statistical consideration. Randomization was only limited to the selected of communities. Consideration was not given to ensure the inclusion of all necessary parameters of the larger population. Another limitation is the inability to make statistical conclusions on the occurrence of the perception. However, this study provides data that could form the basis of a study using a more rigorous statistical and mixed method design. It provides a range of perceptions that would form used categories in developing structured data capture tool for quantification in future.

The findings here confirm the theoretical basis of this study. Based on the health belief model, one can conclude that pregnant women in Enugu State would adopt malaria preventive measures if these measures were available and if they are sufficiently educated on the values of these measures. However, the health workers who should educate the women to use these intervention are themselves short of world expected standard. The health workers also need to be trained on appropriate communication skills so as to act as motivators, rather than inhibitors. It is thus recommended that stakeholders ensure the availability of the commodities in adequate quantity and quality with health education to promote effective access among pregnant women as well as target health workers to create more friendly environment for the clients.

Competing interests
The authors have no competing interest.

Authors' contributions
All authors read and approved the final manuscript.

Author details
[1]Department of Sociology/Anthropology, University of Nigeria Nsukka, Nsukka 410001, Nigeria. [2]Humanities Unit, School of General Studies, University of Nigeria, Enugu Campus, Enugu, Nigeria.

References
1. Federal Ministry of Health (FMoH) [Nigeria], and National Malaria Control Programme (NMCP). Strategic plan 2009-2013: a road map for malaria control in Nigeria; abridged version. Abuja: Yaliam Press Ltd; 2009. p. 34.

2. National Population Commission (NPC) [Nigeria] & National Malaria Control Programme (NMCP) [Nigeria], and ICF International. Nigeria malaria indicator survey 2010. Abuja: NPC, NMCP, and ICF International; 2012. p. 29.

3. Federal Ministry of Health. Malaria desk situation analysis. Abuja: Abuja National Malaria Control Program, Federal Ministry of Health; 2000. p. 13–5.

4. Idowu OA, Mafiana CF, Sotiloye D. Traditional birth home attendance and its implications for malaria control during pregnancy in Nigeria. Trans R Soc Trop Med Hyg. 2008;102(7):679–84.

5. Federal Ministry of Health (FMOH). Malaria situation analysis document. Nigeria: Federal Ministry of Health; 2004. p. 14.

6. Idowu O, Mafiana C, Dapo S. Malaria among pregnant women in Abeokuta, Nigeria. Tanzan Health Res Bull. 2006;8(1):28–31.

7. National Population Commission Nigeria & ICF Macro. Nigeria: DHS, 2008—final report (English). Calverton: Macro International; 2009. p. 29.

8. Wilcox AJ. On the importance—and the unimportance—of birthweight. Int J Epidemiol. 2001;30(6):1233–41.

9. Rijken MJ, Moroski WE, Kiricharoen S, Karunkonkowit N, Stevenson G, Ohuma EO, et al. Effect of malaria on placental volume measured using three-dimensional ultrasound: a pilot study. Malar J. 2012;11:5.

10. Center for Disease Control and Prevention. Alternatives for pregnant women and treatment: severe malaria. Atlanta: CDC; 2007. p. 1–10.

11. Murphy SC, Breman JG. Gaps in the childhood malaria burden in Africa: cerebral malaria, neurological sequelae, anemia, respiratory distress, hypoglycemia, and complications of pregnancy. Am J Trop Med Hyg. 2001;64(1):57–67.

12. Guyatt HL, Snow RW. Impact of malaria during pregnancy on low birth weight in sub-Saharan Africa. Clin Microbiol Rev. 2004;17:760–9.

13. Igwe PC, Ebuchi OM, Imem V, Afolabi BM. Effects of the use of insecticide treated bednets on birth outcomes among primigravidae in a per-urban slum settlement in South East Nigeria. SA Fam Pract. 2007;49(6):15.

14. Ajayi IO, Falade CO, Olley BO, Yusuf B, Gbotosho S, Iyiola O, et al. A qualitative study of the feasibility and community perception on the effectiveness of artemether-lumefantrine use in the context of home management of malaria in South-west Nigeria. BMC Health Serv Res. 2008;8:119.

15. FMOH. National integrated community case management of malaria. Abuja, Nigeria: NMCP/FMOH; 2012. p. 1.

16. WHO/UNICEF. Lives at risk: malaria in pregnancy. Africa Malaria Report: 2003, p. 13.

17. Fegan GW, Noor AM, Akhwale WS, Coussens S, Snow RW. Effect of expanded insecticide-treated bednet coverage on child survival in rural Kenya: a longitudinal study. Lancet. 2007;370:1035–9.

18. WHO. World malaria report. Geneva: WHO; 2010. p. 17.

19. Jhpiego. MCH programme spotlight; a few steps forward on a long, winding road: Jhpiego's work in malaria in pregnancy in Nigeria. 2005. Available at http://www.jhpiego.org/content/maternal-newborn-and-child-health.

20. Garner P, Gulmezoglu A. Drugs for preventing malaria in pregnant women. Cochrane Database Syst Rev. 2006;18(4):CD000169.

21. World Health Organization, (WHO). A strategic framework for malaria prevention and control during pregnancy in Africa regions. Report AFR/MAL/04/01. Brazzaville: Democratic Republic of Congo, WHO Regional Office for Africa; 2004. p. 34–7.

22. World Health Organization (WHO). Lives at risk: malaria in pregnancy. Africa malaria report: 2003. p. 43.

23. Roberts MJ, Hsiao W, Berman P, Reich MR. Getting health reform right: a guide to improving performance and equity. New York: Oxford University Press; 2008.

24. Frost LJ, Reich MR. Access: how do good health technologies get to poor people in poor countries? Cambridge: Massachussetts, Harvard Centre for Population and Development Studies; 2008.

25. Singh H, Haqq ED, Nustapha N. Patients' perception and satisfaction with health care professional at primary care facilities in Trinidad and Tobago. Bull World Health Organ. 1999;77(4):356–60.

26. Dowler E, Green J, Bauer M, Gasperoni G. Assessing public perceptions: issues and methods. In: Carlos D, editor. Health hazard and public debate: lessons for risk communication from BSE/CJD saga. Geneva: World Health Organization; 2006. p. 40–60.

27. Njama D, Dorsey G, Guwatudde D, Kigonya K, Greenhouse B, Musisi S, et al. Urban malaria: primary caregivers' knowledge, attitudes, practices and predictors of malaria incidence in a cohort of Ugandan children. Trop Med Int Health. 2003;8(8):685–92.

28. Okeibunor JC, Orji BC, Brieger W, Ishola G, Otolorin E, Rawlins B, et al. Preventing malaria in pregnancy through community-directed interventions: evidence from Akwa Ibom State, Nigeria. Malar J. 2001;10:227.

29. Onyeneho NG, Orji BC, Okeibunor JC, Brieger WB. Characteristics of women who takes sulphadoxine-pyrimethamine twice in preventing malaria during pregnancy in Nigeria. Int J Gynaecol Obstet. 2013;123(2):101–4.

30. Onyeneho NG, Idemili-Aronu N, Okoye I, Ugwu C, Iremeka FU. Compliance with intermittent presumptive treatment and insecticide treated nets use during pregnancy in Enugu State, Nigeria. Matern Child Health J. 2013. doi:10.1007/s10995-013-1347-1.

31. Pell C, Straus L, Andrew EV, Meñaca A, Pool R. Social and cultural factors affecting uptake of interventions for malaria in pregnancy in Africa: a systematic review of the qualitative research. PLoS One. 2011;6(7):e22452. doi:10.1371/journal.pone.0022452.

32. Mbonye AK, Neema S, Magnussen P. Perceptions on use of sulfadoxine-pyrimethamine in pregnancy and the policy implications for malaria control in Uganda. Health Policy. 2006;77:279–89.

Predictors of maternal health services utilization by poor, rural women: a comparative study in Indian States of Gujarat and Tamil Nadu

Kranti Suresh Vora[1*], Sally A. Koblinsky[2] and Marge A. Koblinsky[3]

Abstract

Background: India leads all nations in numbers of maternal deaths, with poor, rural women contributing disproportionately to the high maternal mortality ratio. In 2005, India launched the world's largest conditional cash transfer scheme, *Janani Suraksha Yojana* (JSY), to increase poor women's access to institutional delivery, anticipating that facility-based birthing would decrease deaths. Indian states have taken different approaches to implementing JSY. Tamil Nadu adopted JSY with a reorganization of its public health system, and Gujarat augmented JSY with the state-funded *Chiranjeevi Yojana* (CY) scheme, contracting with private physicians for delivery services. Given scarce evidence of the outcomes of these approaches, especially in states with more optimal health indicators, this cross-sectional study examined the role of JSY/CY and other healthcare system and social factors in predicting poor, rural women's use of maternal health services in Gujarat and Tamil Nadu.

Methods: Using the District Level Household Survey (DLHS)-3, the sample included 1584 Gujarati and 601 Tamil rural women in the lowest two wealth quintiles. Multivariate logistic regression analyses examined associations between JSY/CY and other salient health system, socio-demographic, and obstetric factors with three outcomes: adequate antenatal care, institutional delivery, and Cesarean-section.

Results: Tamil women reported greater use of maternal healthcare services than Gujarati women. JSY/CY participation predicted institutional delivery in Gujarat (AOR = 3.9), but JSY assistance failed to predict institutional delivery in Tamil Nadu, where mothers received some cash for home births under another scheme. JSY/CY assistance failed to predict adequate antenatal care, which was not incentivized. All-weather road access predicted institutional delivery in both Tamil Nadu (AOR = 3.4) and Gujarat (AOR = 1.4). Women's education predicted institutional delivery and Cesarean-section in Tamil Nadu, while husbands' education predicted institutional delivery in Gujarat.

Conclusions: Overall, assistance from health financing schemes, good road access to health facilities, and socio-demographic and obstetric factors were associated with differential use of maternity health services by poor, rural women in the two states. Policymakers and practitioners should promote financing schemes to increase access, including consideration of incentives for antenatal care, and address health system and social factors in designing state-level interventions to promote safe motherhood.

Keywords: Maternal health services, Poor rural women, India, Cash transfer schemes

* Correspondence: kvora@iiphg.org
[1]Indian Institute of Public Health Gandhinagar, Drive-in-Road, Ahmedabad, Gujarat 380054, India
Full list of author information is available at the end of the article

Background

India has implemented national and state-level strategies and programs to improve women's use of maternal health services, including Child Survival Safe Motherhood (CSSM) and Reproductive Child Health I and II. With a focus on supply-side interventions, these programs enhanced health infrastructure, skilled personnel availability, referral linkages, and blood transfusion accessibility during childbirth [1]. Yet, India continues to lead globally in numbers of maternal deaths, with poor women in rural areas at greatest risk for maternal mortality [2, 3]. Limited uptake of maternity health services among this group of women threatens the country's ability to reach Millennium Development Goals four and five [3].

Under the National Rural Health Mission (NRHM), India introduced schemes to increase demand for maternal health care [1]. In 2005–06, the nation launched the world's largest conditional cash transfer scheme for maternal health, *Janani Suraksha Yojana* (JSY), or a "scheme to protect mothers." JSY aims to reduce maternal and neonatal deaths by providing cash incentives to mothers who give birth in a health institution [1, 3]. The overall framework for JSY is similar throughout India, but states have different eligibility criteria and incentives based on their institutional birth data when the scheme was created [4]. In states with high maternal mortality and low institutional deliveries (low performing states), women receive cash incentives for institutional births in public or accredited health facilities regardless of socioeconomic status, age, or parity. In states with better maternal and institutional delivery data (high performing states), cash incentives are limited to the first two live births of women below the poverty line (BPL) and from scheduled castes and tribes [4].

Another maternal healthcare financing scheme in India is *Chiranjeevi Yojana* (CY), or "scheme for long life." This state-level public-private partnership is administered and currently funded by the Gujarat government, although initially supported by JSY funds. Implemented throughout Gujarat by 2007, the "voucher like" scheme provides tribal and BPL women with free delivery in an accredited private facility and reimbursement for transport. CY has both demand- and supply-side components, increasing women's demand for services while providing incentives to private providers for treating eligible mothers. CY was developed because three-quarters of Gujarati obstetricians worked in private health facilities, with large numbers in rural areas [5–7].

A growing number of studies have examined the impact of JSY and CY in increasing women's use of maternity services [5–11]. However, many have focused on low performing states, limited geographic regions, and the processes involved in implementing JSY [3, 5, 8]. Thus, researchers have called for studies of high performing states that take different approaches to demand-side financing schemes, such as Gujarat and Tamil Nadu. Tamil Nadu's introduction of JSY followed a period in the 1990s when its government increased the availability of round-the-clock obstetrical and newborn care through strategically located primary health facilities. Tamil Nadu uses federal funds to implement JSY, providing a cash incentive to BPL mothers who deliver in public health facilities. The state also offers women a small amount of cash for home births under another scheme to cover nutrition and lost wages [12]. In contrast, Gujarat has relied heavily on the CY scheme to provide poor, rural women with private maternity health services [6, 7], although eligible Gujarati women may also elect to deliver in government facilities under JSY.

Neither JSY nor CY incentivized antenatal care (ANC) in 2007–08 when the DLHS-3 was carried out. Both schemes provide small incentives to Accredited Social Health Activists (ASHAs) or health workers to accompany women to deliver in a health facility. Cesarean-sections (C-sections) are handled differently by the two schemes. Tamil Nadu's JSY scheme provides obstetricians and anesthesiologists with an additional payment to perform C-sections in public facilities, whereas Gujarat's CY scheme makes a flat rate payment to private physicians for 100 deliveries to cover normal and complicated births, thus removing the incentive to conduct surgical procedures [5–7].

Despite different financing mechanisms, JSY and CY both aim to reduce financial barriers to institutional deliveries among poor women. Other health system factors are also likely to influence women's use of maternal health services, particularly in poor, rural populations [13–15]. One such health system factor is the availability of a primary health center that provides 24-hour basic emergency obstetric care [16]. Geographic access to a health facility may also impact service use because 40 % of Indian villages lack all-weather roads, 2.7 million kilometers of rural roads are in poor condition, and 33 % of Indian villages are often cut off from major services by monsoon flooding [17, 18]. Socio-demographic and obstetrical factors have likewise been found to influence maternal health services utilization, including women's education, husbands' education, women's age at first birth, and parity [19, 20]. Given multiple factors that may influence use of maternity services, including financing schemes, this study sought to examine the role of JSY, CY and selected health system, socio-demographic, and obstetric factors in predicting use of adequate ANC, institutional delivery, and C-section among poor, rural women in Gujarat and Tamil Nadu.

Methods

Study setting and sample

This cross-sectional study utilized India's District Level Household Survey (DLHS)-3 Ever-married Women and

Village datasets [21]. The analytic sample included all ever-married women, ages 15–49, in the lowest two wealth quintiles (1st and 2nd) in rural areas of Gujarat and Tamil Nadu, who gave birth between January 2006 and December 2007. The total analytic sample of 2185 included 1584 Gujarati and 601 Tamil women.

Data collection
DLHS-3 (2007–08) data were collected by the International Institute for Population Sciences (IIPS), Mumbai, on behalf of the Indian Government's Ministry of Health and Family Welfare [21]. DLHS-3 was the third in a series of district-level, national surveys in India that provided estimates of important indicators of reproductive, maternal, and child health; it is the latest national-level demographic survey that includes maternal health indicators. About 644,000 ever-married Indian women were surveyed in DLHS-3. Details concerning data collection, weights, and handling of missing data are described on the DLHS-3 website [22].

DLHS-3 definitions were adopted for all study variables. For dependent variables, adequate ANC was defined as having an ANC visit in the first trimester, at least three total antenatal visits, and at least 100 iron folic acid tablets taken during the last pregnancy, as reported by women participants. Institutional delivery was defined as delivery in a public institution (government hospital, dispensary, urban health centre/post/family welfare centre, community health centre/rural hospital, PHC, sub centre, and Ayurveda, Yoga, Unani, Siddha, and Homeopathy (AYUSH) hospital/clinic) or in a private hospital/clinic or private AYUSH hospital/clinic. C-section was defined as a delivery by this operation.

Independent variables included health financing scheme, health system, socio-demographic, and obstetric variables. JSY/CY assistance was defined as a woman's report of receiving financial assistance for delivery care under either scheme. Health system variables were the village leader's report of women having access to a primary health centre (PHC) with 24–7 services in the area (yes or no) and village access to a health facility via an all-weather road (yes or no). Socio-demographic variables included the woman's education and her husband's education, defined as each spouse's total years of schooling. Obstetrical variables included age of the woman's first birth (in years) and parity (primipara, multipara, grand multipara). The control variables of religion (Hindu or non-Hindu) and caste (scheduled caste or non-scheduled caste) were defined as the religion or caste of the household head.

Ethical standards
Following the DLHS-3 protocol, informed consent was obtained from all participants before their participation. All identifiable information was removed from the dataset. The de-identified version of the DLHS-3 is available in the public domain [21, 22]. Ethical clearance was also obtained from the Institutional Research Board at the University of Maryland, where the data analyses were conducted.

Statistical analyses
Survey data were analyzed using primary sampling units and state weights for ever-married women and households, determined by DLHS-3. Descriptive statistics summarized characteristics of the sample and women's use of maternal health services in Gujarat and Tamil Nadu. Comparisons were made of these variables in the two states using Chi squares or a t-test (age of first birth). Relationships among all independent and dependent variables were examined using binary logistic regression. All independent variables were at least moderately ($p < 0.10$) correlated with one or more measures of maternity services utilization in each state. Multicollinearity was also assessed; all independent variables that remained in the final models had acceptable tolerance values. Multiple logistic regression analyses were then used to determine the degree to which independent variables predicted adequate ANC, institutional delivery, and C-section, controlling for religion and caste. Religion and caste were controlled because the literature indicates that both are predictors of Indian women's use of maternal health services [19, 23]. Three separate regression analyses were carried out in each state, one for each dependent variable. Strength of association between study variables was estimated by calculating adjusted odds ratios (AORs) with 95 % confidence intervals (CIs); a p value of .05 or below was considered statistically significant. Hosmer-Lemeshow goodness of fit tests revealed that models for all dependent variables were a good fit for data in both states ($p > 0.05$). A complete case analysis was conducted for each of the dependent variables since some data were differentially missing for adequate ANC in the two states. Missing data for adequate antenatal care were 3.1 % in Gujarat and 0.5 % in Tamil Nadu. Statistical analyses were carried out with IBM SPSS 19.

Results
Results revealed significant differences between samples of poor, rural Gujarati and Tamil women who gave birth in calendar years 2006 and 2007 with respect to JSY/CY participation, health care system, socio-demographic, and obstetric variables, as well as use of maternity services. Table 1 presents descriptive data for mothers in the analytic sample, including 1584 Gujarati and 601 Tamil women. During the birth years studied, Tamil women (28 %) were three times more likely than Gujarati women (9 %) to receive JSY/CY assistance for their most recent birth. Tamil women (74 %) reported greater availability of a primary health care center operating round-the-clock

Table 1 Descriptive statistics for women from Gujarat and Tamil Nadu

Independent variables	Gujart (n = 1584) weighted %	Tamil Nadu (n = 601) weighted %	p-Value
Financial assistance from JSY or CY	08.8 %	28.3 %	0.00**
Availability of PHC providing 24/7 services	58.3 %	73.5 %	0.00**
Access to a health facility by an all-weather road	80.0 %	96.8 %	0.00**
Woman's education			
Uneducated	71.3 %	31.8 %	0.00**
Less than 5 years	9.9 %	10.1 %	
5-9 years	16.5 %	44.7 %	
10 or more years	02.4 %	13.4 %	
Husband's education			
Uneducated	40.1 %	28.0 %	0.00**
Less than 5 years	12.9 %	10.6 %	
5-9 years	32.9 %	46.3 %	
10 or more years	14.1 %	15.1 %	
Woman's age at first birth			
Mean	19.5 yrs	21.0 yrs	0.00**
Minimum	10.0 yrs	14.0 yrs	
Maximum	35.0 yrs	37.0 yrs	
Parity			
Primipara	22.1 %	36.4 %	0.00**
Multipara	42.1 %	52.6 %	
Grand multipara	35.8 %	11.0 %	
Control variables			
Religion			
Hindu	95.8 %	96.4 %	0.51
Non-Hindu	04.2 %	03.6 %	
Caste			
Scheduled caste	53.8 %	95.4 %	0.00**
Non-scheduled caste	46.2 %	04.6 %	
Outcome variables			
Receipt of adequate antenatal care[a]	7.5 %	24.4 %	0.00**
Institutional delivery	30.9 %	85.3 %	0.00**
Percentage of private facility deliveries	52.0 %	19.0 %	0.00**
Percentage of public facility deliveries	48.0 %	81.0 %	
Cesarean section delivery	03.6 %	14.8 %	0.00**

**p < 0.01
[a]Antenatal care data were missing for 50 Gujarati women and 3 Tamil women

than Gujarati women (58 %), and Tamil women (97 %) had greater access to a health facility by an all-weather road than their Gujarati peers (80 %). Although both Tamil Nadu and Gujarat are high-performing states, Gujarati women (71 %) were twice as likely to be uneducated as Tamil women (32 %). Husbands in both states were more educated than their wives, but Gujarati husbands (40 %) were more likely to be uneducated than Tamil husbands (28 %). Tamil women's mean age at first birth (21.0 years) was significantly higher than that of Gujarati women (19.5 years), and there were also significant differences in parity, with a higher percentage of primipara and multipara women in Tamil Nadu and a higher percentage of grand multipara women in Gujarat. The vast majority (96 %) of women in both states were Hindu, but more Tamil women (95 %) than Gujarati women (54 %) were in the scheduled caste.

Examination of women's use of maternal health services in the two states revealed significant differences for all three outcome variables. Tamil women (24 %) were three times as likely as Gujarati women (8 %) to report adequate ANC. Tamil women (85 %) were almost three times more likely to have delivered their last child in a health care facility than Gujarati women (31 %); however, it is notable that 52 % of institutional deliveries in Gujarat were in a private facility as compared to 19 % in Tamil Nadu. C-section deliveries were significantly more prevalent among Tamil (15 %) than Gujarati (4 %) women.

Predictors of maternal health services utilization among women in the two states, based on multivariate analyses, are summarized in Table 2.

Adequate ANC

Receipt of JSY/CY financial assistance, availability of a PHC with 24/7 services, and access to a health facility via an all-weather road failed to significantly predict adequate ANC in Gujarat or Tamil Nadu. None of the socio-demographic or obstetric variables were significant predictors of ANC in either state, except maternal education in Gujarat. The odds of a Gujarati woman receiving adequate ANC were 2.8 times higher among women who had 10 or more years of education compared to uneducated women; however, the association was not significant at other levels of education.

Institutional delivery

Participation in CY/JSY significantly predicted institutional delivery in Gujarat. The odds of delivering in an accredited health facility were 3.9 times higher among Gujarati participants in CY/JSY compared to non-participants in the schemes. No such relationship was found in Tamil Nadu. The odds of having an institutional delivery were 1.4 times higher among Gujarati women and 3.4 times higher among Tamil Nadu women when they could access a

Table 2 Adjusted odds ratios and confidence intervals for use of maternal health services by Gujarati women and Tamil women[a]

Predictors	Adequate antenatal care				Institutional delivery				Cesarean section			
	Gujarat (n=1534)		Tamil Nadu (n=598)		Gujarat (n=1584)		Tamil Nadu (n=601)		Gujarat (n=1584)		Tamil Nadu (n=601)	
	AOR	95 % CI	AOR	95 % CI	AOR	95 % CI	AOR	95 % CI	AOR	95 % CI	AOR	95 % CI
Financial assistance from JSY or CY	0.83	0.42-1.63	0.92	0.61-1.39	3.93***	2.68-5.77	1.60	0.87-2.93	1.11	0.48-2.54	1.66*	1.01-2.70
Availability of PHC providing 24/7 services	0.70	0.44-1.11	0.90	0.59-1.38	1.04	0.83-1.31	1.04	0.62-1.75	1.16	0.93-2.34	1.59	0.90-2.81
Access to a health facility by an all-weather road	1.02	0.49-2.11	NA[b]	NA	1.42*	1.06-1.90	3.42*	1.24-9.47	0.71	0.38-1.34	0.44	0.14-1.31
Woman's education												
Uneducated	Ref		Ref		Ref		Ref		Ref		Ref	
Less than 5 years	1.25	0.63-2.50	0.93	0.47-1.84	0.85	0.58-1.25	1.18	0.43-1.67	0.80	0.30-2.11	2.44*	1.05-5.66
5-9 years	1.32	0.74-2.34	1.12	0.70-1.78	1.01	0.74-1.38	2.34***	1.32-4.15	0.99	0.48-2.02	1.57	0.78-3.18
10 or more years	2.78*	1.08-7.14	1.09	0.56-2.10	0.85	0.43-1.69	2.97*	1.08-8.21	0.86	0.17-4.45	1.99	0.83-4.79
Husband's education												
Uneducated	Ref		Ref		Ref		Ref		Ref		Ref	
Less than 5 years	1.87	0.99-3.54	1.36	0.71-2.62	0.72	0.50-1.06	1.15	0.49-2.72	0.67	0.22-2.01	0.83	0.31-2.22
5-9 years	0.94	0.53-1.68	1.01	0.62-1.64	0.99	0.76-1.30	1.17	0.64-2.13	1.20	0.62-2.32	0.93	0.49-1.79
10 or more years	1.72	0.91-3.26	0.97	0.51-1.86	1.44*	1.03-2.02	1.07	0.45-2.55	1.69	0.77-3.71	1.85	0.84-4.10
Age at first birth	1.07	0.99-1.16	1.04	0.98-1.09	1.05*	1.01-1.09	1.08†	1.00-1.17	0.94	0.83-1.06	1.08*	1.01-1.16
Parity												
Primipara	Ref		Ref		Ref		Ref		Ref		Ref	
Multipara	1.18	0.69-2.01	0.79	0.53-1.18	0.54***	0.41-0.72	0.65	0.51-1.10	0.44***	0.24-0.81	0.58*	0.36-0.96
Grand multipara	0.70	0.37-1.33	0.77	0.39-1.54	0.54***	0.40-0.72	0.43*	0.19-0.97	0.23***	0.10-0.51	0.18*	0.04-0.80

*$p < 0.05$, **$p < .01$, ***$p < 0.001$
[a]All analyses controlled for religion and caste
[b]NA. Variable removed from the model due to multicollinearity

health facility via an all weather road compared to their peers without such access. Although woman's education did not predict institutional delivery in Gujarat, it was a significant predictor in Tamil Nadu. The odds of delivering in a health facility for Tamil women with 5–9 years of education were 2.3 times higher and with 10+ years of education were 3.0 times higher compared to uneducated women. In Gujarat, husband's education was significantly related to his wife's institutional delivery for husbands with 10 + years of education; the odds of institutional delivery for Gujarati women whose husbands had completed secondary or higher education were 1.4 times higher compared to women whose husbands were uneducated. Age at first birth significantly predicted institutional delivery in Gujarat; with each 1 year increase in a woman's age at first birth, the odds of having an institutional delivery increased by 5 %. Parity significantly predicted institutional delivery in both states; the odds of Gujarati multipara and grand multipara women having institutional deliveries were 46 % lower and Tamil grand multipara women were 57 % lower compared to primipara women in their states.

C-section delivery

Receipt of JSY significantly predicted C-section in Tamil Nadu. The odds of having a C-section delivery were 1.7 times higher among JSY participants compared to non-participants. There was no significant association between CY/JSY and C-section in Gujarat. Woman's education significantly predicted C-section for Tamil women but not for Gujarati women. Specifically, the odds of a C-section delivery were 2.4 times higher for Tamil women with 1–4 years of education compared to uneducated women. Age of first birth predicted C-section in Tamil Nadu but not Gujarat. With each 1-year increase in a Tamil woman's age at first birth, the odds of a C-section increased by 8 %. Parity predicted C-sections in both states; the odds of Gujarati multipara women having a C-section were 56 % lower and grand multipara woman 77 % lower compared to primipara women. The odds of Tamil multipara women delivering by C-section were 42 % lower and grand multipara women were 82 % lower compared to primipara women.

Discussion

Our study extends existing research on India's health financing schemes by examining their operation in two high-performing states, and by including consideration of selected health system, socio-demographic, and obstetric factors in predicting use of maternity health services. Of key interest was women's use of JSY or CY to cover the cost of their institutional births. Relatively low percentages of poor, rural women were beneficiaries of the schemes, with Tamil women three times more likely to report receiving government assistance than Gujarati women. Tamil women were also more likely than their Gujarati peers to report adequate ANC or have a C-section birth. Several contextual factors likely contributed to these findings. Tamil Nadu launched JSY in 2005, building on its former Muthulakshmi Reddy Maternity Benefit Scheme established in 1989, while Gujarat's CY scheme was not implemented statewide until January 2007 [6, 12, 24]. Moreover, Tamil Nadu has long been recognized as a national leader in maternal health policy and public health system administration [25]. Annual per capita public health care expenditures are higher for Tamil Nadu at 200 INR compared to approximately 166 INR for Gujarat [26]. Lower government spending increases out-of-pocket healthcare expenses for items such as transportation that contribute to the full cost of institutional deliveries [27, 28].

A major study objective was to examine financial, health system, socio-demographic, and obstetric factors that predicted poor, rural women's use of maternity services in the targeted states. None of the factors under investigation predicted women's adequate ANC in Tamil Nadu, and a high level of maternal education was the only significant predictor of adequate ANC in Gujarat. The general failure of JSY/CY to predict adequate ANC after adjusting for socio-demographic factors was not surprising given that ANC was not incentivized during the study; women received no payments or vouchers for ANC and providers received no scheme incentives to provide the service. ASHAs received a one-time payment for women's institutional deliveries regardless of whether they scheduled any ANC visits for these same women [29]. Another study examining the impact of JSY throughout India also found the program to have little or no impact on antenatal care [30]. It has been argued that JSY and CY should link incentives to ANC, institutional delivery, and postnatal care, providing a continuum of care for mother and child [6, 29]. Currently, few studies have examined the impact of incentivizing ANC [31]; one Honduran study estimated that a conditional cash transfer incentive significantly increased ANC [32] and a Kenyan study found that provision of free bed nets at an ANC clinic greatly increased uptake of prenatal services [33]. Another study revealed no impact of the Mexican conditional cash transfer scheme on ANC, but this finding was attributed to very high baseline rates [34].

Receipt of CY/JSY significantly predicted institutional delivery among poor, rural women in Gujarat, with the odds of women delivering in a health facility almost four times higher among those participating in either scheme compared to non-participants. This finding is consistent with previous research linking CY and other financial schemes to increased institutional deliveries [3, 5–7, 10]. In contrast, a recent study that collected retrospective information from a statewide sample of Gujarati women who delivered since January 2005, as well as DLHS-3 data (2005–2007), concluded that CY has not increased women's probability of having an institutional delivery [11]. The latter study included both urban and rural Gujarati women and the retrospective component made no attempt to identify households with BPL status. Moreover, it was limited by respondents' recall of their ANC and deliveries over a 5-year period (versus the maximum 2-year look back of DLHS-3), suggesting the potential for recall bias. These findings suggest that CY may have a differential impact on particular segments of the Gujarat population, an issue deserving of future research. Notably, an evaluation of JSY throughout India found the scheme to be most effective in increasing institutional deliveries among poor, less educated, and ethnically marginalized women [35].

Receipt of JSY did not predict institutional delivery among Tamil women in the study, the vast majority (85 %) of whom delivered their last child in a health facility. Tamil Nadu's practice of providing some financial assistance to pregnant women even prior to JSY, regardless of whether they delivered in a facility or at home, may have contributed to this finding. The differential payment of INR 500 between institutional and home delivery suggests a relatively weak incentive for those who preferred a home birth [12, 24].

Access to a health facility by an all-weather road significantly predicted institutional deliveries in both Indian states, supporting the importance of addressing this variable in initiatives aimed at motivating rural women to deliver in health facilities. All-weather road access directly affects whether a woman can reach a facility for delivery, and indirectly affects her decision to pursue a facility delivery in the first place. Contrary to expectations, availability of a PHC with 24–7 services did not predict institutional delivery in either state. A number of supply-side constraints linked to PHCs, including unreliable staffing, supply shortages, and problematic referral transport for emergency complications, especially at centers below the district hospital level, may have diminished women's motivation to deliver in some facilities [36–38].

Findings further revealed that JSY participation significantly predicted C-section deliveries in Tamil Nadu, but not in Gujarat. Almost 15 % of poor, rural Tamil women reported a C-section for their last birth, compared to less than 4 % of their Gujarati peers. The significant role of the financing scheme in predicting C-section deliveries in

Tamil Nadu may be influenced by the state's availability of health facilities providing comprehensive emergency care and JSY's additional payment to obstetricians and anesthesiologists for C-section deliveries [12]. The CY scheme factors in an estimated proportion of C-sections in the flat rate payment to obstetricians for delivery care, and thus, does not incentivize surgical intervention. Notably, the Gujarat C-section rate (3.6 %) for women in this study was below WHO's optimal range of 5-15 % for all births in a country and below India's rural C-section rate of 6 % [39]. Thus, the risk with CY may be that there is little incentive for private obstetricians to accept women with complications as patients [5]. One recent study found that Gujarat's C-section rate had increased to 6 % for CY beneficiaries between 2006 and 2010, but these data were not disaggregated for urban and rural, poor women [40]. The researchers noted that private obstetricians tended to be concentrated in Gujarat's cities and small towns, and thus rural women were likely to experience greater barriers in accessing comprehensive emergency obstetric care.

Differential patterns were also found for sociodemographic predictors of women's use of health services in the two states. For example, woman's education was a significant predictor of institutional delivery and C-section in Tamil Nadu, while higher levels of husband's education predicted institutional delivery in Gujarat. Previous research has found woman's education to be a consistent predictor of institutional delivery in rural India [20]. Current findings further suggest that more educated husbands in Gujarat also understood the potential benefits of institutional deliveries. With respect to obstetric factors, age at first birth significantly predicted institutional delivery in Gujarat and C-section in Tamil Nadu; in both cases, older women were more likely to deliver in a health facility or obtain a C-section than their younger peers, suggesting that adolescent women may be underserved. Finally, parity significantly predicted institutional delivery and C-section in both states, with multiparous women less likely to utilize these maternity services. Possible contributors to this finding include JSY's policy of incentivizing only the first two live births [4, 5], limited financial resources of larger families, greater confidence of multiparous women with a history of uncomplicated births, and/or women's possible dissatisfaction with health facilities.

Limitations

Several limitations of our study must be noted. The DLHS-3 collected data on births in 2006 and 2007, with most births occurring in 2007 [21]. Given the frequent time lag between the launch of new policies and effective implementation at the grass roots level, findings may not reflect the current influence of the schemes. Another limitation is the possibility of recall bias, both on the part of women who were asked to remember details of

their antenatal and delivery care, and village heads who reported on access to a PHC and an all-weather road. However, the recall period in this study was relatively short (two years) and DLHS-3 field interviewers were well trained to collect retrospective data.

Additionally, the study's cross-sectional design precludes concluding causality from observed relationships. Our investigation of poor, rural women in two high-performing states likewise prevents generalizing the findings to all Gujarati or Tamil women, or to all low-income, rural women in India. Future research, including studies with longitudinal designs in high- and low-performing states, are needed to assess the impact of financial schemes, health system, and other social factors on Indian women's use of maternal health services, including ANC. Future research might also examine how the relationship between financial assistance from JSY or CY and women's use of institutional delivery is modified by various health system factors such as referral transport and availability of skilled human resources, and various social factors such as women's autonomy.

Policy and program implications

Based on our findings, we recommend that policy makers, program planners, and practitioners consider the following strategies for improving access, use, and quality of maternal health services for poor, rural women in the target states and throughout India.

First, efforts should be made to increase the use of demand-side maternal health financing schemes in the targeted states through health information, education, and communication campaigns aimed at the literate and non-literate, rural poor. ASHAs and community health workers play key roles in enrolling women in the schemes early in their pregnancies and require training. Given the link between incentives and service use, Tamil Nadu might consider eliminating the cash payment for home births to provide a stronger incentive for institutional delivery. States should also consider assigning part of the JSY payment for ANC, with the goal of educating women about fetal growth and nutrition, detecting high risk pregnancies, and developing advance plans for delivery/emergency care.

Second, states should augment promotion of demand-side financing schemes with improvements in the quality of maternal health services for poor, rural women. Enhancements in facility infrastructure, human resources, transport systems, referral coordination, supply chain systems and respectful evidence-based care are likely to improve health outcomes, as well as increase patient satisfaction and future service use.

Third, states should increase geographic access to health care facilities by supporting government investment in rural road infrastructure, including construction of all-weather roads. Such efforts may reduce both direct

Predictors of maternal health services utilization by poor, rural women: a comparative study...

87

transportation costs and opportunity costs of seeking care in facilities that are far from rural women's homes.

Fourth, support for increasing the education and literacy levels of poor, rural women may enhance their ability to make wise decisions about appropriate reproductive care. Health educational campaigns targeting women, husbands, and key household members may increase women's access to valuable maternity services.

Finally, researchers should use both qualitative and quantitative methods to explore poor, rural women's experiences with existing financing schemes, their opinions about the quality of health facilities, and their unmet obstetric needs. Similarly, health impact evaluations should collect qualitative data from health care professionals and managers about contextual factors that influence provision and use of maternity services, with the goal of strengthening understanding of quantitative outcomes.

Conclusion

Differential patterns of findings for the Indian states of Gujarat and Tamil Nadu underscore the complexity of designing interventions to enhance poor, rural women's use of maternity services. Findings suggest the need for both states to increase women's participation in health financing schemes that incentivize institutional delivery, as well as improve women's access to ANC. States should conduct careful contextual analyses and leverage existing resources to develop policies and programs that enhance the quality, use, and equity of maternal health services. Additional evaluation of JSY, CY, health system and social factors may strengthen interventions aimed at reducing India's maternal mortality ratio and influence maternal health schemes for poor women throughout the world.

Competing interests
The authors declare that they have no competing interests.

Authors' contributions
All authors read and approved the final manuscript.

Author details
[1]Indian Institute of Public Health Gandhinagar, Drive-in-Road, Ahmedabad, Gujarat 380054, India. [2]University of Maryland, College Park,, Prince George's. [3]USAID, Washington D.C, USA.

References
1. Vora KS, Mavalankar DV, Ramani KV, Upadhyay M, Sharma B, Iyengar S, et al. Maternal health situation in India: a case study. J Health Popul Nutr. 2009;27(2):184–201.
2. WHO, UNICEF, UNFPA. World Bank: trends in maternal mortality: 1990–2008. WHO library cataloguing-in-publication data. Geneva: WHO; 2010.
3. Randive B, Diwan V, de Costa A. India's conditional cash Transfer programme (the JSY) to promote institutional birth: is there an association between institutional birth proportion and maternal mortality? PLoS One. 2013;8(6):e67452.
4. Ministry of Health and Family Welfare, Government of India (MoHFW). Janani Suraksha Yojana: Revised Guidelines for implementation. New Delhi: MoHFW; 2006. (http://www.ilo.org/dyn/travail/docs/683/Janani%20 Suraksha%20Yojana%20-%20Guidelines%20for%20implementation%20-% 20Ministry%20of%20Health%20and%20Family%20Welfare.pdf, accessed 25 May 2014).
5. Jehan K, Sidney K, Smith H, de Costa A. Improving access to maternity services: an overview of cash transfer and voucher schemes in South Asia. Reprod Health Matters. 2012;20(39):142–54.
6. Bhat R, Mavalankar DV, Singh PV, Singh N. Maternal healthcare financing: Gujarat's Chiranjeevi scheme and its beneficiaries. J Health Popul Nutr. 2009;27(2):249–58.
7. Singh A, Mavalankar DV, Bhat R, Desai A, Patel SR, Singh PV, et al. Providing skilled birth attendants and emergency obstetric care to the poor through partnership with private sector obstetricians in Gujarat, India. Bull World Health Organ. 2009;87:960–4.
8. United Nations Population Fund (UNFPA)-India. Concurrent assessment of Janani Suraksha Yojana (JSY) in selected states: Bihar, Madhya Pradesh,Orissa, Rajasthan, Uttar Pradesh. New Delhi: UNFPA; 2009.
9. Devadasan N, Elias MA, John D, Grahacharya S, Ralte L. A conditional cash assistance programme for promoting institutional deliveries among the poor in India: process evaluation results. Studies in HSO&P. 2008;24:257–73.
10. Lim SS, Dandona L, Hoisington JA, James SL, Hogan MC, Gakidou E. India's Janani Suraksha Yojana, a conditional cash transfer programme to increase births in health facilities: an impact evaluation. Lancet. 2010;375(9730):2009–23.
11. Mohanan M, Bauhoff S, La Forgia G, Singer Babiarz K, Singh K, Miller G. Effect of Chiranjeevi Yojana on institutional deliveries and neonatal and maternal outcomes in Gujarat, India: a difference-in-differences analysis. Bull World Health Organ. 2014;92:187–94.
12. WHO. Safer pregnancy in Tamil Nadu: from vision to reality. New Delhi, India: WHO SEARO; 2009.
13. Gabrysh S, Campbell OMR. Still too far to walk: literature review of the determinants of delivery service use. BMC Pregnancy Childbirth. 2009;9(34):9–34.
14. Morgan L, Stanton ME, Higgs ES, Balster RL, Bellows BW, Brandes N, et al. Financial Incentives and maternal health: where do we go from here? J Health Popul Nutr. 2013;31 Suppl 2:8–22.
15. Stephenson R, Tsui AO. Contextual influences on reproductive health service use in Uttar Pradesh. India Stud Fam Plann. 2002;33(4):309–20.
16. Dalal K, Dawad S. Non-utilization of public healthcare facilities: examining the reasons through a national study of women in India. Rural and Remote Health [Internet]. 2009; 9: 1178. Available from: http://www.rrh.org.au/asia/defaultnew.asp.
17. Mazumdar PG, Kanjilal B, Barman D, Mandal A. Revisiting the role of geographical accessibility in women's access to healthcare. Jaipur, India: Indian Institute of Health Management Research; 2009. Working paper IV: India Series. (http://r4d.dfid.gov.uk/pdf/outputs/futurehealth_rpc/wp-iv.pdf accessed 1 April 2015).
18. New all-weather roads boost rural income: IDA at work: India [Internet]. Washington D.C., USA: International Development Association; 2012. (http://web.worldbank.org/WBSITE/EXTERNAL/EXTABOUTUS/IDA/0,,contentMDK: 22311357~menuPK:4754051~pagePK:51236175~piPK:437394~theSitePK: 73154,00.html, accessed 22 March 2014).
19. Say L, Raine R. A systematic review of inequalities in the use of maternal health care in developing countries: examining the scale of the problem and the importance of context. Bull World Health Organ. 2007;85:812–19.
20. Govindasamy P, Ramesh B. Maternal education and the utilization of maternal and child health services in India. Mumbai, India: International Institute of Population Sciences; 1997 (http://www.eastwestcenter.org/sites/default/files/filemanager/Research_Program/NFHS_Subject_Reports/subj-5.pdf accessed 1 April 2015).
21. District Level Household and Facility Survey 2007–08: India. Mumbai, India: International Institute for Population Sciences; 2009.
22. Introduction. National Report. District Level Household and Facility Survey 2007–08: India. Mumbai, India: International Institute for Population Sciences; 2009. (http://www.rchiips.org/pdf/INDIA_REPORT_DLHS-3.pdf, accessed 12 December 2014).
23. Pallikadavath S, Foss M, Stones RW. Antenatal care: provision and inequality in rural north India. Soc Sci Med. 2004;59(6):1147–58.
24. Padmanaban P, Raman PS, Mavalankar DV. Innovations and challenges in reducing maternal mortality in Tamil Nadu. India J Health Popul Nutr. 2009;27(2):202–19.
25. Smith SL. Political Contexts and maternal health policy: insights from a comparison of south Indian states. Soc Sci Med. 2014;100:46–53.

26. Guruswamy M, Mazumdar S, Mazumdar P. Public financing of health services in India: an analysis of central and state government expenditure. J Healthc Manag. 2008;10(1):49–85.

27. Ghuman BS, Mehta A. Health care services in India: problems and prospects. Paper presented at: International conference on the Asian social protection in comparative perspective. Singapore: National University of singapore; 2009. p. 7–9.

28. Mohanty SK, Srivastava A. Out-of-pocket expenditure on institutional delivery in India. Health Policy Plan. 2013;28:247–62.

29. Lahariya C. Cash incentives for institutional delivery: linking with antenatal and postnatal care may ensure 'continuum of care' in India. Indian J Community Med. 2009;34(2):15–8.

30. Mazumdar S, Mills A. Powell-Jackson, T. Financial incentives in health: new Evidence from India's Janani Suraksha Yojana. London: London School of Hygiene and Tropical Medicine; 2011.

31. Dow WH, White JS. Incentivizing use of health care. Expert Paper No.2013/13. New York: United Nations; 2013.

32. Morris S, Flores R, Olinto P, Medina JM. Monetary incentives in primary health care and effects on use and coverage of preventive health care interventions in rural Honduras: cluster randomized trial. Lancet. 2004;364:2030–37.

33. Dupas P. The impact of conditional in-kind subsidies on preventive health behaviours: evidence from Western Kenya. Paris: EHESS-PSE; 2005 (http://web.stanford.edu/~pdupas/TAMTAMpaper07.11.05.pdf, accessed 30 March 2015).

34. Barber S, Gertler P. The impact of Mexico's conditional cash transfer program, Oportunidades, on birthweight. Trop Med Int Health. 2008;13(11):1405–14.

35. Glassman A, Duran D, Fleisher L, Singer D, Burke R, Angeles G, et al. Impact of conditional cash transfers on maternal and new born health. J Health Popul Nutr. 2013;31(4):548–66.

36. Krupp K, Madhivanan P. Leveraging human capital to reduce maternal mortality in India: enhanced public health system or public-private partnership? Hum Resour Health. 2009;7:18.

37. Gupta M, Mavalankar D, Ramani KV. Referral transport. In: Visaria L, editor. Midwifery and maternal health in India: a situational analysis. Ahmedabad, India: Centre for Management of Health Systems; 2010. p. 90–9.

38. Mavalankar DV, Vora KS, Ramani KV, Raman P, Sharma B, Upadhyaya M. Maternal health in Gujarat, India: a case study. J Health Popul Nutr. 2009;27(2):235–48.

39. Gibbons L, Belizan JM, Lauer JA, Betran AP, Merialdi M, Althabe F. The global numbers and costs of additionally needed and unnecessary Caesarean sections performed per year: overuse as a barrier to universal coverage. World Health Organization;2010. (http://www.who.int/healthsystems/topics/financing/healthreport/30C-sectioncosts.pdf accessed 1 April 2015)

40. De Costa A, Vora KS, Ryan K, Raman PS, Santacatterina M, Mavalankar D. The state-led large scale public private partnership 'Chiranjeevi Program' to increase access to institutional delivery among poor women in Gujarat, India. How has it Done? What can we learn? PLoS One. 2014;9(5):e95704.

Magnitude of undernutrition in children aged 2 to 4 years using CIAF and conventional indices in the slums of Mumbai city

Mitravinda S. Savanur[*] [iD] and Padmini S. Ghugre

Abstract

Conventional indicators – weight-for-age, height-for-age, weight-for-height and mid-upper arm circumference (MUAC) reflect different facets of the nutritional status. Weight-for-age is the most commonly used indicator. When used individually or in combination, conventional indices fail to depict the overall magnitude of undernutrition in the population. Composite Index of Anthropometric Failure (CIAF) is an alternative classification system which attempts to fill this lacuna. Thus, we undertook this study with the objective to compare the prevalence of undernutrition using CIAF and the conventional indices. We included 634 children aged between 2 to 4 years from *anganwadis* located in three areas of Mumbai. Weight, height and MUAC measurements were taken. Z scores were computed for weight-for-age (WAZ), height-for-age (HAZ) and weight-for-height (WHZ) using WHO Anthro software. Children were classified as per the conventional indices and CIAF. The prevalence of underweight, stunting and wasting was 35.7 %, 33.8 % and 18.5 % respectively. None of the children had MUAC < 11.5 cm. About 1 % of the children were moderately wasted according to MUAC. As per CIAF, 47.8 % children were undernourished. According to CIAF, one-third of the undernourished children had single anthropometric failure while half of them had dual failure and 17.1 % had multiple failures. When compared with the conventional indices, CIAF could recognize 12.1 %, 14.0 %, 29.3 % and 46.7 % more undernourished children than WAZ, HAZ, WHZ and MUAC respectively. In conclusion, CIAF is seen to have many advantages over the conventional indices. CIAF is useful in assessing the overall magnitude of undernutrition and identifying children with multiple anthropometric failures. It also recognizes more undernourished children than all the conventional indices. Therefore, CIAF should be used more widely as a tool for nutritional assessment particularly in developing countries where the burden of undernutrition is high.

Keywords: CIAF, Underweight, Stunting, Wasting, Nutritional status, Children, India

Background

Undernutrition among children under five years is traditionally assessed using anthropometric indices such as – weight-for-age, height-for-age, weight-for-height and mid-upper arm circumference (MUAC). Stunting or low height-for-age is an indicator of chronic undernutrition which is manifested as poor skeletal growth. Low weight-for-height reflects wasting or acute undernutrition with loss of lean as well as fat mass [1]. On the other hand, low MUAC (<11.5 cm) is not only suggestive of severe wasting or severe acute malnutrition but also indicative of morbidity and risk of mortality [2, 3]. Underweight or low weight-for-age, on the other hand, is indicative of both acute and chronic undernutrition [1]. These indices reflect different facets of undernutrition. Although underweight, stunting and wasting reflect different facets of undernutrition, they are not mutually exclusive categories. For instance, a child who is found to be stunted can also be underweight and wasted at the same time. Hence, a sum of the children who are underweight, stunted and wasted in a group does not reveal the overall number of undernourished children in a population. The conventional indices therefore fail to provide the overall prevalence of undernutrition in a group.

There is another concern with the use of conventional indices. Weight-for-age is most commonly used to assess

* Correspondence: mitrasav@gmail.com
Department of Food Science and Nutrition, Sir Vithaldas Vihar, S.N.D.T. Women's University, Juhu Road, Mumbai 400049, Maharashtra, India

the nutritional status. This may be because underweight indicates both acute and chronic undernutrition. However, underweight is not the summation of children who are wasted and stunted. As a result, we might tend to miss out on children who are stunted and wasted if underweight is used as a sole indicator of nutritional status.

In the year 2000, Swedish Economist Prof. Peter Svedberg suggested an alternative measure to assess the overall magnitude of undernutrition – Composite Index of Anthropometric Failure (CIAF). CIAF identifies seven groups of children including those without any form of anthropometric failure (Table 1). A summation of the groups B, C, D, E, F and Y gives the total magnitude of undernutrition. At the same time, it can be useful in detecting multiple anthropometric failures [4].

Investigators in Kenya, China and Bangladesh have used CIAF to assess the extent of undernutrition [5–7]. In Kenya, Berger et al estimated the prevalence of undernutrition among children with HIV/AIDS [5]. Khan et al and Pei et al also identified the sociodemographic factors determining overall undernutrition [7, 6]. Nandy and Miranda have used the national data from seven developing countries to calculate the CIAF and compare it with prevalence of underweight in the same areas [8].

In India, Nandy *et al* was the first to use the concept of CIAF on the data of 1998 – 99 National Family Health Survey – 2 (NFHS - 2) [1]. Thereafter most of the Indian studies that have used CIAF have been conducted in rural or tribal areas of West Bengal [9–15]. Only two studies so far have used CIAF in an urban setting i.e. in Coimbatore, Tamil Nadu and Bankura town, West Bengal [16, 17].

In Maharashtra state, the prevalence of underweight, stunting and wasting in under-five children in rural and urban areas was 37 %, 46 % and 17 % respectively. The nutritional status of under-five children in Mumbai was reportedly worse than the other urban areas in the state. The prevalence of underweight and stunting was 40 % and 14 % higher respectively in the slum than the non-slum areas of Mumbai [18]. The overall extent of undernutrition in the children belonging to the slums in Mumbai remains unknown.

We therefore conducted the present study with an objective to compare the prevalence of undernutrition by using CIAF and the conventional indices.

Methods

The study was approved by Independent Ethics Committee (IEC no 09122), Navi Mumbai, Maharashtra, India.

Study design

This cross-sectional study was carried out from July, 2013 to January, 2014 in the slums of Mumbai city, Maharashtra, India. We undertook the study in three urban slum areas located in the western suburbs of the city. Each of these areas had 140 to 150 *anganwadis* each. *Anganwadi* is a child-care and mother-care centre which is run by the Integrated Child Development Service (ICDS) in India. We obtained a list of *anganwadis* in each of these areas from the respective Child Development Project Officers (CDPO). From this list, every sixth *anganwadi* was selected by simple random sampling. Thus, from every area, we selected 25 *anganwadis* each (Fig. 1). Participants: Six hundred and thirty four children aged between 2 to 4 years participated in the study. The inclusion and exclusion criteria for including the children in this study were.

Inclusion criteria

Children who (i) were beneficiaries of the *anganwadi*, (ii) had authentic records of their date of birth and (iii) had completed 24 months of age and were less than or equal to 48 months were included in the study. Age was calculated on the basis of their date of birth to the nearest one month.

Exclusion criteria

Children who were – (i) suffering from any chronic illness that influenced their nutritional status, (ii) born with congenital anomalies, (iii) born extremely premature (<28 weeks of gestational age).

Parents and/or guardians of the children were explained about the study procedure in the local language and an informed consent was obtained from them.

Assessment of nutritional status

Weight and height measurements of all the children were taken using standard procedure [19]. Children were weighed on a digital weighing scale (Dr Gene Health and Wellness; Model no: MS8270) with an accuracy of 0.1 kg. Height was measured using a non-

Table 1 Categories of the composite index of anthropometric failure (CIAF)

Group	Description of the group	Definition
A	No anthropometric failure	Normal WAZ, HAZ and WHZ
B	Wasting only	WHZ < -2SD but normal WAZ and HAZ
C	Wasting and underweight	WHZ and WAZ < -2 SD but normal HAZ
D	Wasting, underweight and stunting	WHZ, WAZ and HAZ < -2 SD
E	Stunting and underweight	HAZ and WAZ < -2 SD but normal WHZ
F	Stunting only	HAZ < -2 SD but normal WAZ and WHZ
Y	Underweight only	WAZ < -2 SD but normal HAZ and WHZ

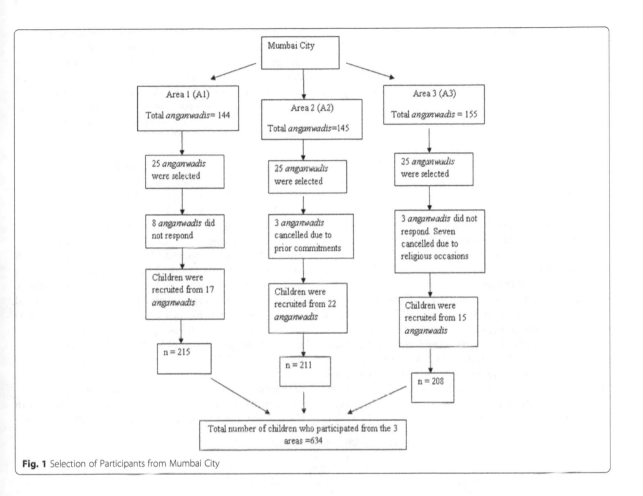

Fig. 1 Selection of Participants from Mumbai City

extensible, flexible measuring tape with an accuracy of 0.1 cm which was calibrated against the standard anthropometric scale. Based on these measurements, weight-for-age Z scores (WAZ), height-for-age Z scores (HAZ) and weight-for-height Z scores (WHZ) were computed. MUAC was measured using a non-extensible, flexible measuring tape at the mid-point between the acromion and olecranon processes of the child's arm flexed at 90° angle. The child was then made to relax the arm so that it hangs just away from the side of the body and the circumference was measured at the mid-point with an accuracy of 0.1 cm [20].

Children with WAZ, HAZ and WHZ scores between – 3.0 to – 2.0 SD were classified as moderately underweight, stunted and wasted respectively. Those with WAZ, HAZ and WHZ scores were < -3.0 SD were classified as severely underweight, stunted and wasted respectively. And, those children who had Z scores > -2.0 SD were classified as 'normal' [21]. MUAC < 11.5 cm and between 11.5 to 12.5 cm were classified as severe acute malnutrition (SAM) and moderate acute malnutrition (MAM) respectively. Those

with MUAC > 12.5 cm were considered 'normal' [3]. Further, children were also classified using CIAF [1].

Statistical analysis

WAZ, HAZ and WHZ scores were computed using WHO Anthro software version 3.2.2. The data was analyzed using SPSS version 20. For WAZ, HAZ, WHZ and MUAC one-way ANOVA was used to analyze the difference in the mean Z scores between boys and girls. Chi-square tests were performed to study the age-wise and gender-wise differences in the prevalence of undernutrition.

Results

There were 53.6 % (n = 340) boys and 46.4 % (n = 294) girls in the study. The mean age of the children was 3.1 ± 0.8 years. The mean anthropometric measurements of children are presented in Table 2. Boys weighed significantly more (F = 12.039, p = 0.001) and had a significantly higher MUAC (F = 4.151, p = 0.042) than the girls.

Table 2 Mean anthropometric measurements of boys and girls (n = 634)

Parameter	Boys (n = 340)	Girls (n = 294)	F	P value
Weight (kg)	11.9 ± 1.8	11.4 ± 1.8	12.039	0.001
Height (cm)	90.1 ± 7.2	89.2 ± 7.0	2.427	0.120
WAZ	-1.6 ± 1.0	-1.7 ± 0.9	2.194	0.139
HAZ	-1.5 ± 1.2	-1.6 ± 1.1	0.921	0.337
WHZ	-1.1 ± 1.0	-1.1 ± 0.9	0.000	0.987
MUAC (cm)	14.9 ± 1.1	14.8 ± 1.1	4.151	0.042

WAZ Weight-for-age Z score, *HAZ* Height-for-age Z score, *WHZ* Weight-for-height Z score, *MUAC* Mid-upper arm circumference

However no statistical differences were seen between boys and girls for the other anthropometric parameters.

Nutritional Status
Using conventional indices
Children were classified as per WHO Growth Standards [3, 21]. One hundred and seventy-six (27.8 %) children were moderately underweight and 50 (7.9 %) were severely underweight (Table 3). One hundred and forty-three (22.6 %) children and 71(11.2 %) were moderately and severely stunted respectively. One hundred and four (16.4 %) children and 13 (2.1 %) children had moderate and severe wasting respectively. None of the children had a MUAC < 11.5 cm. Seven children (1.1 %) had

MAM according to MUAC. There were no significant differences were observed in the prevalence rates in boys and girls. Similarly, no statistical differences were seen in the prevalence of underweight and stunting across the age groups. However, significantly higher number of children in the age group of 3 to 4 years were moderately wasted than children aged 2 to 3 years of age (20.3 % v 12 %; $\chi2 = 7.983$, p = 0.018).

Using composite index of anthropometric failure
According to CIAF classification, 331 children (52.2 %) were well nourished (Table 4). Nearly half the children i.e. 303 (47.8 %) were undernourished. Of all the undernourished children, 101 children (33.3 %) suffered from single anthropometric failure (Group – B, F and Y). Almost half the undernourished children (49.5 %) suffered from dual anthropometric failure (Group – C and E) while fifty-two children i.e. 17.1 % experienced multiple failures i.e. they were underweight, stunted and wasted at the same time. No age-wise ($\chi2 = 11.516$, p = 0.074) and sex-wise ($\chi2 = 10.864$, p = 0.093) differences were noted in the prevalence of single, dual and multiple anthropometric failures.

CIAF v Conventional indices of undernutrition
CIAF could identify more undernourished children than the conventional indices. The prevalence of undernutrition

Table 3 Prevalence of undernutrition according to the conventional indices

Indicator	Classification	Age (years)		Sex		Total % (n)
		2 to 3 % (n)	3 to 4 % (n)	Boys % (n)	Girls % (n)	
WAZ (Underweight)	Normal	64.5 (209)	64.2 (199)	66.8 (227)	61.6 (181)	64.4 (408)
	Moderate underweight	29.6 (96)	25.8 (80)	25.6 (87)	30.3 (89)	27.8 (176)
	Severe underweight	5.9 (19)	10.0 (31)	7.6 (26)	8.2 (24)	7.9 (50)
	$\chi2$	4.273		1.962		
	p	0.118		0.375		
HAZ (Stunting)	Normal	66.0 (214)	66.5 (206)	67.6 (230)	64.6 (190)	66.2 (420)
	Moderate stunting	22.2 (72)	22.9 (71)	20.9 (71)	24.5 (72)	22.6 (143)
	Severe stunting	11.7 (38)	10.6 (33)	11.5 (39)	10.9 (32)	11.2 (71)
	$\chi2$	0.202		1.175		
	p	0.904		0.556		
WHZ (Wasting)	Normal	85.8 (278)	77.1 (239)	79.7 (271)	83.7 (246)	81.5 (517)
	Moderate wasting	12.7 (41)	20.3 (63)	17.9 (61)	14.6 (43)	16.4 (104)
	Severe wasting	1.5 (5)	2.6 (8)	2.4 (8)	1.7 (5)	2.1 (13)
	$\chi2$	7.983		1.688		
	p	0.018		0.430		
MUAC (Acute malnutrition)	Normal (>12.5 cm)	99.1 (321)	98.7 (306)	98.8 (336)	99.0 (291)	98.9 (627)
	MAM (11.5 to 12.5 cm)	0.9 (3)	1.3 (4)	1.2 (4)	1.0 (3)	1.1 (7)
	$\chi2$	0.193		0.035		
	p	0.720		1.000		

WAZ Weight-for-age Z score, *HAZ* Height-for-age Z score, *WHZ* Weight-for-height Z score, *MUAC* Mid-upper arm circumference

Table 4 Prevalence of undernutrition according to CIAF

Group	Description of the group	Age (years)		Sex		Total % (n)
		2 to 3 % (n)	3 to 4 % (n)	Boys % (n)	Girls % (n)	
A	No anthropometric failure	53.7 (174)	50.6 (157)	54.1 (184)	50.0 (147)	52.2 (331)
B	Wasting only	1.2 (4)	4.2 (13)	3.8 (13)	1.3 (4)	2.6 (17)
C	Wasting and underweight	6.2 (20)	8.7 (27)	6.7 (23)	8.5 (25)	7.5 (48)
D	Wasting, underweight and stunting	6.8 (22)	9.7 (30)	9.7 (33)	6.4 (19)	8.2 (52)
E	Stunting and underweight	17.6 (57)	14.8 (46)	13.8 (47)	18.7 (55)	16.1 (102)
F	Stunting only	9.6 (31)	9.4 (29)	8.8 (30)	10.2 (30)	9.4 (60)
Y	Underweight only	4.9 (16)	2.6 (8)	2.9 (10)	4.76 (14)	3.7 (24)
	Total anthropometric failure (B + C + D + E + F + Y)	46.3 (150)	49.4 (153)	45.8 (156)	50.0 (147)	47.8 (303)
	$\chi 2$	11.516		10.864		
	p	0.074		0.093		

according to CIAF was 47.8 %. On the other hand, using conventional indices, 35.7 % were underweight, 33.8 % were stunted and 18.5 % were wasted. Thus, CIAF could recognize 12.1 %, 14.0 % and 29.3 % more undernourished children than WAZ, HAZ and WHZ respectively. CIAF could recognize 46.7 % more children as undernourished than MUAC. Among all the children classified as well nourished by MUAC, 16.1 % had single anthropometric failure while 23.4 % and 7.7 % suffered from dual and multiple failures respectively (Table 5).

Discussion

The present study compared the prevalence of undernutrition by using CIAF and the conventional indices. The prevalence of undernutrition according to CIAF was 47.8 %. On the other hand, according to the conventional indices 35.7 %, 33.8 % and 18.5 % children were underweight, stunted and wasted respectively. Also, about 1 % children were classified as MAM according to MUAC.

Some researchers have used CIAF to assess the prevalence of undernutrition. Nandy and Miranda [8] computed the CIAF using the national data from 1998 to 2001 of seven developing countries - India, Ethopia, Nepal,

Table 5 Distribution of children in MUAC categories across the CIAF

CIAF Classification	MUAC Categories % (n)	
	11.5 to 12.5 cm	>12.5 cm
	(n = 7)	(n = 627)
No failure	0	52.8 (329)
Wasting only	0	2.7 (17)
Wasting and underweight	14.3 (1)	7.3 (46)
Wasting, underweight and stunting	57.1 (4)	7.7 (48)
Stunting and underweight	28.6 (2)	16.1 (101)
Stunting only	0	9.6 (60)
Underweight only	0	3.8 (24)

Tanzania, Zimbabwe, Bolivia and Peru. The prevalence rates in Peru (23.3 %), Bolivia (26.6 %) and Zimbabwe (35.8 %) were lower than that observed our study while in Nepal (56.5 %) and Ethopia (58 %) rates were much higher. Recent reports indicate that 21.4 % children were undernourished in rural China [6] while in rural Bangladesh the prevalence was 58.7 % [7]. On the other hand, the rates were slightly lower in urban Bangladesh (47.9 %) and were comparable to that observed in our study [7].

In India, a total of 59.8 % children were reported to be undernourished using the NFHS – 2 data collected during 1998 – 99 [8]. Other studies in India have been mainly conducted in rural and tribal West Bengal wherein the prevalence rates ranged from 50.2 to 73.0 % which were much higher than those observed in our study [9–14]. Similarly, 59.6 % were reported to be undernourished in rural Wardha, Maharashtra state [22]. Factors associated with undernutrition in these rural and tribal areas were reported to be birth order, low birth weight, breastfeeding practices and mother's education [15]. Only two studies have been reported from urban areas of India, one from Tamil Nadu [16] and another from West Bengal [17]. The prevalence rates in these studies were higher than our study. These differences can be possibly attributed to various factors such as socioeconomic status, educational level, living conditions, maternal health, birth weight, feeding practices and rates of infections. However, we have not studied the factors influencing the overall prevalence of undernutrition as a part of this paper.

In the studies where CIAF and conventional indices were used together, CIAF identified more undernourished children than the latter [8, 14, 16, 23]. Nandy and Miranda [8] found that the use of weight-for-age underestimated the prevalence by 9.7 to 21.7 % as compared to CIAF. Similar findings have been noted by some other researchers in India [14, 16, 23]. However, these workers compared CIAF with only WAZ. We compared CIAF with WAZ, HAZ, WHZ and MUAC. WAZ underestimated the prevalence by 12.1 %, HAZ by 14.0 % and WHZ by 29.3 % as compared to CIAF. Also, MUAC identified 1.1 % children as MAM but failed to identify 46.7 % children who had varying degrees of undernutrition. Thus the conventional indices underestimated the prevalence of undernutrition and erroneously classified a sizeable section of the population as 'normal'.

Further, conventional indicators do not give a holistic picture of the nutritional status of a population. For instance, by using conventional indices we can find out how many children are underweight. But, there could be some children who are wasted as well as underweight. Such groups of children suffering from two or more anthropometric failures remain unidentified when conventional measures are used. In view of this, Svedberg added three categories to the existing conventional indicators (Group C: wasting and underweight, D: underweight, stunting and wasting and E: underweight and stunting) [4]. In this study, only 33 % of the undernourished children exhibited single anthropometric failure while the remaining had either dual or multiple anthropometric failures which was not revealed with the use of conventional indices. These children exhibiting multiple anthropometric failures will require regular counseling and monitoring than those having single anthopometric failure.

In India, ICDS is the national programme that aims at reducing undernutrition and improving the nutritional status of children up to six years of age. Presently, the ICDS uses weight-for-age and MUAC as the indicators of nutritional status. WAZ identifies underweight children while MUAC recognizes those with extreme wasting. Stunted and moderately/severely wasted children are not identified as undernourished. As a result, a significant proportion of children suffering from dual or multiple failures are missed out. These vulnerable children fail to receive adequate attention and appropriate counseling from the *anganwadi* workers. This can further increase the burden of undernutrition and risk for morbidity. Thus, with the use of CIAF all the undernourished children can be identified.

The ICDS routinely weighs the children. If height is also measured then CIAF can be easily used. Using CIAF will not incur any extra financial burden on the government machineries. The use of CIAF will not only help in assessment but also in monitoring the growth of these children suffering from various degrees of anthropometric failure. Parents can be sensitized and appropriately counseled regarding their child's nutritional status. Such steps can help reduce the overall burden of undernutrition and also pave the path towards attaining the Millennium Development Goals (MDGs).

The strength of the present study is that this is the first study to have used CIAF to estimate the overall prevalence of undernutrition in the slums of Mumbai. Also, the study compares the prevalence rates of CIAF with all the conventional indices including MUAC. The limitation of our study was that it was carried out in three slum areas of Mumbai city. It would have been worthwhile if similar data was gathered from the non-slum areas where people across the socioeconomic spectrum reside. Also, we used only anthropometric indices and did not include any biochemical parameters for the assessment of nutritional status.

Conclusion

CIAF is a useful tool which provides a holistic picture of the overall prevalence of undernutrition. Conventional indicators when used individually grossly underestimate the extent of undernutrition. ICDS should thus, consider using CIAF at the national level as a step towards reducing the overall burden of undernutrion in children.

Competing interests
The authors declare that they have no competing interests.

Authors' contributions
MSS and PSG conceptualized and designed the study. MSS collected and analyzed the data. MSS drafted the manuscript. PSG provided critical inputs to the manuscript. All authors read and approved the final manuscript.

Acknowledgement
We wish to acknowledge the continuous support and co-operation of the CDPOs, *anganwadi* workers and helpers.

References
1. Nandy S, Irving M, Gordon D, Subramaniun SV, Smith GD. Poverty, child undernutrition and morbidity: new evidence from India. Bull World Health Organ. 2005;83(3):210–6.
2. Berkley J, Mwangi I, Griffiths K, Ahmed I, Mithwani S, English M, et al. Assessment of severe malnutrition among hospitalized children in Rural Kenya: comparison of weight for height and mid upper arm circumference. J Am Med Assoc. 2005;294:591–7.
3. World Health Organization and UNICEF. WHO child growth standards and the identification of severe acute malnutrition in infants and children. A Joint Statement by the World Health Organization and the United Nations Children's Fund. Geneva: World Health Organization; 2009.
4. Svedberg P. Poverty and undernutrition: theory, measurement and policy. New Delhi: Oxford India Paperbacks; 2000.
5. Berger MR, Fields-Gardner C, Wagle A, Hollenbeck CB. Prevalence of malnutrition in human Immunodeficiency virus/acquired immunodeficiency syndrome orphans in the Nyanza Province of Kenya: a comparison of conventional indexes with a composite index of anthropometric failure. J Am Diet Assoc. 2008;108:1014–7.
6. Pei L, Ren L, Yan H. A survey of undernutrition in children under three years of age in rural Western China. BMC Public Health. 2014;14:121–31.
7. Khan REA, Raza MA. Nutritional status of children in Bangladesh: measuring composite index of anthropometric failure (CIAF) and its determinants. Pak J Commer Soc Sci. 2014;8(1):11–23.
8. Nandy S, Miranda JJ. Overlooking undernutrition? Using composite index of anthropometric failure to assess how underweight misses and misleads the assessment of undernutrition in young children. Soc Sci Med. 2008;66(9-5):1963–6.

9. Biswas S, Bose K, Mukhopadhyay A, Bhadra M. Prevalence of undernutrition among pre-school children of Chapra, Nadia District, West Bengal, India, measured by composite index of anthropometric failure (CIAF). Anthropol Anz. 2009;67(3):269–79.

10. Mandal GC, Bose K. Assessment of overall prevalence of undernutrition using composite index of anthropometric failure (CIAF) among preschool children of West Bengal, India. Iran J Pediatr. 2009;19(3):237–43.

11. Das S, Bose K. Assessment of nutritional status by anthropometric indices in Santal Tribal Children. J Life Sci. 2011;3(2):81–5.

12. Sen J, Dey S, Mondal N. Conventional nutritional indices and Composite Index of Anthropometric Failure: which seems more appropriate for assessing under-nutrition among children? A cross-sectional study among school children of the Bengalee Muslim Population of North Bengal, India. Italian J Public Health. 2011;8(2):172–84.

13. Sinha NK, Maiti S. Prevalence Of Undernutrition Among Underprivileged Preschool Children (2-6 years) Of Midnapore Town, India Malaysian Journal Of Paediatrics And Child Health Online Early 2012; 18 (1). Available at http://mjpch.com/index.php/mjpch/article/viewFile/201/202.

14. Acharya A, Mandal GC, Bose K. Overall burden of under-nutrition measured by a Composite Index in rural pre-school children in Purba Medinipur, West Bengal, India. Anthropol Rev. 2013;76(1):109–16.

15. Dasgupta A, Parthasarathi R, Prabhakar R, Biswas R, Geethanjali A. Assessment of under nutrition with composite index of anthropometric failure (CIAF) among under-five children in a Rural Area of West Bengal, Indian. J Community Health. 2014;26(2):132–8.

16. Seetharam N, Chacko TV, Shankar SLR, Mathew AC. Measuring malnutrition – The role of Z-scores and composite index of anthropometric failure (CIAF). Indian J Community Med. 2007;1(1):35–9.

17. Shit S, Taraphdar P, Mukhopadhyay DK, Sinhababu A, Biswas AB. Assessment of nutritional status by composite index for anthropometric failure: a study among slum children in Bankura, West Bengal. Indian J Public Health. 2012;56:305–7.

18. International Institute for Population Sciences (IIPS) and Macro International. National Family Health Survey (NFHS-3), India, 2005-06. Maharashtra. Mumbai: IIPS; 2008.

19. Fidanza F, Keller W. Anthropometric Methodology. In: Fidanza F, editor. Nutritional Status Assessment - A Manual for Population Studies. London: Champman & Hall; 1991. p. 6–11.

20. Heymsfield S. Anthropometric methodology. In: Fidanza F, editor. Nutritional status assessment - A manual for population studies. London: Chapman & Hall; 1991. p. 24–8.

21. World Health Organization. The WHO Child Growth Standards. WHO website. http://www.who.int/childgrowth/standards/en/ Accessed on July 4, 2013.

22. Deshmukh PR, Dongre AR, Sinha N, Garg BS. Acute childhood morbidities in rural Wardha: some epidemiological correlates and health care seeking. Indian J Med Sci. 2009;63:345–54.

23. Anjum F, Pandit MI, Mir AA, Bhat IA. Z score and CIAF – A comprehensive measure of magnitude of under nutrition in a rural school going population of Kashmir, India. Glob J Med Public Health. 2012;1(5):46–9.

Is there a value for probiotic supplements in gestational diabetes mellitus? A randomized clinical trial

Neda Dolatkhah[1], Majid Hajifaraji[2*], Fatemeh Abbasalizadeh[3], Naser Aghamohammadzadeh[4], Yadollah Mehrabi[5] and Mehran Mesgari Abbasi[6]

Abstract

Background: Although several studies have found probiotics encouraging in prevention of gestational diabetes mellitus (GDM), the evidence for the use of probiotics in diagnosed GDM is largely limited. The aim of this study was to assess the effect of a probiotic supplement capsule containing four bacterial strains on glucose metabolism indices and weight changes in women with newly diagnosed GDM.

Methods: Sixty-four pregnant women with GDM were enrolled into a double-blind placebo-controlled randomized clinical trial. They were randomly assigned to receive either a probiotic or placebo capsule along with dietary advice for eight consecutive weeks. The trend of weight gain along with glucose metabolism indices was assayed.

Results: During the first 6 weeks of the study, the weight gain trend was similar between the groups. However, in the last 2 weeks of the study, the weight gain in the probiotic group was significantly lower than in the placebo group ($p < 0.05$). Fasting blood sugar (FBS) decreased in both intervention (from 103.7 to 88.4 mg/dl) and control (from 100.9 to 93.6 mg/dl) groups significantly, and the decrease in the probiotic group was significantly higher than in the placebo group ($p < 0.05$). Insulin resistance index in the probiotic group had 6.74 % reduction over the study period ($p < 0.05$). In the placebo group, however, there was an increase in insulin resistance index (6.45 %), but the observed change in insulin resistance was not statistically significant. Insulin sensitivity index was increased in both groups. The post-intervention insulin sensitivity index in the probiotic group was not significantly different from placebo when adjusted for the baseline levels.

Conclusions: The probiotic supplement appeared to affect glucose metabolism and weight gain among pregnant women with GDM. This needs to be confirmed in other settings before a therapeutic value could be approved.

Keywords: Probiotics, Gestational diabetes mellitus, Nutrition, Randomized clinical trial

Background

Gestational diabetes mellitus (GDM) is a condition in which the pregnant woman has high serum glucose levels during the gestation. It is defined as carbohydrate intolerance first diagnosed during pregnancy [1]. It is characterized by maternal insulin resistance and is associated with inflammation through the gestation [2]. GDM is shown to be associated with a range of adverse pregnancy outcomes such as preeclampsia and abnormal delivery. The newborns may also suffer from some health problems as a consequence. GDM rates are increasing both in high-income as well as the low- and middle-income countries as a consequence of increasing rates of overweight and obesity [3]. Both women with GDM and their infants are at increased risk of diabetes mellitus and metabolic dysfunction later in life [4, 5]. It has been confirmed that treatment of GDM improves pregnancy outcomes with significant reductions in the rate of serious perinatal problems such as macrosomia, dystocia and inevitable caesarean section deliveries.

* Correspondence: m.hajifaraji@nnftri.ac.ir
[2]Nutrition Society, National Nutrition and Food Technology Research Institute, Faculty of Nutrition and Food Technology, Beheshti University of Medical Sciences, Baran 3, West Arghavan, Farahzadi Blvd., Shahrak Qods, 19395-4741, istanbul 1981619573, turkey
Full list of author information is available at the end of the article

Generally, the treatment includes diet with or without medication [6].

Probiotics are known to be the good bacteria usually consumed as capsules or drinks to supplement the bowl bacteria. As narrated by Salmin, currently, the most commonly used definition for probiotics is given by Fuller as "Probiotics are live microbial feed supplements which beneficially affect the host animal by improving its intestinal microbial balance" [7, 8]. They are shown to affect the consumer's metabolism. The use of probiotics has been investigated on various infectious or noninfectious conditions [9–13]. Probiotics have also been investigated for their effect on type 2 diabetes or prevention of gestational diabetes [14–21]. Although several studies have found probiotics encouraging in prevention of GDM, the evidence for use of probiotics for those with diagnosed GDM is largely limited. The aim of this study was to assess the effect of a probiotic supplement capsule containing four bacterial strains in comparison with placebo on glucose metabolism indices and weight changes in women with newly diagnosed GDM.

Methods

In a double-blind placebo-controlled randomized clinical trial, 64 subjects with GDM referred to Alzahra University Hospital in Tabriz, Northwest of Iran, were enrolled during the spring and summer months in 2014. The patients were randomly allocated to receive either probiotic supplement or placebo capsules once daily for 8 weeks.

Each probiotic capsule of four bacterial strains (4 biocap $> 4 \times 10^9$ CFU) in standard freeze-dried culture included *Lactobacillus acidophilus* LA-5, *Bifidobacterium* BB-12, *Streptococcus thermophilus* STY-31 and *Lactobacillus delbrueckii bulgaricus* LBY-27 plus dextrose anhydrous filler and magnesium stearate lubricant produced by CHR HANSEN, Denmark, packed and gelatin covered in Tehran Darou drug industries.

The eligible subjects to be enrolled included all nulliparous women with GDM screened during 24–28 weeks of gestation who were referred to the specialty and subspecialty gynaecology or endocrinology clinics of Tabriz University of Medical Sciences.

The inclusion criteria were as follows: Nulliparity; Gestational diabetes between 24 and 28 week (+6 days) of gestation newly diagnosed through screening done by either a gynaecologist or an internal medicine specialist; Age range of 18–45 years; Fasting blood sugar range of 92 to 126 mg/dl early at the diagnosis; Body mass index (BMI) above 18.5 kg/m^2; No history of type 2 diabetes mellitus; No history of chronic diseases; No smoking and alcohol consumption; Not using probiotic food products during the 2 weeks before intervention; Not using antibiotics during the month before intervention;

Lack of acute gastrointestinal problems a month before trial and Not using Glucocorticoids (GCs) and immunosuppressive drugs. The exclusion criteria were the following: Needing to use insulin of other diabetes drugs through the study period; Use of antibiotics through the study period and Use of GCs and immunosuppressive drugs through the study period.

At baseline, the purpose and method of study were described in detail for the patients, and a trained practitioner provided similar diet recommendations for patients in both groups. Written informed consent was obtained from all the patients for being enrolled into this study. Then, during an interview with the participants, a general questionnaire and a dietary recall questionnaire were completed. The general questionnaire was used to collect data on demographic information, weight before pregnancy, physical activity, past medical history, drug history over the past month and use of probiotic food products over the past 2 weeks before the study. Physical activity was only measured at baseline. Subjects were categorized into three groups: those with low physical activity (those with a sedentary life and physical activity limited to chores such as cooking, sewing, working with computer and so on); those with moderate physical activity whose activity is limited to works such as cleaning or taking care of children and other works needing small amounts of movement or bodily movements and those with high physical activity who used to have brisk walking, running, biking and swimming regularly [22]. A 24-h dietary recall questionnaire was completed at sessions of three nonconsecutive days each (two weekdays and one in weekend) once at the baseline, and then after 4 weeks and also at the end of study. To obtain the nutrient intake of participants based on these 3-day food diaries, we used Nutritionist IV software (First Databank, San Bruno, Calif., USA) modified for Iranian foods. Weight, height and blood pressure were measured, and some information about their dietary habits and weight before pregnancy were also taken. Seca 206 wall-mounted stadiometer and Seca 813 digital scale were used to measure weight and height. Body mass index (BMI) was then calculated and categorized according to the world health organization guidelines [23].

After taking blood samples and randomly allocating them into one of two study groups, subjects were given a 2-week package of either probiotic or placebo capsules. Fasting blood samples (10 ml) before and after the intervention were collected from forearm vein by a laboratory technician for measurement of fasting blood glucose and fasting insulin at Alzahra Hospital laboratory. Plasma glucose levels were assessed using a glucose oxidase/peroxidase method as an enzymatic colorimetric (GOD-PAP) methodology [24] by Pars Azmoon test kits (Pars Azmoon Inc, Tehran, Iran). Serum insulin levels were measured by ELISA method using Monobind kit [25]. Homeostasis model assessment insulin resistance (HOMA-IR) was used to assess insulin resistance [26]. A HOMA-IR value above 3.8 is defined as insulin resistance [27]. QUICKI index (quantitative insulin sensitivity check) was used in present study to assess insulin sensitivity [28]. Details of data collection methodology and laboratory testing are published in the trial protocol elsewhere [29].

HOMA-IR was used as the main outcome for estimating the sample size. Sample size was estimated using parameters from the study by Asemi et al. assuming a maximum type 1 error of 0.05 and 90 % statistical power, HOMA-IR index standard deviation equal to 31 % and an effect size equal to 0.2; a total number of 32 subjects were estimated to be enrolled for each group

taking into account 10 % attrition rate [30]. A total of 64 pregnant women with GDM were randomly allocated using block randomization techniques stratified according to the prepregnancy fasting blood sugar (FBS) and BMI groups. To ensure double blinding, a coder anonymously labelled the capsules packages as "A" or "B" and therapist assigned them according to the random sequence generated through a computer program [31]. Patients were visited in obstetrics and gynaecology clinics of Alzahra University Hospital in Tabriz. Weight and blood pressure measurements were also done every 2 weeks. Through the study course, in order to improve the compliance, the participants were contacted by telephone each week asked about any problems they may have and about gastrointestinal symptoms as well as use of any drugs through the period.

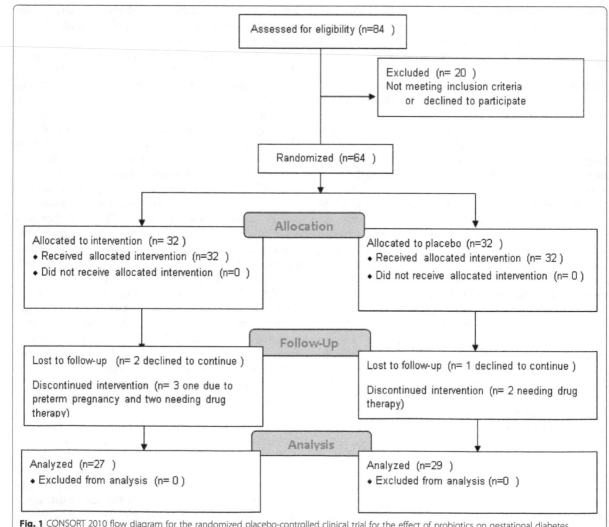

Fig. 1 CONSORT 2010 flow diagram for the randomized placebo-controlled clinical trial for the effect of probiotics on gestational diabetes mellitus (GDM)

Data were analyzed using SPSS statistical software package version 22. Mean response scales measured over the 8-week study period were analyzed using appropriate statistical methods including independent samples t test, repeated measurements analysis of variance, one-way analysis of variance and analysis of covariance. Energy-adjusted nutrient intakes were calculated as the residuals from the regression model, with absolute nutrient intake as the dependent variable and total energy intake as the independent variable. A p value below 0.05 was considered as statistically significant.

Results

A total of 64 nulliparous pregnant women with gestational diabetes participated in the study, data from the 29 patients in the probiotic group and 27 in the placebo group were finally analyzed (see CONSORT flow diagram in Fig. 1). Mean age of the patients was 27.3 (SD: 5.8) years. Comparison of the baseline characteristics for both groups of pregnant women under study are presented in Table 1.

Comparing the frequency of blood glucose levels at baseline in pregnant women showed that in probiotic group, 69 % of mothers had fasting plasma sugar between 92 and 104 mg/dl and among 31 % of them, FBS ranged 105–126 mg/dl. The values in the placebo group were 66.7 and 33.3 %, respectively. There was no statistically significant difference between the groups in terms of classification of blood glucose at baseline. Mean weight change over the study period is compared between the groups in Fig. 2.

The weight gain over the study period, adjusted also for energy intake, is given in Table 2. It shows that no significant differences between the intervention and control groups were observed in weight gain measures among the pregnant women within 2-week intervals during the first 6 weeks of the study. However, in the last 2 weeks of the study, the weight gain in pregnant women in the probiotic group was significantly lower than in the placebo group. The results stayed statistically significant after adjusting for the changes in daily energy intake between the two groups, ($p < 0.05$).

Fasting blood sugar levels, fasting insulin level, insulin resistance index (HOMA-IR) and insulin sensitivity index (QUICKI index) were not found to be different between the probiotic supplement and placebo groups at baseline. According to the results of the analysis of covariance, FBS in both the intervention and control groups decreased significantly (14.66 and 7.38 %, respectively), both of which were statistically significant ($p < 0.05$). Post-intervention comparison, after adjustment for baseline values, showed that decrease in the probiotic group was significantly higher than in the placebo group ($p < 0.05$). Insulin resistance index in the probiotic

Table 1 Baseline comparison of demographic and anthropometric characteristics of the pregnant women with gestational diabetes mellitus enrolled either to receive probiotic or placebo

Baseline measures	Intervention ($N = 29$)	Placebo ($N = 27$)	p value
Maternal age	28.14 ± 6.24	26.48 ± 5.23	0.36
Family history of DM			
Yes	16 (55.2 %)	12 (44.4 %)	0.59
No	13 (44.8 %)	15 (55.6 %)	
Educational level			
Under graduate diploma	4 (13.8 %)	5 (18.5 %)	0.91
High school diploma	17 (58.6 %)	15 (55.6 %)	
Academic education	8 (27.8 %)	7 (25.9 %)	
Employment			
Employed	10 (34.5 %)	9 (33.3 %)	1.00
Unemployed or housewife	19 (65.5 %)	18 (66.7 %)	
Residence			
Urban			
Rural	17 (58.6 %)	15 (55.6 %)	1.00
	12 (41.4 %)	12 (44.4 %)	
Physical activity			
Low	22 (75.9 %)	17 (63.0 %)	
Moderate	7 (24.1 %)	10 (37.0 %)	0.38
High	0	0	
Weight (kg)	83.27 ± 12.06	78.67 ± 11.09	0.14
Height (cm)	162.68 ± 5.65	162.14 ± 5.93	0.72
Body mass index (kg/m^2)	31.41 ± 3.92	29.86 ± 3.39	0.12

Numeric scales are reported as mean ± standard deviation, and categorical measures are reported as frequency (percent)

group significantly decreased over the study period (6.74 % reduction), which was statistically significant ($p < 0.05$). In the placebo group, however, there was an increase in insulin resistance (6.45 %), but the change was not statistically significant. Insulin sensitivity index was increased in both groups. These changes in the probiotic group (5.76 %) were statistically significant. The post-intervention insulin sensitivity index in the probiotic group was not significantly different from that in the placebo group when adjusted for the baseline levels. Detailed information on changes in glucose metabolism indices are provided in Table 3.

Discussion

It was observed in present study that the weight gain did not change during the first 6 weeks of the study, but, in the last 2 weeks of the study, the weight gain in pregnant women in the probiotic group was significantly lower than in the placebo group. With respect to glucose metabolism indices, probiotic supplementation was also

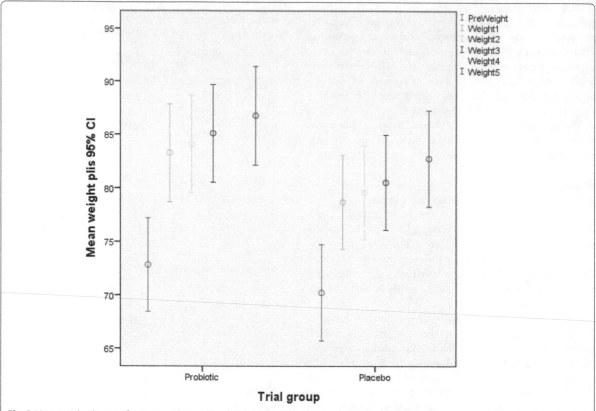

Fig. 2 Mean weight change of women with gestational diabetes mellitus (GDM) over the 8-week study period compared between the probiotic and placebo groups

effective. FBS decreased in the probiotic group significantly more than in the placebo group. Insulin resistance index in the probiotic group significantly decreased over the study period (6.74 % reduction), which was statistically significant while the increase in insulin resistance (6.45 %) in the placebo group was not statistically significant. Insulin sensitivity index was increased in both groups, but the post-intervention insulin sensitivity index in the probiotic group was not significantly different from the placebo group.

Although several studies have been done on effect of probiotics on preventing GDM and some studies have been done on general glucose patterns among normal pregnant populations, studies are scarce investigating the effect of probiotics when taken after diagnosis of GDM. One very recent double-blind randomized clinical trial on women with a new diagnosis of GDM and impaired glucose tolerance assigned them to a daily probiotic (Lactobacillus salivarius UCC118) or placebo capsule. Among the 149 women enrolled, no difference

Table 2 Weight gain trend over the 8-week study period comparing women gestational diabetes mellitus receiving probiotic supplement versus placebo capsules

Weight gain	Probiotic (n = 29)	Placebo (n = 27)	Mean difference (95 % CI)	p value*	p value**
First 2 weeks (mean ± SE)	0.83 ± 0.08	0.89 ± 0.07	−0.61 (−0.29,0.17)	0.59	0.34
Second 2 weeks (mean ± SE)	0.98 ± 0.07	0.93 ± 0.06	0.05 (−0.14,0.25)	0.60	0.69
Third 2 weeks (mean ± SE)	0.91 ± 0.06	1.00 ± 0.05	−0.09 (−0.27,0.08)	0.31	0.19
Fourth 2 weeks (mean ± SE)	0.74 ± 0.14	1.22 ± 0.11	−0.48 (−0.85,−0.10)	0.01	0.02
First 4 weeks (mean ± SE)	1.82 ± 0.12	1.82 ± 0.12	−0.008 (−0.37,0.35)	0.96	0.62
Second 4 weeks (mean ± SE)	1.65 ± 0.13	2.22 ± 0.13	−0.57 (−0.95,−0.19)	0.004	0.004

* Independent samples t test
**One-way ANOVA with differences in energy intake as covariate

Table 3 Changes in glucose metabolism indices among women with gestational diabetes receiving probiotic supplement versus placebo

Glucose metabolism indices	Probiotic (n = 29)	Placebo (n = 27)	p value (Independent samples t test)	p value (ANCOVA)
Fasting blood sugar (mg/dl)				
Before trial	103.65 (1.34)	100.89 (1.52)	0.17	0.02
After trial	88.37 (2.05)	93.59 (3.61)	0.20	
P (paired samples t test)	<0.001	0.02		
Absolute change	−15.27 (1.83)	−7.30 (3.04)	0.02	
Relative change	−14.66 (1.77)	−7.38 (15.09)	0.03	
Fasting serum insulin (µIU/ml)				
Before trial	5.95 (0.50)	5.60 (0.37)	0.58	0.09
After trial	5.15 (0.41)	6.12 (0.50)	0.14	
P (paired samples t test)	0.16	0.30		
Absolute difference	−0.80 (0.56)	0.52 (0.49)	0.08	
Relative difference	10.55 (18.55)	14.55 (9.21)	0.85	
HOMA-IR index				
Before trial	1.52 (0.12)	1.38 (0.08)	0.41	0.03
After trial	1.11 (0.09)	1.40 (0.11)	0.06	
P (paired samples t test)	0.007	0.93		
Absolute difference	−0.40 (0.13)	0.01 (0.12)	0.03	
Relative difference	−6.74 (14.84)	6.45 (9.22)	0.46	
QUICKI index				
Before trial	0.15 (0.00)	0.15 (0.00)	0.92	0.11
After trial	0.16 (0.00)	0.16 (0.00)	0.11	
P (paired samples t test)	0.02	0.46		
Absolute difference	0.008 (0.003)	0.002 (0.002)	0.16	
Relative difference	5.76 (2.16)	1.38 (1.69)	0.12	

HOMA-IR homeostasis model assessment insulin resistance, *QUICKI* quantitative insulin sensitivity check

was observed between the probiotic and placebo groups in post-intervention fasting glucose levels. However, they found a likely effect for the probiotic on lipid profile of the patients [32]. Regardless of the differences in study design and population, the main characteristic possibly describing the reason for positive results in present study may be attributed to different probiotic contents of the supplement in two studies. Observing the effect of probiotics in present study with a smaller sample size while yielding reasonably narrower confidence interval justifies a promising effect for the intervention used in our study. Aside from the different probiotic in present study and the magnitude of potential random error attributable to the sample size, other issues may affect the results either such as the variations in normal weight gain through the pregnancy, variations in gut flora, physical activity and diet. Normally, such variations are controlled through randomization, but this cannot be fully guaranteed unless the study is large enough to ensure the efficacy of randomization [33]. No doubt physical

activity is a major risk indicator in several noncommunicable diseases including diabetes. In present study, the physical activity was measured only at baseline, and we recommend to consider it as a time-dependent variable in future clinical trial studies assessing the role of probiotics on GDM. Studies like present study conducted specifically on patients diagnosed with GDM are quite rare; however, there are bunches of studies on role of probiotics on prevention of GDM or its related pregnancy outcomes. Generally, the effect of probiotics in prevention of GDM and poor pregnancy outcomes have been shown to be promising [6, 20, 21, 34–39]. Probiotics have also been investigated when combined with diet recommendations. In a study from Finland, 256 pregnant women were randomized early through the gestation to receive nutrition counselling or not to receive it as controls; the group with dietary intervention was further randomized to receive probiotics (Lactobacillus rhamnosus GG and Bifidobacterium lactis Bb12; diet/probiotics) or placebo (diet/placebo). It was found that blood glucose levels as well as HOMA-IR and QUICKI indices were lowest in the diet/probiotics group concluding that improved blood glucose control could be reached by dietary counselling combined with probiotics even in normoglycaemic pregnant women [40]. A recent review on dietary interventions, lifestyle changes and dietary supplements in preventing GDM has concluded that trials in which only intake or expenditure has been the target of interventions may not achieve positive efficacy results, whereas combined interventions and dietary and lifestyle interventions could show better efficacy in the reduction of GDM prevalence. The same review has stated the results of probiotic studies to be promising and has recommended future larger scale studies [41]. Although, the cost-effectiveness of probiotics has not been well documented in literature, probiotic supplements have been shown to have acceptability among patients [42, 43].

About 95 % of the intestinal microbiome in healthy people with normal weight consists of the species belonging to three phyla of the bacteria including *Bacteroidetes, Firmicutes* and *Actinobacteria*. The plausibility of the observed effect of probiotics is not much hard to be approved considering the available evidence on role of healthy gut microbiome on carbohydrate metabolism and the synergistic relationships of probiotic foods and supplements with the host gut microbiome [21, 44, 45]. To complete the plausibility pattern, the changes in gut microbiome during diabetes mellitus should also be considered. A new theory suggests that gut microbiota have a role in the regulation of the energy homeostasis and causing metabolic diseases and insulin resistance [46]. It has been shown that type 2 diabetes is associated with changes in gut microbiome. For instance, it has been shown that the ratio of *Bacteroidetes* to *Firmicutes* species is associated with diabetes type 2 and FBS, especially that the changes in gut microbiome are different from what is observed during obesity and a larger number of opportunistic pathogens along with a lower number of butyrate-producing bacteria are attributed to presence of diabetes [21, 47–51].

Conclusions

The probiotic supplement appeared to affect glucose metabolism and weight gain among pregnant women with GDM.

Ethical issues

Study protocol was approved by the Research Ethics committee of International branch of Shahid Beheshti University of Medical Sciences as a thesis proposal for PhD degree in Nutrition Sciences. Written informed consent was taken from all participants.

The clinical trial was registered in the Iranian Registry of Clinical Trials with reference number IRCT201405181597N3, available at: http://www.irct.ir, accessible through world health organization database of clinical trial registries.

Statement of human and animal rights

All procedures followed were in accordance with the ethical standards of the responsible committee on human experimentation (institutional and national) and with the Helsinki Declaration of 1975, as revised in 2008 (5).

Competing interests
The authors declare that they have no conflict of interest.

Authors' contributions
ND was the PhD student doing her thesis and contributed A-Z of research conduct and reporting. MH was the main supervisor and contributed A-Z of research conduct and reporting. FA, NA and YM contributed in clinical examinations and data collection as well as interpretation of the results. MA contributed in laboratory assays. All the authors contributed in drafting or reviewing the manuscript. All authors read and approved the final manuscript.

Acknowledgement
This paper is taken from PhD Thesis of Nutrition Sciences, International Branch of Shahid Beheshti University of Medical Sciences, Tehran, Iran. We are grateful to all the participants who helped us to conduct this study and Tehran Darou Pharmaceuticals, Tehran, Iran, for providing 4-Biocap (a probiotic supplement) for the present study. The authors would like to thank the staff of the Alzahra Obstetrics and Gynecology Clinic (Tabriz, Iran) for their assistance with this project during the study.

Author details
[1]Department of Nutrition Sciences, Shahid Beheshti University of Medical Sciences (SBUMS), International Branch, tehran, iran. [2]Nutrition Society, National Nutrition and Food Technology Research Institute, Faculty of Nutrition and Food Technology, Beheshti University of Medical Sciences, Baran 3, West Arghavan, Farahzadi Blvd., Shahrak Qods, 19395-4741, istanbul 1981619573, turkey. [3]Department of Obstetrics & Gynecology, Tabriz University of Medical Sciences, tabriz, iran. [4]Section of Endocrinology & Metabolism, Department of Internal Medicine, Tabriz University of Medical Sciences, Tabriz, Iran. [5]Department of Biostatistics & Epidemiology, Shahid Beheshti University of Medical Sciences, Tehran, Iran. [6]Drug Applied Research Center, Tabriz University of Medical Sciences, Tabriz, Iran.

References

1.   Hadar E, Oats J, Hod M. Towards new diagnostic criteria for diagnosing GDM: the HAPO study. J Perinat Med. 2009;37:447–9.
2.   Kuhl C. Etiology and pathogenesis of gestational diabetes. Diabetes Care. 1998;21 Suppl 2:B19–26.
3.   Ma RC, Chan JC. Pregnancy and diabetes scenario around the world: China. Int J Gynaecol Obstet. 2009;104:S42–5.
4.   Hossain P, Kawar B, El NM. Obesity and diabetes in the developing world—a growing challenge. N Engl J Med. 2007;356:213–5.
5.   Moore TR. Fetal exposure to gestational diabetes contributes to subsequent adult metabolic syndrome. Am J Obstet Gynecol. 2010;202:643–9.
6.   Barrett HL, Dekker NM, Conwell LS, Callaway LK. Probiotics for preventing gestational diabetes. Cochrane Database Syst Rev. 2014;2, CD009951.
7.   Salminen, Ouwehand A, Benno Y, Lee YK. Probiotics: how should they be defined? Trends Food Sci Technol. 1999;10:107–10.
8.   Fuller R. Probiotics in man and animals. J Appl Bacteriol. 1989;66:365–78.
9.   Saez-Lara MJ, Gomez-Llorente C, Plaza-Diaz J, Gil A. The role of probiotic lactic acid bacteria and bifidobacteria in the prevention and treatment of inflammatory bowel disease and other related diseases: a systematic review of randomized human clinical trials. Biomed Res Int. 2015;2015:505878.
10. Allen SJ. The potential of probiotics to prevent Clostridium difficile infection. Infect Dis Clin North Am. 2015;29:135–44.

11. Guandalini S. Are probiotics or prebiotics useful in pediatric irritable bowel syndrome or inflammatory bowel disease? Front Med (Lausanne). 2014;1:23.

12. Tang RB, Chang JK, Chen HL. Can probiotics be used to treat allergic diseases? J Chin Med Assoc. 2015;78:154–7.

13. Ruggiero P. Use of probiotics in the fight against Helicobacter pylori. World J Gastrointest Pathophysiol. 2014;5:384–91.

14. Mazloom Z, Yousefinejad A, Dabbaghmanesh MH. Effect of probiotics on lipid profile, glycemic control, insulin action, oxidative stress, and inflammatory markers in patients with type 2 diabetes: a clinical trial. Iran J Med Sci. 2013;38:38–43.

15. Alokail MS, Sabico S, Al-Saleh Y, Al-Daghri NM, Alkharfy KM, Vanhoutte PM, et al. Effects of probiotics in patients with diabetes mellitus type 2: study protocol for a randomized, double-blind, placebo-controlled trial. Trials. 2013;14:195.

16. Frontiers in Endocrinology Editorial Office. Retraction: colonic flora, probiotics, obesity and diabetes. Front Endocrinol (Lausanne). 2013;4:110.

17. Gomes AC, Bueno AA, de Souza RG, Mota JF. Gut microbiota, probiotics and diabetes. Nutr J. 2014;13:60.

18. Sekhar MS, Unnikrishnan MK. Probiotic research for diabetes prevention. Nutrition. 2015;31:248.

19. Panwar H, Rashmi HM, Batish VK, Grover S. Probiotics as potential biotherapeutics in the management of type 2 diabetes—prospects and perspectives. Diabetes Metab Res Rev. 2013;29:103–12.

20. Nitert MD, Barrett HL, Foxcroft K, Tremellen A, Wilkinson S, Lingwood B, et al. SPRING: an RCT study of probiotics in the prevention of gestational diabetes mellitus in overweight and obese women. BMC Pregnancy Childbirth. 2013;13:50.

21. Barrett HL, Callaway LK, Nitert MD. Probiotics: a potential role in the prevention of gestational diabetes? Acta Diabetol. 2012;49 Suppl 1:S1–S13.

22. Mahan LK, Escott-Stump S, Raymond JL. Krause's food & the nutrition care process. 13th ed. 2012.

23. Diet, nutrition and the prevention of chronic diseases. World Health Organ Tech Rep. Ser. 2003;916:i-viii, 1–149. 2003. Ref Type: Report

24. Barham D, Trinder P. An improved colour reagent for the determination of blood glucose by the oxidase system. Analyst. 1972;97:142–5.

25. MacDonald MJ, Gapinski JP. A rapid ELISA for measuring insulin in a large number of research samples. Metabolism. 1989;38:450–2.

26. Matthews DR, Hosker JP, Rudenski AS, Naylor BA, Treacher DF, Turner RC. Homeostasis model assessment: insulin resistance and beta-cell function from fasting plasma glucose and insulin concentrations in man. Diabetologia. 1985;28:412–9.

27. Bodlaj G, Berg J, Pichler R, Biesenbach G. Prevalence, severity and predictors of HOMA-estimated insulin resistance in diabetic and nondiabetic patients with end-stage renal disease. J Nephrol. 2006;19:607–12.

28. Hrebicek J, Janout V, Malincikova J, Horakova D, Cizek L. Detection of insulin resistance by simple quantitative insulin sensitivity check index QUICKI for epidemiological assessment and prevention. J Clin Endocrinol Metab. 2002; 87:144–7.

29. Dolatkhah N, Hajifaraji M, Abbasalizadeh F, Aghamohammadzadeh N, Mehrabi Y, Megari Abbasi M: Effect of probiotics in gestational diabetes mellitus: study protocol. Journal of Clinical Research & Governance 2015, Unpublished.

30. Asemi Z, Samimi M, Tabassi Z, Naghibi RM, Rahimi FA, Khorammian H, et al. Effect of daily consumption of probiotic yoghurt on insulin resistance in pregnant women: a randomized controlled trial. Eur J Clin Nutr. 2013;67:71–4.

31. Asghari-Jafarabadi M, Sadeghi-Bazargani H. Randomization: techniques and software-aided implementation in medical studies. J Clin Res Gov . 2014;3.

32. Lindsay KL, Brennan L, Kennelly MA, Maguire OC, Smith T, Curran S, et al. Impact of probiotics in women with gestational diabetes mellitus on metabolic health: a randomized controlled trial. Am J Obstet Gynecol. 2015.

33. Hajebrahimi S, Mostafaie A, Sadeghi-Bazargani H. Evidence for the future—designing a clinical trial. Indian J Urol. 2011;27:494–7.

34. Luoto R, Laitinen K, Nermes M, Isolauri E. Impact of maternal probiotic-supplemented dietary counselling on pregnancy outcome and prenatal and postnatal growth: a double-blind, placebo-controlled study. Br J Nutr. 2010; 103:1792–9.

35. Luoto R, Laitinen K, Nermes M, Isolauri E. Impact of maternal probiotic-supplemented dietary counseling during pregnancy on colostrum adiponectin concentration: a prospective, randomized, placebo-controlled study. Early Hum Dev. 2012;88:339–44.

36. Lindsay KL, Walsh CA, Brennan L, McAuliffe FM. Probiotics in pregnancy and maternal outcomes: a systematic review. J Matern Fetal Neonatal Med. 2013;26:772–8.

37. Lindsay KL, Kennelly M, Culliton M, Smith T, Maguire OC, Shanahan F, et al. Probiotics in obese pregnancy do not reduce maternal fasting glucose: a double-blind, placebo-controlled, randomized trial (Probiotics in Pregnancy Study). Am J Clin Nutr. 2014;99:1432–9.

38. Gomez Arango LF, Barrett HL, Callaway LK, Nitert MD. Probiotics and pregnancy. Curr Diab Rep. 2015;15:567.

39. Rogozinska E, Chamillard M, Hitman GA, Khan KS, Thangaratinam S. Nutritional manipulation for the primary prevention of gestational diabetes mellitus: a meta-analysis of randomised studies. PLoS One. 2015,10, e0115526.

40. Laitinen K, Poussa T, Isolauri E. Probiotics and dietary counselling contribute to glucose regulation during and after pregnancy: a randomised controlled trial. Br J Nutr. 2009;101:1679–87.

41. Facchinetti F, Dante G, Petrella E, Neri I. Dietary interventions, lifestyle changes, and dietary supplements in preventing gestational diabetes mellitus: a literature review. Obstet Gynecol Surv. 2014;69:669–80.

42. Lindsay KL, Brennan L, McAuliffe FM. Acceptability of and compliance with a probiotic capsule intervention in pregnancy. Int J Gynaecol Obstet. 2014; 125:279–80.

43. Arslan S, Durak AN, Erbas M, Tanriverdi E, Gulcan U. Determination of microbiological and chemical properties of probiotic boza and its consumer acceptability. J Am Coll Nutr. 2015;34:56–64.

44. Arumugam M, Raes J, Pelletier E, Le PD, Yamada T, Mende DR, et al. Enterotypes of the human gut microbiome. Nature. 2011;473:174–80.

45. Greiner T, Backhed F. Effects of the gut microbiota on obesity and glucose homeostasis. Trends Endocrinol Metab. 2011;22:117–23.

46. Moreno-Indias I, Cardona F, Tinahones FJ, Queipo-Ortuno MI. Impact of the gut microbiota on the development of obesity and type 2 diabetes mellitus. Front Microbiol. 2014;5:190.

47. Sun Q, Wedick NM, Pan A, Townsend MK, Cassidy A, Franke AA, et al. Gut microbiota metabolites of dietary lignans and risk of type 2 diabetes: a prospective investigation in two cohorts of U.S. women. Diabetes Care. 2014;37:1287–95.

48. Larsen N, Vogensen FK, van den Berg FW, Nielsen DS, Andreasen AS, Pedersen BK, et al. Gut microbiota in human adults with type 2 diabetes differs from non-diabetic adults. PLoS One. 2010;5, e9085.

49. Burcelin R, Serino M, Chabo C, Blasco-Baque V, Amar J. Gut microbiota and diabetes: from pathogenesis to therapeutic perspective. Acta Diabetol. 2011; 48:257–73.

50. Qin J, Li Y, Cai Z, Li S, Zhu J, Zhang F, et al. A metagenome-wide association study of gut microbiota in type 2 diabetes. Nature. 2012;490:55–60.

51. Esteve E, Ricart W, Fernandez-Real JM. Gut microbiota interactions with obesity, insulin resistance and type 2 diabetes: did gut microbiote co-evolve with insulin resistance? Curr Opin Clin Nutr Metab Care. 2011;14:483–90.

Antiretroviral therapy adherence strategies used by patients of a large HIV clinic in Lesotho

Johanna Maria Axelsson[1*], Sofie Hallager[2] and Toke S. Barfod[3]

Abstract

A high degree of adherence to antiretroviral therapy (ART) in patients infected with *human immunodeficiency virus* (HIV) is necessary for long term treatment effects. This study explores the role of timing of ART intake, the information patients received from health workers, local adherence patterns, barriers to and facilitators of ART among 28 HIV-positive adults at the Senkatana HIV Clinic in Maseru, Lesotho. This qualitative, semi-structured interview study was carried out during February and March of 2011 and responses were analyzed inspired by the Grounded Theory method. Results were then compared and discussed between the authors and the main themes that emerged were categorized. The majority of the respondents reported having missed one or more doses of medicine in the past and it was a widespread belief among patients that they were required to skip the dose of ART if they were "late". The main barriers to adherence were interruptions of daily routines or leaving the house without sufficient medicine. The use of mobile phone alarms, phone clocks and support from family and friends were major facilitators of adherence. None of the patients reported to have been counseled on family support or the use of mobile phones as helpful methods in maintaining or improving adherence to ART. Being on-time with ART was emphasized during counseling by health workers. In conclusion, patients should be advised to take the dose as soon as they remember instead of skipping the dose completely when they are late. Mobile phones and family support could be subjects to focus on during future counseling particularly with the growing numbers of mobile phones in Africa and the current focus on telemedicine.

Keywords: Adherence, Antiretroviral Therapy, Barriers, Facilitators, HIV/AIDS, Lesotho, Sub-Saharan Africa

Background

The prevalence of infections with the human immunodeficiency virus (HIV) in Lesotho among adults was estimated to be 23.1 %, the second highest HIV prevalence in the world, with an estimated 15,000 AIDS related deaths per year in 2012 [1]. Fifty-nine percent of eligible patients in Lesotho were estimated to receive antiretroviral therapy (ART) in 2012 [1].

The introduction of ART has changed HIV from a deadly to a chronic infection for people living with HIV (PLWH). Research has shown that there is a relationship between the level of adherence to ART and disease progression [2] and mortality [3]. Current ART can supress viral load at moderate adherence levels (70–90 % of prescribed doses taken over a given time), to receive

the best outcomes, however, ART should be taken correctly as prescribed [4].

Non-adherence increases the risk of development of resistance [5, 6] and since the cost of second-line therapy is considerably higher than first-line therapy, high levels of adherence is important for cost control and improved survival especially in resource-limited countries [7].

Self-reported adherence is the most widely used method to estimate adherence although it is prone to overestimate the level of adherence [8]. In a meta-analysis of 27 Sub-Saharan African studies conducted prior to 2006, 23 % of the patients receiving ART had sub-optimal levels of adherence, defined by local thresholds [9]. Sub-optimal adherence is caused by different barriers to treatment adherence and frequently reported barriers in Sub-Saharan Africa include: transport costs [10–12]; lack of social support (financial and emotional) [13, 14]; service-related factors [10–14]; pill burden and side-effects [11–14]; poor knowledge about HIV; stigma [10–12]; non-disclosure of

---
* Correspondence: jm.axelsson@gmail.com
[1]Department of Medicine, Copenhagen University Hospital Glostrup, Glostrup, Denmark
Full list of author information is available at the end of the article

HIV status[10, 12, 14]; and a lack of food [12, 14]. Furthermore, adherence tend to decline over time [15–17] and a major challenge in resource poor settings is yet to provide ART to all eligible patients [18, 19].

To our knowledge no previous studies have been conducted exploring the information obtained during counselling on the timing of ART intake. In more affluent countries, it is suggested that HIV-positive patients are advised to take their daily ART in conjuction with daily routines, such as eating dinner or brushing their teeth [20]. However, it is our personal experience from clinical work in Lesotho and Botswana and from discussions with Sub-Saharan African colleagues that patients are often told to take their ART *"on time"*. *"On time"* in this setting indicates to take the daily doses of ART at the exact same time every day. This practice may cause patients who discover that they are late, to completely skip the dose. Thus, the aims of this study was to explore adherence patterns, describe barriers to and facilitators of adherence to ART, and to investigate the role of "timing of doses" and information received at the clinic about "timing of doses".

Methods

Participants, procedures and settings

The Senkatana HIV clinic had two physicians and three nurse practitioners employed. The number of patients visiting the clinic regularly was estimated to be within the range of 6000–9000 patients. The clinic in Maseru were in 2011 one of over 30 publicly funded clinics in the city. The clinic provided counseling, ART and a few other drugs for free but not travels expenses or nutritional supplements. Prior to initiation of ART, patients were counseled by adherence counselors (nurse practitioners). Patients were given medication for one month at a time. For adherence control, patients provided their remaining medication and an adherence calendar ("mokoko") every month to the pharmacists. If patients had been non-adherent, they were told by the pharmacists to take their medicine. The pharmacists referred patients to a physician for adherence counselling if necessary. Patients were offered brief counselling during a follow-up with a physician every 3 months.

PLWH at the Senkatana HIV Clinic in Maseru, Lesotho, were purposefully selected by non-random sampling as they were awaiting their monthly clinic visit, during February and March of 2011. Patients were approached by the author, T.B., and two local research assistants. Our sampling goal was to obtain a variety among patients in terms of gender and age. Eligible patients were 18 years of age and older, HIV-positive and receiving ART. They were orally informed and gave oral consent to participation in the study. No financial compensation

was given. It was emphasized that participation was entirely voluntary, all interviews were confidential and that whether the patients participated or not would not affect their treatment at the clinic. A total of 30 patients were approached for participation, however, two patients declined to participate. Both gave as reason that they wished to be financially compensated. The interview-guide consisted of 17 semi-structured questions and 14 demographic, structured questions. The author T.B. created the questionnaire based on his experience with qualitative research conducted in Denmark among PLWH and on clinical experience in low-and middle income countries. Originally written in English, the interview-guide was translated into the local language Sesotho and double checked by three independent translators. The set of questions were constructed to be comprehensive with respect to the relevant themes of adherence in an everyday setting. Each individual interview followed its own path and depended on the patient's answers. The casual form of the interviews gave the interviewer the opportunity to ask the informant to further specify certain answers. Questions regarding adherence were focused on facilitators and barriers to adherence, such as what made it difficult or easy to take the daily ART. Patients were asked about demographics including age, gender, and language, names of medicine, duration on ART, ART regimen, education and monthly household income. Patients were asked whether they had ever missed a dose of ART and how many days they had missed ART in the past month and year. Fifteen interviews were carried out by the senior author, T.B. A local translator was used in cases where the patient did not speak English. The remaining 13 interviews were carried out by two local research assistants fluent in both Sesotho and English and carefully instructed in interviewing techniques. The response to each question was written down in English during the interview, the phrasing as close to the spoken words as possible, in a slightly abbreviated form. All interviews were discussed with the author, T.B., on the same day to clarify any misunderstandings and ambiguous answers. The research protocol was approved by the Director General of Health Services in Maseru, Lesotho.

Data analysis and management

All handwritten answers were manually converted into digital forms using Microsoft Words 2010 and grouped according to specific questions in a Microsoft Excel 2010 spreadsheet by two research assistants and co-authors, J.M.A. and S.H. All digitized answers were read and approved as being identical to the original by the author T.B. The grouped responses were subsequently analyzed, inspired by the Grounded Theory method [21], by coding each answer in Microsoft Excel 2010. Results were then compared and discussed between the authors and the main themes emerging during the coding and analyzing process were categorized. Since this was a qualitative study and due to the small, non-random sample size, no statistical analyses were carried out.

Results

Demographics and ART regimen

Demographic data are presented in Table 1 *and ART regimens in Table* 2. Seventeen women and eleven men were interviewed. Residence was both urban settings in Maseru, and rural with up to 1 day's travelling distance to the clinic. The majority of respondents had some degree of schooling (89.3 %). A wide range in household income was seen, with a substantial part of respondents reporting dependence on a family member's income. Duration on ART varied between 2 months and 6 years with a mean of approximately 3 years, and the majority of patients were on a once daily (OD) ART regimen with one Nucleoside Analogue Reverse-Transcriptase Inhibitor (NRTI), one Nucleotide Analogue Reverse-Transcriptase Inhibitor (NtRTI) and one Non-Nucleoside Reverse-Transcriptase Inhibitor (NNRTI).

Information received during counseling

The respondents reported that they received adherence counseling when they initiated ART but no one reported explicitly having received education, counseling or advice since then. One patient reported not having received any counseling since 2004, another patient reported not having received any counseling at all and a third patient could

Table 1 Demographic data on respondents (n = 28)

Characteristics	Value
Age, mean	39.8 years (range 22–56 years)
Sex	17 females (60.7 %), 11 males (39.3 %)
Years of schooling, mean	6.96 years (10.7 % had no education)
Household income per month (RSA Rands)[a]	Mean: 759, Median: 600 (Range: 0–3000)
Number of people per household	Some are living together with their siblings, parents or older relatives and others have their own families with a partner and typically 1–2 children. A few patients lived on their own and the main reason was that their partner had passed away.
Treatment duration, months	Mean: 35.9, Median: 36 (Range: 2–72)
Type of treatment	OD: 19 (67.9 %), BD: 9 (32.1 %)
CD4-cell count (cells/mm³), mean	442 (Range: 9–1300)

[a]Mean income was calculated based on the household's total reported income, regardless of whether the patient contributed or the number of individuals in the household. A few reported no income. Three participants were excluded, one because the patient had not responded to the question and two because of uncertainty about the amount of income

Table 2 ART regimen

Drugs[a]	OD	BD	n = 28 (%)
TDF, 3TC, EFV	12	1	13 (46.4)
TDF, 3TC, NVP	1	4	5 (17.9)
AZT, 3TC, EFV		1	1 (3.6)
AZT, 3TC, rtv/LPV		1	1 (3.6)
D4t, 3TC, EFV		1	1 (3.6)
Cannot remember the name of the drug	6	1	7 (25)
Total	19	9	28 (100)

[a]Nucleoside analog reverse-transcriptase inhibitors (NRTIs): 3TC (Lamivudine), AZT (Zidovudine), d4T (Stavudine); Nucleotide analog reverse-transcriptase inhibitors (NtRTIs): TDF (Tenofovir); Non-nucleoside reverse-transcriptase inhibitors (NNRTIs): EFV (Efavirenz), NVP (Nevirapine); Protease inhibitors (PIs): rtv/LPV (Ritonavir/Lopinavir)

not remember what he was counseled about because he was very ill at the time.

"I don't know because I was very ill. Cannot remember about how and when to take the medicine." 44-year old male

The message many patients recalled from their counseling was to take the medicine at the exact same time every single day, eat well and keep good hygiene, not to drink alcohol and the importance of monthly pill-refills.

"Yes, they told me that I had to take the pill at the same time and eat well and live in a clean place." 54-year old female

Patients were informed that alcohol had negative effects on adherence and health. A couple of patients mentioned being advised against traditional medicine.

"I was counseled and asked to stop taking traditional medicine because it would lower CD4 and rise viral load. Because the virus comes up I will lose weight and get other diseases." 24-year old female

Patients were recommended to use the "Mokoko" ("Mokoko" is the word for rooster in Sesotho), which is a 1-sheet, 1-month diary with symbols (e.g. a rooster for the morning, a sun for midday and a moon for evening), to help remember their doses. The patient can then check-off every time a dose has been taken on any given day. It was also used by the clinicians at the monthly clinic visits for adherence control.

"They told me to mark mokoko at same time every day. Stop beer and smoke. Stop thinking stress. Exercise every day." 49-year old male.

It appeared that not all patients knew about their possibility to send friends or family members to refill ART at the Senkatana HIV clinic.

"We must be allowed to send other people to pick up med's. The service is slow…when picking of files [medical records]. There are three sick-leaves in a month sometime! Better if all together." 35-year old female

Missed doses and the role of timing of doses

Patients were asked what they would do if the time of correct dosing had been surpassed (Table 3). Sixteen out of 26 (61.5 %) patients (two patients did not respond) reported that they had missed one or more doses of medicine during their time on ART (mean time on ART: 35.5 months). Only seven patients responded to the specific questions about how many days they had missed their ART during the last month (mean: 4.7 days, range: 0–17) and year (mean: 15.6 days, range: 1–72).

The majority of patients had been advised by clinic staff to take the medicine either at 7 A.M. or at 7 A.M. and 7 P.M, but a few was informed to choose the time of dosage on their own.

"How and when [at the pharmacy] to take med's, choose time myself, every day, not wait with refill until finished." 36-year old male

"Stick to the chosen time and be punctual." 42-year old female

One patient explained that she had been told by a clinician to skip her daily dose, if she was more than 30 minutes late.

"Take them daily at the same hour, not after 30 minutes. Take them for the rest of life." 29-year old female

Several patients admitted that they would skip doses of ART if they came in a situation of being just a few hours late (*Table 3*) and two patients had skipped doses of ART in the past because they were late.

"I stay with my nephews and when they fight I forget to take the pills. They fight with fists. They were in the bedroom, I was in the kitchen. I keep the pills in the bedroom. I am not afraid but forget. I remember later but was told [by clinic staff] to skip [ART] if too late." 34-year old female

"Leave it, even if only 1 hour late, and ask counselor. It happened once when my wife passed away, never again." 47-year old male

Barriers to adherence

Barriers to ART-adherence reported by two or more respondents are shown in Table 4. The reason most frequently listed by the patients as a barrier to adherence was a **change in routines or an unpredicted event**, which could cause the patient to miss doses for various time periods, ranging from days to weeks.

"The cows were stolen and I took a week looking for them and had forgotten the medicine. 15 cows in the mountains were missing – I walked to get them." 42-year old male

"I was stressed because attackers wanted to kill my son at my home, and I forgot to pick up the medicine. I was forgetting everything even to eat for at least 3 weeks.

Table 3 Consequences of delayed doses

Question	Answer	OD (n = 19)	BD (n = 9)
After how many hours would you skip a dose if you were late?	I would skip if I was 1 hour late	1	2
	I would skip if I was 3 hours late	2	1
	I would skip if I was 4 hours late	4	
	I would skip if I was 5 hours late	1	
	I would skip if I was 6 hours late	6	3
	I would skip if I was 8 hours late	1	
	I would skip if I was 12 hours late	1	
	I would take it even if 12 hours late	3	1
	I don't know what to do if I am late		2

Table 4 Barriers to ART-adherence

Answer[a]	n = 28[b]
Change in routine or an unpredicted event	10
Not bringing pills along when leaving the house	6
Running out of pills or being prevented from picking up refills	5
Alcohol	4
Work	4
Water and/or food were not available	3
Skipping doses of ART as told by clinic staff when he/she was late	2

[a]Barriers mentioned by two respondents or more were included in the table
[b]Respondents were allowed to mention as many options as preferred. Thus the number of response categories per person to each question could be higher than one

Others have already been killed at night with guns, and animals are stolen." 47-year old female

Similarly, one woman said she attended a funeral, another had to take a sick child to the hospital, and a man was prevented from leaving his job because of a flood that made medicine unavailable at dose time.

The issue of **not bringing pills along when leaving the house** was mentioned as a reason for having missed one or more doses of medicine.

"I was in a hurry to work. The past 3 months I have been working in a factory, I get up at five and meet at seven. I carry [ART] in my pocket, but sometimes I forget to bring it along with me." 32-year old male

"I can forget it, if I am busy at work. It happens sometimes. I am a farmer, and in the morning and in evening the doses can be missed. I work 2 hours away. I bring the tablets along if I know I will be busy... but sometimes I did not know I would be busy, or I was travelling, and there was no water. I cannot take it without water." 52-year old male

"I am a driver. They can ask me to go to RSA or other countries and not sleep at home. Sometimes I could not take [ART]." 43-year old male

Another problem was **running out of pills or being prevented from picking up refills**. In some cases the reason for why a patient had not managed to refill in time was simply forgetfulness. Others mentioned being out of town or unable to pick up refills. In the following example the patient arrived late at the clinic and could not refill her pill bottle because the clinic was closed for the day.

"This last Friday I came after 12 [A.M.] and the reception was closed. The people were there but did not want to unlock. I was late because I had problems with the taxi. I have been told to be here at 11, but the taxi broke on the way. I missed [taking ART] Sunday through Monday and Tuesday morning." 46-year old female

Alcohol was a barrier mentioned by a few patients. One patient explained that he would skip his medicine when he had been drinking due to concerns about interactions with alcohol. Another patient missed several doses due to forgetfulness caused by alcohol.

"Yes, I was drinking beer, and was forgetting an entire week. Then I was taken to the counselor by the grandmother. It happened for only 1 week." 25-year old male

Work (meetings, long and busy working days or advice to take ART during working hours) would cause patients to postpone or miss one or more doses of ART.

"Once I postponed for three hours because I was in a meeting." 42-year old female

Another barrier to adherence was that **water and/or food were not available** when it was time to take the medicine. Some patients felt that the medicine made them hungry and when food was not available they would skip a dose. Another patient would not be able to swallow the pills without water.

"I was not forgetting but I defaulted because I had nothing to eat, and pills make me hungrier." 33-year old female

"I missed a dose of medicine 2 weeks ago. I was on a journey, and I had no water, but I had the tablets in my pocket." 52-year old male

Two patients reported **skipping doses of ART as told by clinic staff when he/she was late** with a dose. (See citations in *Missed Doses and the role of Timing of Doses*.)

A few reported that they missed daily doses of medicine because they **simply forgot** or **slept over** and one patient explained that the night-dose in a bi-daily (BD) ART regimen was the most difficult to remember.

Facilitators of adherence

The facilitators of ART-adherence reported by two or more respondents are shown in Table 5. A large number of respondents listed the **mobile phone alarm and/or mobile phone clock** as the primary tool to help remember taking ART. Not all patients had a mobile phone of their own, but most households had access to one. The mobile phone often belonged to a younger family member.

"I am reminded by my husband and by our phone alarm. The alarm rings at seven when I take it, and eight, when he takes it." 36-year old female

"My children say:" Daddy it is time to take the medicine" when they hear the phone alarm." 43-year old male

Support from family and/or friends was a frequently reported facilitator of ART-adherence.

"My sister reminds me, we live together, she is HIV-unknown, but looks sick. Puts them [the pills] where I can see them." 33-year old female

Table 5 Facilitators of ART-adherence

Answer[a]	n = 28[b]
Mobile phone alarm and/or mobile phone clock	18
Support from family and/or friends	17
TV and Radio	12
Regular clock or alarm clock	9
HIV-positive partner, relative or friend	7
Remember the medication pontaneously	5
Previous severe symptoms of HIV infection	3
Mokoko[c]	2
Planning ahead	2
Disclosure of HIV serostatus	2

[a]Facilitators mentioned by two respondents or more were included in the table
[b]Respondents were allowed to state/mention as many options as preferred. Thus the number of response categories per person to each question could be higher than one
[c]Mokoko (meaning "rooster" In Sesotho), is a markable 1-sheet 1-month calendar built up by symbols (e.g. A rooster for the morning, a sun for the day and a moon for the evening) to help patients remember their doses

"My children. They made a song called Sogum [the medicine] – "Mummy it is time for Sogum"." 45-year old female

"Wife or children [remind him] if phone battery is charged far away from home." 44-year old male

TV and radio or using a **regular clock or alarm clock** also played a dominant role in helping patients remember to take the medicine on time.

"Radio. I am a babysitter, listens all the time." 39-year old female

"Radio. I do not know how to read the clock." 32-year old female

"Watch, no alarm, or TV. I have no cell phone." 22-year old female

"Looks at the clock on the wall. If not home – I have another watch. Have no cell phone. Takes it after meal or if no food just takes them." 56-year old female

Another facilitator of adherence was to have an **HIV-positive partner, relative or friend** to share the experience with or get reminders and support from.

"My wife reminds me, she is also on ARV's, also takes them seven, but BD." 41-year old male

"My neighbor, who is also positive – asks: "now it is 7 o'clock, did you take it?"." 39-years old female

Several patients stated that they would **remember their medication spontaneously.** Three patients mentioned **previously severe symptoms of HIV infection**, which motivated them to stay adherent to ART. After initiating ART one patient began to feel better and explained:

"I have the interest in taking them [the pills] because I was very sick and got better after taking them." 47-year old female

Two patients used the **mokoko** to remember their daily doses of ART and two other patients were **planning ahead**, typically by bringing ART along when leaving the house. For example a 36-year old male always made sure he was home when it was time to take the 7 P.M. dose and he would bring ART along on travels.

Two respondents reported predominantly positive emotions and feed-back when they **disclosed their HIV serostatus** to family members and co-workers.

"It helps that I have disclosed to boss and all co-workers." 32-year old male

Discussion

In this qualitative study we discovered "surpassed medication intake time" as an issue, and mapped obstacles and facilitators of adherence to treatment. A change in routine, an unpredicted event or leaving home without pills was often mentioned as obstacles to ART-adherence. Use of mobile phones and social support appear to be key factors in ensuring adherence to ART.

The non-randomly selected group of adult respondents had a majority of women and an education level slightly higher than the overall estimated mean years of schooling in Lesotho, (6.9 vs. 5.9 years (2012)) [22], in congruence with the higher HIV prevalence in women [23], the slightly higher prevalence of women in Lesotho and the urban–rural disparities in school attendance [24].

The interviews indicated that the patients did not receive adherence counseling as frequently as would be optimal. It is known that adherence is not static, but is a dynamic process and tends to decline over time [15–17]. Increasing the frequency of education and counseling could therefore be an area of intervention to improve adherence in this setting, as shown in earlier Sub-Saharan studies [25].

We found that the respondents were generally told by the counselors to take their medication "on time" and unfortunately, several patients were willing to skip their medication, if they discovered they were late by just a few hours. Two patients were **skipping doses of ART as told by clinic staff when he/she was late**. This iatrogenic barrier has to our knowledge not been explored elsewhere, although it has been reported as a barrier to ART adherence by a health care provider and three patients who were failing second-line ART in a small study from RSA [26]. In more affluent countries, forgetfulness has shown to be an important barrier to ART adherence and it has been suggested to advice patients to link the daily dosage with a daily routine such as tooth brushing or having breakfast [20]. However, patients reported that inconsistency in daily routines was a primary barrier to adherence. Therefore, coupling medication intake with daily routines may be sub-optimal in this setting. There are no large randomized controlled trials which compare regimens of "on time" with "routine coupled" dosage of ART in Sub-Saharan Africa. In a small pilot study viral suppression was maintained at 24 and 48 weeks on intermittent treatment with an Efavirenz-based regimen (5 days on and 2 days off) [27]. In contrast, studies of longer (≥1 week) ART interruptions have resulted in increased viral load [28, 29]. We suggest that physicians should emphasize to patients the importance of taking a delayed dose as soon as they remember, instead of skipping the dose completely.

The main barriers to adherence in this study were related to hassles of daily life, such as a **change in routine or an unpredicted event. Not bringing pills along when leaving the house** was also a frequently mentioned barrier. Other researchers have reported being away from medicine at dose time as the main reasons for non-adherence [30]. Patients should be advised to maintain a travel kit filled with sufficient medication for the duration of their absence from home. Pill burden was not reported as a barrier to ART adherence in this setting but one patient found the night dose in a BD regimen as more difficult to remember than the morning dose. The majority of patients were on a OD ART regimen which could improve adherence as opposed to BD regimens [31].

A few patients had skipped doses of ART because **water and/or food were not available** at dose time. Lack of food [12, 14] and hunger [30, 32–34] have previously been reported as barriers to adherence to ART in sub-Saharan Africa. Cantrell et al. conducted a pilot study in Zambia, showing improved adherence with food supplements delivered to HIV patients on ART [35]. Other solutions could be to advice patients to always carry a bottle of water and a snack together with the daily ART. **Alcohol** is a problem in Sub-Saharan Africa, especially with its unfortunate effects on HIV transmission rates and ART adherence [36]. In our sample of patients, alcohol was reported as a barrier to ART adherence by four patients. The majority of patients recalled being counselled not to drink alcohol. Some patients **were running out of pills or being prevented from picking up refills**. At the Senkatana HIV clinic in Lesotho it is an option to send friends or family members to pick up ART at the clinic, but this was not known to all of the respondents.

In this study the **mobile phone alarm and/or mobile phone clock** was often used by patients or their friends and family as medication reminders. A recent qualitative study from Ethiopia report the same use of mobile phones as a reminder tool [37]. Other studies have found positive evidence with supportive text messages and other reminder devices [25, 38, 39]. At the clinic in Maseru, reminding patients by sending text messages was not an option at the time of the study. With an estimated 86.3 mobile-phone subscriptions per 100 inhabitants in Lesotho in 2013 [40] and the growing number of mobile phones in Africa [41–43], this practice could face widespread application. Most respondents had access to a mobile phone in this setting and thus, using Short Message Service in ART-clinics could be a future option. **Support from family and/or friends** facilitated adherence, for example the children of the person taking ART. The literature suggests school education programs for children to strengthen their role as treatment supporters [38]. Recommending patients to bring family members along to counseling and to treat family members together has shown to have a positive impact on adherence [15]. We saw a tendency to form alliances with an **HIV-positive partner, relative or friend** and peer-counseling has been shown to have a positive effect on adherence [44]. Several patients in this setting used the **TV or radio** as a reminder and other studies confirm this method's frequent use [38]. We suggest that clinicians discuss with the patient the preferred facilitators, and encourage its use.

One of the major obstacles to improvement of HIV/AIDS health care in Sub-Saharan Africa is to ensure that all patients eligible for ART have access to ART. In 2012 an estimated 59 % of all eligible patients received ART in Lesotho [1]. Once ART is initiated an estimated 72 % of the patients in Lesotho are still on ART 12 months after commencement [1]. Thus retention to ART and accessibility are important issues to address. Addressing these issues may have a greater impact on survival than simply focusing on individual adherence.

To address these major challenges we suggest: introducing more flexible refill-practices, telling patients that family members are allowed to pick up medicine, introducing rations that last for more than a month, group sessions to encourage peer-support, more frequent counseling including education about disease and treatment, and sending text messages in advance to remind patients that it is time for a refill. Actions costing money like additional counseling sessions or text message services may not be realistic to implement in HIV-clinics of recourse limited countries. However, the existing counseling may be improved concerning the information given. Adherence and quality of life may be improved by allowing the patients to be more flexible with regard to timing of doses, for instance by taking the medicine in combination with a daily routine or to take the dose as soon as they remember instead of skipping it completely if they are delayed, and informing the patients about the potentials of mobile phones and support from family and friends. Specifically, counselors could focus on the scenario of an upcoming unexpected event or a change in routines and how to prepare patients for these situations. Finally we believe that it is of great importance that counselors are attentive towards patients' preferred methods of remembering their ART doses and try to facilitate their good behavior.

Strengths and limitations

A strength of this study is that we explored in depth the barriers and facilitators, and that the issue of "surpassed medication intake time" was discovered. The in-depth interviews in native language enhance trustworthiness of the findings. However, there are also some limitations to our study. The relatively few respondents, the fact the researchers did not speak the local language, and the lack of taped interviews. Another limitation to our study is that only patients were interviewed in depth. It would have been optimal to be able to compare patients' and clinicians' point of views. Finally, the findings of this study cannot necessarily be generalized to other countries or parts of Lesotho due to the small, non-randomly design. However, the issues of timing of doses of ART and the widespread use of mobile phones may well be useful in other Sub-Saharan African HIV clinics. This study confirms the complexity of barriers to and facilitators of adherence to ART.

Conclusions

Our findings suggest that patients are often told by clinicians to be strictly on time with their doses of ART and unfortunately several patients would skip a dose if they came in a situation of being only a few hours late. Patients should be advised to take their medicine immediately when they remember, instead of skipping it altogether when late. We hypothesize, that in some settings it may be easier for patients to be adherent to ART if the medication is linked to daily routines, for example tooth-brushing, but the literature lacks large randomized clinical trials comparing medication intake at exactly the same time each day with medication intake linked to daily routines. A major barrier to ART adherence was interruptions of daily routines and therefore coupling medication intake to daily routines may be unsuitable in this setting. Leaving the house without sufficient medicine was also listed as an important barrier and patients should be advised to maintain a travel kit. Mobile phone alarms and family support were major facilitators of adherence and is supported in the literature. None of the patients reported to have been counseled on family support or the use of mobile phones as helpful methods to improve adherence to ART. These areas could be subjects of focus during counseling particularly with the growing numbers of mobile phones in Africa and the current focus on telemedicine.

Abbreviations
ART: Antiretroviral therapy; BD: Bi-daily; HIV: Human immunodeficiency virus; NRTI: Nucleoside analog reverse-transcriptase inhibitor; NtRTI: Nucleotide analog reverse-transcriptase inhibitor; NNRTI: Non-nucleoside reverse-transcriptase inhibitor; OD: Once daily; PI: Protease inhibitor; PLWH: People living with HIV; RSA: Republic of South Africa.

Competing interests
The authors declare that they have no competing interests.

Authors' contributions
TB designed the project, created the questionnaire and led the work with conducting the interviews. JMA and SH processed the data, performed the analysis and wrote the manuscript with support from TB. All authors read and approved the final manuscript.

Acknowledgements
We would like to especially thank the study participants, the translators and the local research assistants for their contribution. Special thanks to Dr. Pearl Ntseke as the Chief Physician at the Senkatana clinic for her great support.

Author details
[1]Department of Medicine, Copenhagen University Hospital Glostrup, Glostrup, Denmark. [2]Department of Infectious Diseases, Hvidovre University Hospital, Hvidovre, Denmark. [3]Department of Medicine, Roskilde University Hospital, Roskilde, Denmark.

Reference List
1. Joint United Nations Programme on HIV/AIDS. Global Report: UNAIDS Report on the Global AIDS Epidemic 2013. Geneva: UNAIDS; 2013.
2. Bangsberg DR, Perry S, Charlebois ED, Clark RA, Roberston M, Zolopa AR, et al. Non-adherence to highly active antiretroviral therapy predicts progression to AIDS. AIDS. 2001;15(9):1181–3.
3. Wood E, Hogg RS, Yip B, Harrigan PR, O'Shaughnessy MV, Montaner JS. Effect of medication adherence on survival of HIV-infected adults who start highly active antiretroviral therapy when the CD4+ cell count is 0.200 to 0.350 x 10(9) cells/L. Ann. Intern. Med. 2003;139(10):810–6.
4. Nachega JB, Mills EJ, Schechter M. Antiretroviral therapy adherence and retention in care in middle-income and low-income countries: current status of knowledge and research priorities. Curr. Opin.HIV. AIDS. 2010;5(1):70–7.
5. Sethi AK, Celentano DD, Gange SJ, Moore RD, Gallant JE. Association between adherence to antiretroviral therapy and human immunodeficiency virus drug resistance. Clin Infect Dis. 2003;37(8):1112–8.
6. Harrigan PR, Hogg RS, Dong WW, Yip B, Wynhoven B, Woodward J, et al. Predictors of HIV drug-resistance mutations in a large antiretroviral-naive cohort initiating triple antiretroviral therapy. J Infect Dis. 2005;191(3):339–47.
7. Bennett DE, Bertagnolio S, Sutherland D, Gilks CF. The World Health Organization's global strategy for prevention and assessment of HIV drug resistance. Antivir Ther. 2008;13 Suppl 2:1–13.
8. Berg KM, Arnsten JH. Practical and conceptual challenges in measuring antiretroviral adherence. J AcquirImmune Defic Syndr. 2006;43 Suppl 1:S79–87.
9. Mills EJ, Nachega JB, Buchan I, Orbinski J, Attaran A, Singh S, et al. Adherence to antiretroviral therapy in sub-Saharan Africa and North America: a meta-analysis. JAMA. 2006;296(6):679–90.
10. Duff P, Kipp W, Wild TC, Rubaale T, Okech-Ojony J. Barriers to accessing highly active antiretroviral therapy by HIV-positive women attending an antenatal clinic in a regional hospital in western Uganda. J Int AIDS Soc. 2010;13:37.

11. Kip E, Ehlers VJ, van der Wal DM. Patients' adherence to anti-retroviral therapy in Botswana. J Nurs Scholarsh. 2009;41(2):149–57.

12. Murray LK, Semrau K, McCurley E, Thea DM, Scott N, Mwiya M, et al. Barriers to acceptance and adherence of antiretroviral therapy in urban Zambian women: a qualitative study. AIDS Care. 2009;21(1):78–86.

13. Dahab M, Charalambous S, Hamilton R, Fielding K, Kielmann K, Churchyard GJ, et al. "That is why I stopped the ART": patients' & providers' perspectives on barriers to and enablers of HIV treatment adherence in a South African workplace programme. BMC Public Health. 2008;8:63.

14. Sanjobo N, Frich JC, Fretheim A. Barriers and facilitators to patients' adherence to antiretroviral treatment in Zambia: a qualitative study. SAHARA J. 2008;5(3):136–43.

15. Byakika-Tusiime J, Crane J, Oyugi JH, Ragland K, Kawuma A, Musoke P, et al. Longitudinal antiretroviral adherence in HIV+ Ugandan parents and their children initiating HAART in the MTCT-Plus family treatment model: role of depression in declining adherence over time. AIDS Behav. 2009;13 Suppl 1:82–91.

16. Liu H, Miller LG, Hays RD, Golin CE, Wu T, Wenger NS, et al. Repeated measures longitudinal analyses of HIV virologic response as a function of percent adherence, dose timing, genotypic sensitivity, and other factors. J Acquir Immune Defic Syndr. 2006;41(3):315–22.

17. Parruti G, Manzoli L, Toro PM, D'Amico G, Rotolo S, Graziani V, et al. Long-term adherence to first-line highly active antiretroviral therapy in a hospital-based cohort: predictors and impact on virologic response and relapse. AIDS Patient Care STDS. 2006;20(1):48–56.

18. Joint United Nations Programme on HIV/AIDS (UNAIDS). Global report: UNAIDS report on the global AIDS epidemic 2012. Geneva, Switzerland. 2012. http://www.unaids.org/sites/default/files/media_asset/20121120_UNAIDS_Global_Report_2012_with_annexes_en_1http://www.unaids.org/sites/default/files/en/media/unaids/contentassets/document.

19. WHO, UNICEF, UNAIDS. Global update on HIV treatment 2013: Results, impact and opportunities. Geneva, Switzerland. 2013 Jun. http://apps.who.int/iris/bitstream/10665/85326/1/9789241505734_eng.pdf?ua=1.

20. Barfod TS, Sørensen HT, Nielsen H, Rodkjær L, Obel N. 'Simply forgot' is the most frequently stated reason for missed doses of HAART irrespective of degree of adherence. HIV Med. 2006;7(5):285–290.

21. Corbin J, Strauss A. Basics of Qualitative Research: Techniques and Procedures for Developing Grounded Theory. 3rd ed. Los Angeles: SAGE Publications; 2007.

22. United Nations Development Programme (UNDP). Human Development Report 2013 - The Rise of the South: Human Progress in a Diverse World. New York, USA. 2013. http://hdr.undp.org/sites/default/files/reports/14/hdr2013_en_complete.pdf.

23. Ministry of Health and Social Welfare (MOHSW) [Lesotho] and ICF Macro. Lesotho Demographic and Health Survey 2009. Maseru: MOHSW and ICF Macro; 2010.

24. Liang X, Tan J-P, Mutumbuka DB. Primary and secondary education in Lesotho - a Country Status Report for education. Africa Region Human Development working paper series. Washington: World Bank; 2005.

25. Barnighausen T, Chaiyachati K, Chimbindi N, Peoples A, Haberer J, Newell ML. Interventions to increase antiretroviral adherence in sub-Saharan Africa: a systematic review of evaluation studies. Lancet Infect Dis. 2011;11(12):942–51.

26. Barnett W, Patten G, Kerschberger B, Conradie K, Garone DB, van Cutsem G, et al. Perceived adherence barriers among patients failing second-line antiretroviral therapy in Khayelitsha, South Africa. South Afr J HIV Med. 2013;14(2013):166–9.

27. Cohen CJ, Colson AE, Sheble-Hall AG, McLaughlin KA, Morse GD. Pilot study of a novel short-cycle antiretroviral treatment interruption strategy: 48-week results of the five-days-on, two-days-off (FOTO) study. HIV.Clin. Trials. 2007;8(1):19–23.

28. Ananworanich J, Nuesch R, Le BM, Chetchotisakd P, Vibhagool A, Wicharuk S, et al. Failures of 1 week on, 1 week off antiretroviral therapies in a randomized trial. AIDS. 2003;17(15):F33–7.

29. Dybul M, Nies-Kraske E, Daucher M, Hertogs K, Hallahan CW, Csako G, et al. Long-cycle structured intermittent versus continuous highly active antiretroviral therapy for the treatment of chronic infection with human immunodeficiency virus: effects on drug toxicity and on immunologic and virologic parameters. J Infect Dis. 2003;188(3):388–96.

30. Senkomago V, Guwatudde D, Breda M, Khoshnood K. Barriers to antiretroviral adherence in HIV-positive patients receiving free medication in Kayunga. Uganda AIDS Care. 2011;23(10):1246–53.

31. Parienti JJ, Bangsberg DR, Verdon R, Gardner EM. Better adherence with once-daily antiretroviral regimens: a meta-analysis. Clin Infect Dis. 2009;48(4):484–8.

32. Nagata JM, Magerenge RO, Young SL, Oguta JO, Weiser SD, Cohen CR. Social determinants, lived experiences, and consequences of household food insecurity among persons living with HIV/AIDS on the shore of Lake Victoria. Kenya AIDS Care. 2012;24(6):728–36.

33. Weiser SD, Tuller DM, Frongillo EA, Senkungu J, Mukiibi N, Bangsberg DR. Food insecurity as a barrier to sustained antiretroviral therapy adherence in Uganda. PLoS One. 2010;5(4):e10340.

34. Hardon AP, Akurut D, Comoro C, Ekezie C, Irunde HF, Gerrits T, et al. Hunger, waiting time and transport costs: time to confront challenges to ART adherence in Africa. AIDS Care. 2007;19(5):658–65.

35. Cantrell RA, Sinkala M, Megazinni K, Lawson-Marriott S, Washington S, Chi BH, et al. A pilot study of food supplementation to improve adherence to antiretroviral therapy among food-insecure adults in Lusaka. Zambia J Acquir Immune Defic Syndr. 2008;49(2):190–5.

36. Hahn JA, Woolf-King SE, Muyindike W. Adding fuel to the fire: alcohol's effect on the HIV epidemic in Sub-Saharan Africa. CurrHIV/AIDS Rep. 2011;8(3):172–80.

37. Bezabhe WM, Chalmers L, Bereznicki LR, Peterson GM, Bimirew MA, Kassie DM. Barriers and facilitators of adherence to antiretroviral drug therapy and retention in care among adult HIV-positive patients: a qualitative study from Ethiopia. PLoS One. 2014;9(5):e97353.

38. Hardon A. World Health Organization. From access to adherence the challenges of antiretroviral treatment: studies from Botswana, Tanzania and Uganda. Geneva, Switzerland. 2006. 0 AD. http://whqlibdoc.who.int/publications/2006/9241563281_eng.pdf.

39. Horvath T, Azman H, Kennedy GE, Rutherford GW. Mobile phone text messaging for promoting adherence to antiretroviral therapy in patients with HIV infection. Cochrane Database Syst Rev. 2012;3:CD009756.

40. ITU (International Telecommunication Union). Lesotho Profile (Latest data available: 2013). http://www.itu.int/net4/itu-d/icteye/Geneva,Switzerland.

41. Africa's mobile economic revolution Killian Fox, The Guardian. 2011 Jul 24.

42. Vital Wave Consulting. mHealth for Development: The Opportunity of Mobile Technology for Healthcare in the Developing World. Washington, D.C. and Berkshire, UK: UN Foundation-Vodafone Foundation Partnership. Web adress: http://www.globalproblems-globalsolutions-files.org/unf_website/assets/publications/technology/mhealth/mHealth_for_Development_full.pdf.

43. Africa's mobile phone industry 'booming' BBC News Africa. 2011 Nov 9.

44. Gusdal AK, Obua C, Andualem T, Wahlstrom R, Chalker J, Fochsen G. Peer counselors' role in supporting patients' adherence to ART in Ethiopia and Uganda. AIDS Care. 2011;23(6):657–62.

Caesarean delivery and its correlates in Northern Region of Bangladesh: application of logistic regression and cox proportional hazard model

Mostafizur Rahman[1*], Asma Ahmad Shariff[2], Aziz Shafie[3], Rahmah Saaid[4] and Rohayatimah Md. Tahir[2]

Abstract

Background: Caesarean delivery (C-section) rates have been increasing dramatically in the past decades around the world. This increase has been attributed to multiple factors such as maternal, socio-demographic and institutional factors and is a burning issue of global aspect like in many developed and developing countries. Therefore, this study examines the relationship between mode of delivery and time to event with provider characteristics (i.e., covariates) respectively.

Methods: The study is based on a total of 1142 delivery cases from four private and four public hospitals maternity wards. Logistic regression and Cox proportional hazard models were the statistical tools of the present study.

Results: The logistic regression of multivariate analysis indicated that the risk of having a previous C-section, prolonged labour, higher educational level, mother age 25 years and above, lower order of birth, length of baby more than 45 cm and irregular intake of balanced diet were significantly predict for C-section. With regard to survival time, using the Cox model, fetal distress, previous C-section, mother's age, age at marriage and order of birth were also the most independent risk factors for C-section. By the forward stepwise selection, the study reveals that the most common factors were previous C-section, mother's age and order of birth in both analysis. As shown in the above results, the study suggests that these factors may influence the health-seeking behaviour of women.

Conclusions: Findings suggest that program and policies need to address the increase rate of caesarean delivery in Northern region of Bangladesh. Also, for determinant of risk factors, the result of Akaike Information Criterion (AIC) indicated that logistic model is an efficient model.

Keywords: Caesarean delivery, Risk factors, Logistic regression, Cox model, AIC, Bangladesh

Background

Delivery may occur either by caesarean or non-caesarean. A multiple factors associated with safe delivery practices, ranging from demographic to socio-economic [1]. More than 70 % of the deliveries took place at home, and only 32 % birth in Bangladesh were under safe and hygienic conditions [2]. In recent years, caesarean delivery is one of the most common surgical procedures. Caesarean sections (C-section) are more common among first births (12.7 %), births in urban areas (15.9 %), and especially among births in the private sector (67.3 %), whereas the public sector

was (34.6 %) [2]. The rate of C-sections is increasing in Bangladesh. In 2001, only 2.6 % of births were delivered by C-section, compared with 12.2 % in 2010 [3]. The number of caesarean delivery has also been growing in many developed and developing countries [4, 5] and this increase has not been clinically justified [6]. Over the last few years, the rates of C-section have risen substantially in many countries such as Brazil (30 %), [7] Chile (40 %), [8] USA (24.4 %) [9] and Malaysia (15.7 %) [10]. According to WHO, there is no justification for any region to have a caesarean rate higher than 10–15 %. This signifies a serious cause for concern in most of the countries in the world and due to several investigations into

* Correspondence: mos_pshd@yahoo.com
[1]University of Rajshahi, Rajshahi, Bangladesh
Full list of author information is available at the end of the article

the reasons for the rising rates in caesarean delivery, it is now identified as emerging "global epidemic" [11, 12].

The increase in caesarean deliveries has been attributed to multiple factors ranging from maternal, socio-demographic and institutional factors. Caesarean delivery rates are known to vary widely among different population groups, with known risk factors including maternal age, [13–15] order of birth, [16] baby weight, [17] socioeconomic status, [18] high levels of maternal education, [19–23] previous c-section, [24–26] obstetric complications, [24, 28] maternal request (refers to a primary caesarean delivery performed because the mother requests this method of delivery in the absence of conventional medical or obstetrical indications) [27–29] and high income level [18, 22, 30–33]. The increase in caesarean delivery rates has also raised questions in Bangladesh like in most other countries. Though increased caesarean rates have been questioned and emphasized, for the lack of reliable administrative records, no early studies were carried out to identify the possible risk factors associated with C-section in this country. However, some related studies have been conducted in other countries. This study presents the most recent estimate of C-section delivery in northern region of Bangladesh and examines the association of reported complications around delivery as well as socio-demographic and relevant characteristics of women with C-section using data from sample survey. To investigate the significant relationship between mode of delivery (that is, caesarean or non-caesarean) and covariates (independent variables), most of the studies carried out logistic regression model [16, 18, 26, 34]. On the other hand, time (it is measured as after marriage to getting one child or previous child to current child) is one of the factors that may play an important role in C-section but it is not yet considered in other studies. From this point of view, the study also examined the relationship between time to event (that is, caesarean or non-caesarean) and covariates. In these cases, Cox's model is considered to be the most used procedure for modelling the relationship of covariates to a survival or other censored outcomes [35]. Consequently, to obtain a more complete assessment of risk factors, this study considered time as a dependent variable and the concomitant variables (covariates) as independent variables and compared the results of empirical data analyzed by logistic regression and Cox proportional hazard model.

Methods
Study area
The study sample comprised of 1142 women who had delivery either by caesarean or non-caesarean delivery at four private and four public hospitals maternity wards in the northern region of Bangladesh during the period of January to March 2010. Among the 1142 delivery cases,

652 were caesarean and the remaining 490 were non-caesarean. The northern region is the part of north in Bangladesh, where the hospitals were situated. The hospitals involved in the study are Islamic bank hospital, Shapla, Rangpur and city clinic which are the private hospitals, while Rajshahi, Bogra, Rangpur and Dinajpur medical college hospitals are expressed as public hospitals. Also, the terms private and public patients refer to respondents, who were admitted in maternity wards for safe delivery in the respective hospitals.

Study population
Pregnant women in the Northern region of Bangladesh.

Sampling design
The study followed a cross-sectional design where data were collected by direct interviews. Before delivery, the participants were selected by simple random sampling and proportion to the estimated load of deliveries, which accounted for 60 % of all deliveries during the survey period. Most of the questions were close-ended and the answers chosen by the respondents were indicated by the tic mark. The response rate was 100 %.

Measurement of variables
Dependent variables
The dependent variables considered as (i) the types of delivery coded as dichotomous (caesarean = 1, non-caesarean = 0) and (ii) duration of time (that is, after marriage to getting one child or from previous child to current child) to event (that is, mode of delivery).

Independent variables
The maternal variables included prolonged labour (more than 12 h), fetal distress (it is commonly used to describe fetal hypoxia that is low oxygen levels in the fetus, which can result in fetal damage if the fetus is not promptly delivered), previous c-section, breathing difficulty, child aborted around delivery, multiple births; head circumference, length and weight of babies.

For the analysis of data, the category related to prolonged labour, fetal distress, previous C-section, breathing difficulty, child aborted around delivery and multiple births were assessed as yes or no. The head circumference of newborns was classified into two categories: <32 cm and more than 32 cm. The length and weight of baby were categorized into: <45 cm or more than 45 cm and <2.5 kg or more than 2.5 kg respectively. The socio-demographic variables included maternal age at birth, age at marriage, parity (order of birth), and maternal educational level. Maternal age was categorized into four broad groups (years): <20, 20–24, 25–29 and more than 30. The age at marriage was classified into three categories: <18 years, 18–22 years and 23 years and above. The parity was divided into three groups: 1, 2, and ≥ 3. Education status is the highest level of schooling attained, measured as primary and below (0–5 years), secondary (6–10 years) and higher (11 years and above). Place of residence and duration of taking balance diet (it refers to milk, fish, egg, fruit and vegetables that contains adequate amounts of all the necessary nutrients required for healthy growth and activity and those diets were taken a woman in pregnancy period) were also considered as the other related variables in the study. Additionally, place of residence was classified as rural verses urban and duration of taking balance diet was measured as a categorical variable: often, once a week and rarely.

Statistical analysis

An initial bivariate analysis was performed to identify significant associations between types of delivery (caesarean vs. non-caesarean) and a series of independent variables. Dichotomous variables were analysed by the χ^2 test or Fisher exact test, where appropriate. To determine the risk factors which are associated with the C-section, based on the different criteria, two multivariate techniques were used. They are logistic regression model and Cox proportional hazard model. Logistic Regression and Cox proportional hazard models are the most frequently used for analysing data in epidemiological and clinical studies [38]. The logistic regression is analogous to multiple linear regressions where the dependent measure is dichotomous in nature (coded by the values 0 and 1); whereas the Cox proportional regression model assumes that the effects of the predictor variables (names of variables that we expect to predict survival time) are constant over time. For both techniques, maternal, socio-demographic and other relevant variables were treated as independent variables, while the dependent variables were already mentioned in the above section. The most influential risk factors were estimated separately for overall, public and private hospital by stepwise selection. The value of $P < 0.05$ was considered statistically significant. Finally, to identify and measure the risk factors for caesarean delivery, that is, how well the model fits the data, Akaike Information Criterion (AIC) is used. Generally, the AIC formula is $-2 \log(L) + 2$ k, where, L is the maximized value of the likelihood function for the estimated model and k is the number of parameters in the statistical model. Lower AIC indicates a better likelihood.

Ethical clearance

We obtained informed verbal consent from the respondents before conducting the interview.

The study was approved by the ethical board and research review committee of the Dept. of Population

Science & Human Resource Development, University of Rajshahi, Bangladesh.

Results

Patient characteristics and significant variables are listed in Table 1. The sample comprised of 1142 mothers with the aggregate caesarean section (C-section) rate among the participants being 57.09 %. The C-section rate in the public hospital was 30.28 % ($n - 199$), while the C-section rate in private hospital was 93.47 % ($n = 453$). Caesarean rates varied by level of maternal complications. The significant rate was highest among women having previous C-section (94.8 %). Similarly, the rate was highest among women with higher education level (76.8 %, compared to 44.8 % for mothers with primary and below level of education) followed by higher maternal ages (30 years and above) as compared to lower age groups (less than 20 years). The same pattern was also observed in age at marriage. Residence and nutritional status were among the factors associated with the likelihood of having C-section. C-section deliveries were of low frequency in urban areas as compared to rural areas. The highest Caesarean rate was observed for those who rarely take a balanced diet (76.0 %). Out of 15 variables examined, eight were statistically significant while the remaining eight were statistically not associated with the type of delivery.

Figure 1 displays the survival for mean values for selected covariates in the Cox model over time by health facilities. The survival curve represents the probability of mothers who have delivery by caesarean at any given time. During the period of below 2 years, the probability of getting first child from the women in private hospital is greater than those who delivered by caesarean in public hospital. Figure 1 also shows that the rate of caesarean cases over time is relatively constant and approximately below 1 % after the duration time of 6 years and above.

The adjusted odds ratios (ORs) and hazard ratios (HRs) (with 95 % confidence intervals) for a C-section are shown in Tables 2, 3 and 4 at overall, private and public hospitals respectively. As shown in Table 2 within overall delivery cases, the binary logistic regression of multivariate analysis indicated that the risk of having previous C-section (OR = 20.18, CI = 10.46–25.58), prolonged labour (OR = 0.17, CI = 0.12–0.23), higher educational level (OR = 2.68, CI = 1.58–4.54), mother's age > 25 years (OR = 2.74, CI = 1.58–4.72), lower order of birth (OR = 0.74 CI = 0.49–1.12), length of baby > 45 cm (OR = 1.45, CI = 1.04–2.02), and irregular intake of balance diet (OR = 1.87 CI = 1.24–2.81) significantly predict C-section delivery. The odds ratio 20.18 indicated that the odds of being C-section to the women were seen 20.18 times greater in previous C-section as compared to those were not in previous C-section. The others odds ratio can be explained in the same way. In a Cox's regression

Table 1 Percentage distributions of maternal, socio-demographic and other characteristics by type of delivery and their significance level in northern region of Bangladesh

Selected variables	Delivery type				P-Value
	Caesarean delivery		Non-Caesarean delivery		
	N	%	N	%	
Fetal Distress					0.829
No	588	57.2	440	42.8	
Yes	64	56.1	50	43.9	
Previous C-Section					<0.001
No	561	53.6	485	46.4	
Yes	91	94.8	5	05.2	
Multiple Birth					0.945
No	643	57.1	483	42.9	
Yes	9	56.3	7	43.8	
Pregnancy-Induced Breathing Difficulty					0.993
No	612	57.1	460	42.9	
Yes	40	57.1	30	42.9	
Prolonged Labour					<0.001
No	541	70.0	232	30.0	
Yes	111	30.1	258	69.9	
Mother's Education					<0.001
Primary and below	147	44.8	181	55.2	
Secondary	310	55.4	250	44.6	
Higher	195	76.8	59	23.2	
Mother's Age: years					<0.001
<20	185	44.5	231	55.5	
20–24	160	55.2	130	44.8	
25–29	198	69.0	89	31.0	
30+	109	73.2	40	26.8	
Age at Marriage: years					<0.001
<18	344	50.3	340	49.7	
18–22	188	61.2	119	38.8	
23+	120	79.5	31	20.5	
Order of Birth					0.062
1	369	54.7	306	45.3	
2	199	62.6	119	37.4	
3+	84	56.4	65	43.6	
Length of Baby: cm					0.029
<45	457	55.1	372	44.9	
45+	195	62.3	118	37.7	
Weight of Baby: kg					0.894
<2.5	214	57.4	159	42.6	
2.5+	438	57.0	331	43.0	
Head Circumferences: cm					0.180
<32	486	56.0	382	44.0	
32+	166	60.6	108	39.4	
Residence					<0.001
Rural	244	67.6	117	32.4	
Urban	408	52.2	373	47.8	
Ever had a Child Aborted					0.817
No	631	57.2	473	42.8	
Yes	21	55.3	17	44.7	
Duration of Taking Balanced Diet					<0.001
Often	363	51.2	346	48.8	
Once a week	74	49.3	76	50.7	
Rarely	215	76.0	68	24.0	

(Table 1 Percentage distributions of maternal, socio-demographic and other characteristics by type of delivery and their significance level in northern region of Bangladesh (Continued))

model, the multivariate analysis indicated that fetal distress, previous C-section, mother's age, age at marriage and lower order of birth were significantly independent risk factors for C-section. The risk of having fetal distress and previous C-section had a higher risk as compared to those who did not. The hazard ratios of C-section for older mothers were higher than their younger counterparts. Women who married at the age

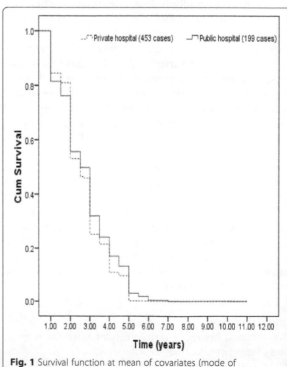

Fig. 1 Survival function at mean of covariates (mode of delivery: caesarean)

Table 2 Logistic and Cox's regression results of the effects of selected characteristics on C-section: Overall cases

Selected variables	Results of logistic regression analysis		Results of Cox's regression analysis	
	Odds ratio [Exp (β)]	95 % CI	Hazard ratio [Exp (β)]	95 % CI
Fetal Distress				
(No)	1.00		1.00	
Yes	1.08	0.67 1.76	1.01*	0.52–1.51
Previous C-section				
(No)	1.00		1.00	
Yes	20.18*	10.46–25.58	9.80*	7.11–12.36
Multiple Birth				
(No)	1.00		1.00	
Yes	1.12	0.35–3.58	1.01	0.54–2.78
Pregnancy-Induced Breathing Difficulty				
(No)	1.00		1.00	
Yes	1.06	0.55–2.03	1.02	0.45–2.35
Prolonged Labour				
(No)	1.00		1.00	
Yes	0.17*	0.12–0.23	0.95	0.45–1.89
Mother's Education				
(Primary and below)	1.00		1.00	
Secondary	2.19*	1.55–3.11	1.15	0.57–2.47
Higher	2.68*	1.58–4.54	1.53	0.78–2.41
Mother's Age: years				
(<20)	1.00		1.00	
20–24	1.39	0.92–2.11	1.12*	0.75–2.31
25–29	2.74*	1.58–4.72	1.48*	0.85–2.59
30+	5.07*	2.31–11.12	2.05*	1.02–3.52
Age at Marriage: years				
(<18)	1.00		1.00	
18–22	0.93	0.64–1.35	0.57*	0.31–1.95
23+	1.06	0.54–2.05	1.01*	0.54–2.01
Order of Birth				
(1)	1.00		1.00	
2	0.74*	0.49–1.12	0.43*	0.16–1.57
3+	0.33	0.17–0.64	0.28	0.07–1.47
Length of Baby: cm				
(<45)	1.00		1.00	
45+	1.45*	1.04–2.02	1.07	0.45–2.07
Weight of Baby: kg				
(<2.5)	1.00		1.00	
2.5+	0.74	0.54–1.02	0.49	0.17–1.31
Head Circumferences: cm				
(<32)	1.000		1.00	

Table 2 Logistic and Cox's regression results of the effects of selected characteristics on C-section: Overall cases *(Continued)*

32+	1.084	0.76–1.54	1.02	0.57–1.89
Residence				
(Rural)	1.00		1.00	
Urban	0.854	0.61–1.91	0.51	0.28–1.18
Ever had a Child Aborted				
(No)	1.00		1.00	
Yes	0.57	0.25–1.33	0.34	0.16–1.51
Duration of Taking Balance Diet				
(Often)	1.00		1.00	
Once a week	1.45*	0.95–2.22	1.20	0.54–2.22
Rarely	1.87*	1.24–2.81	1.45	0.69–2.07
Intercept	−0.25		−2 log likelihood	13765.19
−2 log likelihood	2997.81		Modelchi-square	398.94*
Cox &Snell R²	0.54		Degrees of freedom	21
Nagelkerke R²	0.57			
AIC	3031.82		AIC	13799.19

*P < 0.05, significant risk factors in the model; CI = confidence interval; parentheses indicate the reference categories

of 18–22 years had a lower risk of C-section as compared to women who married at an early age (<18 years) and married at an older age (23 years and above). Similarly, increased parity (order of birth) had a lower risk as compared to lower parity (first order of birth) for C-section.

To examine the Caesarean delivery with associated risk factors by types of health facilities, separate models were constructed for deliveries in private and public hospitals (Tables 3 and 4). Based on the results of logistic regression alone, it was found that women who have related complications around delivery (previous C-section, prolonged labour) and delivered in public hospitals tend to have higher risk of C-section than those who delivered in private hospitals. In public hospitals, the highest odds ratios for caesarean delivery were seen in women aged 30 years and above (OR = 2.96, CI = 0.94–7.32) as compared to those aged 25 years and below. Similarly, first and second-born babies had higher odds of being delivered by C-section (OR = 0.52, CI = 0.16–1.83) as compared to third or above for deliveries occurring in private hospitals. For the length of baby, compared between the two facilities, it is found that this determinant factor was also less important in public hospitals as compared to private hospital. By comparing the place of delivery, it was a significant determinant of C-section for women delivering in private hospitals, with the

Table 3 Logistic and Cox's regression results of the effects of selected characteristics on C-section: Private hospitals

Selected variables	Private hospitals			
	Odds ratio [Exp (β)]	95 % CI	Hazard ratio [Exp (β)]	95 % CI
Fetal Distress				
(No)	1.00		1.00	
Yes	1.32	1.04–2.51	1.03	0.82–1.71
Previous C-section				
(No)	1.00		1.00	
Yes	6.72	3.48–12.05	2.21	1.01–4.03
Multiple Birth				
(No)	1.00		1.00	
Yes	1.32	0.89–2.91	1.01	0.46–2.27
Pregnancy-Induced Breathing Difficulty				
(No)	1.00		1.00	
Yes	1.25	0.98–2.03	1.13	0.52–2.47
Prolonged Labour				
(No)	1.00		1.00	
Yes	0.02*	0.01–0.08	0.82	0.28–1.48
Mother's Education				
(Primary and below)	1.00		1.00	
Secondary	0.49	0.13–1.48	0.24	0.07–1.41
Higher	0.71	0.38–1.93	0.49	0.09–1.78
Mother's Age: years				
(<20)	1.00		1.00	
20–24	1.01	0.22–2.57	1.01*	0.68–2.14
25–29	1.94	0.38–3.58	1.21*	0.75–3.15
30+	4.69	0.54–11.01	2.04*	1.30–4.21
Age at Marriage: years				
(<18)	1.00		1.00	
18–22	1.00	0.22–3.57	1.52*	1.03–2.23
23+	1.05	0.23–5.89	2.14*	1.14–3.24
Order of Birth				
(1)	1.00		1.00	
2	0.52*	0.16–1.83	0.27*	0.05–1.20
3+	0.13	0.03–1.84	0.12*	0.04–1.05
Length of Baby's: cm				
(<45)	1.00		1.00	
45+	0.11	0.03–0.38	0.18	0.08–1.48
Weight of Baby's: kg				
(<2.5)	1.00		1.00	
2.5+	2.26	0.58–6.32	1.99	0.59–2.81

Table 3 Logistic and Cox's regression results of the effects of selected characteristics on C-section: Private hospitals *(Continued)*

Head Circumferences: cm				
(<32)	1.00		1.00	
32+	0.56	0.19–1.45	0.38	0.15–1.38
Residence				
(Rural)	1.00		1.00	
Urban	4.60*	1.27–12.10	1.93	0.47–2.41
Ever had a Child Aborted				
(No)	1.00		1.00	
Yes	0.34	0.03–1.83	0.23	0.05–1.12
Duration of Taking Balance Diet				
(Often)	1.00		1.00	
Once a week	2.45	0.65–9.63	1.28	0.59–2.21
Rarely	8.23	1.18–14.32	3.31	1.42–5.63
Intercept	4.38		−2 log likelihood	5022.35
−2 log likelihood	1123.01		Model chi-square	189.47*
Cox &Snell R²	0.51		Degrees of freedom	21
Nagelkerke R²	0.53			
AIC	1157.01		AIC	5056.35

*P < 0.05, significant risk factors in the model; CI = confidence interval; parentheses indicate the reference categories

strongest risk shown for women residing in urban areas. Finally, a C-section was 1.73 times more likely to occur in public hospitals to women who rarely take a balanced diet. Conversely, to determine independent risk factors for survival time, the Cox's regression model showed that maternal age, age at marriage and parity were only statistically significant with C-section in both health facilities.

To identify the best regression model for caesarean delivery, we carried out a stepwise regression analysis on the variables in Table 2. In the overall and different hospitals, the most influential significant variables are listed in Tables 5 and 6 respectively. By the stepwise selection, the logistic and Cox's regression analysis reveals that seven and five remained significant independent risk factors to predict which patients were at highest risk for caesarean delivery. The most common factors were previous C-section, mother's age and order of birth in both analyses (Table 5). From the different health facilities in Table 6, the logistic regression analysis indicated in a stepwise manner the following risk factors: prolonged labour, length of baby more than 45 cm, urban residence and lower birth order were the most

Table 4 Logistic and Cox's regression results of the effects of selected characteristics on C-section: Public hospitals

Selected variables	Public hospitals			
	Odds ratio [Exp (β)]	95 % CI	Hazard ratio [Exp (β)]	95 % CI
Fetal Distress				
(No)	1.00		1.00	
Yes	1.57	0.82–2.11	1.23*	0.08–2.17
Previous C-section				
(No)	1.00		1.00	
Yes	8.98*	5.21–10.51	3.75	1.25–5.36
Multiple Birth				
(No)	1.00		1.00	
Yes	1.59	0.79–2.74	1.30	0.78–2.58
Pregnancy-Induced Breathing Difficulty				
(No)	1.00		1.00	
Yes	1.52	0.78–2.01	1.20	0.55–1.84
Prolonged Labour				
(No)	1.00		1.00	
Yes	0.20*	0.11–0.28	0.48	0.07–1.62
Mother's Education				
(Primary and below)	1.00		1.00	
Secondary	1.65*	1.14–2.85	1.27	0.72–2.14
Higher	1.81	0.93–4.38	1.46	0.24–2.36
Mother's Age: years				
(<20)	1.00		1.00	
20–24	1.97	1.15–3.42	1.35*	1.02–2.14
25–29	2.79*	1.23–5.36	2.15*	1.28–3.20
30+	2.96*	0.94–7.32	2.37*	1.32–4.17
Age at Marriage: years				
(<18)	1.00		1.00	
18–22	0.89	0.48–1.35	0.51*	0.24–1.50
23+	0.88	0.34–2.23	0.66*	0.41–1.62
Order of Birth				
(1)	1.00		1.00	
2	0.71	0.46–1.34	0.55*	0.22–1.25
3+	0.29*	0.19–1.01	0.22*	0.09–1.06
Length of Baby's: cm				
(<45)	1.00		1.00	
45+	1.49*	0.95–2.47	1.22	0.16–3.29
Weight of Baby's: kg				
(<2.5)	1.00		1.00	
2.5+	0.75	0.46–1.12	0.65	0.13–1.81
Head Circumferences: cm				
(<32)	1.00		1.00	
32+	0.80	0.47–1.27	0.63	0.082
Residence				
(Rural)	1.00		1.00	
Urban	0.82	0.48–1.23	0.78	0.15–1.08
Ever had a Child Aborted				
(No)	1.00		1.00	
Yes	0.48	0.16–1.66	0.31	0.17–1.11
Duration of Taking Balance Diet				
(Often)	1.00		1.00	
Once a week	1.44*	0.82–2.59	1.11	0.41–2.31
Rarely	1.73	0.98–2.83	1.42	0.71–3.21
Intercept	−1.19		−2 log likelihood	7196.24
−2 log likelihood	1665.89		Model chi-square	223.72*
Cox &Snell R2	0.52		Degrees of freedom	21
Nagelkerke R2	0.55			
AIC	1699.89		AIC	7230.24

*P < 0.05, significant risk factors in the model; CI – confidence interval; parentheses indicate the reference categories

significant determinants of caesarean section in private hospitals, while for public hospitals prolonged labour, previous C-section, and higher mother's educational level were the most important risk factors for determinants of caesarean delivery in Northern Region of Bangladesh. In a foregoing study using the Cox's regression model by stepwise method, it is also found that mother's age, age at marriage and order of birth were the common most influential variables among the selected variables in private and public patients. In addition, Table 2, 3 and 4 also shows that the values AIC is lower in parametric (logistic) model as compare to semi parametric (Cox's) model. Therefore, the results indicated that the logistic model is the most efficient than Cox's model for determinant the risk factors for caesarean delivery in multivariable analysis.

Discussion

The findings of this study provide us an insight into the impact of maternal, socio-demographic and relevant factors on C-section in the northern region of Bangladesh. The analysis of the C-section deliveries for the private and public hospitals substantiates this concern. The rate of C-section was higher in private hospitals as compared to public hospitals. Past studies in different countries found that the rate of caesarean delivery in private hospitals is also higher than public hospitals [36, 37]. It seems that the private practice of the doctors and the

Table 5 Stepwise regression results of the effects of selected characteristics on C-section: Overall cases

Results of logistic regression by stepwise selection		
Most influential variables among selected variables	Odds ratio [Exp (β)]	95 % CI
Prolonged Labour		
(No)	1.00	.
Yes	0.17*	0.12–0.23
Previous C-section		
(No)	1.00	
Yes	20.53*	10.23–24.92
Mother's Education		
(Primary and below)	1.00	
Secondary	2.04*	1.49–3.01
Higher	2.50*	1.48–4.31
Mother's Age: years		
(<20)	1.00	
20–24	1.35	0.82–1.82
25–29	2.85*	1.42–4.12
30+	5.76*	2.12–12.41
Order of Birth		
(1)	1.00	
2	0.70	0.48–1.01
3+	0.31*	0.12–0.58
Duration of Taking Balance Diet		
(Often)	1.00	
One day per week	1.50*	1.10–2.52
Rarely	1.87*	1.32–2.85
Length of Baby's: cm		
(<45)	1.00	
45+	1.46*	1.11–2.24
Constant	0.66*	0.23–1.57
Results of Cox's regression by stepwise selection		
Most influential variables among selected variables	Hazard ratio [Exp (β)]	95 % CI
Mother's Age: years		
(<20)	1.00	
20–24	1.32*	1.10–3.23
25–29	1.55*	1.21–2.51
30+	2.25*	1.25–3.35
Age at Marriage: years		
(<18)	1.00	
18–22	0.69*	0.24–1.87
23+	1.10*	0.54–2.56
Order of Birth		
(1)	1.00	

Table 5 Stepwise regression results of the effects of selected characteristics on C-section: Overall cases *(Continued)*

2	0.40*	0.21–1.36
3+	0.34*	0.16–1.53
Fetal Distress		
(No)	1.00	
Yes	1.21*	0.69–2.14
Abdominal Operation		
(No)	1.00	
Yes	10.20*	3.28–18.62

*P < 0.05, significant risk factors in the model; CI = confidence interval; parentheses indicate the reference categories

financial motive of the private hospitals may be playing some important role in determining the caesarean rates. This statement is supported by the previous studies [37]. The result from the logistic regression analysis showed that previous C-section, prolonged labour (more than 12 h), maternal education level, mother's age of more than 25 years, low birth order, length of baby more than 45 cm and irregular intake of a balanced diet were important determinants of C-section. Conversely, two newly independent risk factors (fetal distress and age at marriage) were also found to determinants of C-section by the Cox's regression model. Furthermore, the association of these determinants with C-section varied by the different health facilities. By the stepwise selection in logistic regression analysis, we confirmed that demographic characteristics such as length of baby, place of residence and order of birth were more important in private facilities whereas mothers complication such as prolonged labour, previous C-section were more significant determinants in public facilities. Moreover, the Cox's model found that only one factor which is included in mothers' complication as fetal distress was independent risk factor for C-section in public facilities. Therefore, as shown in these findings, we have expected the rate of C-section will be higher in public patients than in private patients but the observed result shows the inverse.

In the multivariate analysis, educational level, maternal age and parity were found to be the significant non-clinical factors as the ones being the best efficient models in the logistic model. Our results also confirmed by other studies [38, 39]. The findings of the present study may indicate that educated women tend to delay giving birth, thus increasing their likelihood of having C-section. In the previous study, it was found that mother's education is a proxy of socio-economic variable and it is associated with C-section [40]. In 2001, Ecker et al. [14] cited changes in the childbearing population as a significant cause of the increase of Caesarean birth rates. It is also established that age of

Table 6 Stepwise regression results of the effects of selected characteristics on C-section: Private & Public hospitals

Results of logistic regression by stepwise selection

Most influential variables among selected variables	Private hospital		Most influential variables among selected variables	Public hospital	
	Odds ratio [Exp (β)]	95 % CI		Odds ratio [Exp (β)]	95 % CI
Prolonged Labour			Prolonged Labour		
(No)	1.00		(No)	1.00	
Yes	0.03*	0.01–0.08	Yes	0.21*	0.11–0.27
Length of Baby: cm			Previous C-section		
(<45)	1.00		(No)	1.000	
45+	0.17*	0.03–0.41	Yes	7.74*	4.12–9.36
Residence			Mother's Education		
(Rural)	1.00		(Primary and below)	1.00	
Urban	4.07*	1.31–10.11	Secondary	1.43	1.10–2.73
			Higher	2.59*	1.82–5.93
Order of Birth					
(1)	1.00				
2	0.89*	0.23–1.21	Constant	0.36*	0.12–1.67
3+	0.23*	0.12–1.54			
Constant	8.64*	2.54–16.82			

Results of Cox's regression by stepwise selection

Most influential variables among selected variables	Private hospital		Most influential variables among selected variables	Public hospital	
	Hazard ratio [Exp (β)]	95 % CI		Hazard ratio [Exp (β)]	95 % CI
Mother's Age: years			Mother's Age: years		
(<20)	1.00		(<20)	1.00	
20–24	1.04*	0.57–2.14	20–24	1.37*	0.65–2.36
25–29	1.31*	0.45–2.21	25–29	2.17*	1.15–3.87
30+	2.25*	1.20–4.12	30+	2.57*	1.36–4.13
Age at Marriage: years			Age at Marriage: years		
(<18)	1.00		(<18)	1.00	
18–22	1.67*	1.02–3.25	18–22	0.61*	0.32–1.19
23+	2.35*	1.26–4.36	23+	1.21*	0.49–2.58
Order of Birth			Order of Birth		
(1)	1.00		(1)	1.00	
2	0.38*	0.04–1.13	2	0.65*	0.13–1.21
3+	0.23*	0.11–1.10	3+	0.41*	0.18–1.20
Fetal Distress			Fetal Distress		
(No)	Not found		(No)	1.00	
Yes			Yes	1.51*	0.84–3.10

*$P < 0.05$, significant risk factors in the model; CI = confidence interval; parentheses indicate the reference categories

mother is closely related to C-section [40]. Nassar & Sullivan [45] suggested that age and parity (order of birth) alone account for most demographic changes because there is a high primary caesarean rate for first birth to women 30 years age and older. Mothers with low birth order who undergo C-section, explained that the choice were made mainly because of their greater risk of pregnancy and delivery-related complications [37, 43, 44]. Therefore, it has been suggested that delivery by caesarean birth is a complicated health issue on a country level and also a global perspective. In addition, place of residence is one of the most important factors in determining whether to perform a C-section in private or public hospital, which is consistent with the findings of other studies [41, 44] have also found that there is a strong association between C-section and place of residence. It seems that women residing in urban areas of the northern region were more likely to undergo C-section in private hospitals. This indicates the importance of social status in determining the type of delivery and also pertains to issues related to disparities in the distribution of health facilities in the country with respect to several studies [45]. Furthermore, numerous socio-economic and cultural factors influence the decision on pattern of feeding and balance diet that may influence the type of delivery. As a point of view, duration of taking balanced diet was considered as an independent variable and the study found that irregular intake of a balanced diet is a significant determinant for caesarean delivery from logistic regression analysis. As also previously mentioned, the significant non-clinical factor found in this study was age at marriage. Therefore, it may indicate that adding more proteins, carbohydrate, vitamins in daily intake will be more beneficial for pregnant women to avoid C-section and decreasing late marriage of the study population for C-section.

Conclusion

The above discussion leads to the conclusion that delivery by C-section is a complicated health issue. Efforts to reduce C-section birth in developing countries like the northern region of Bangladesh will require a comprehensive approach to address patients' variables, caregiver practices and hospital policies. In order to address the reduction of caesarean rate in the northern region, significant factors such as previous C-section, prolonged labour, maternal educational level, age at marriage, mother's age of more than 25 years, low birth order, length of baby more than 45 cm and irregular intake of a balanced diet can be considered to be predictors for C-section. Finally, from the statistical point of view, this study also suggests that these factors may influence the health-seeking behavior of women. Additionally, for determinants of risk factors, the evaluation criteria on AIC, this study imply that logistic regression model can be lead to more precise results as an alternative for the Cox model. Thus, the following steps may be recommended in view of the observed findings:

i. In the study we found that the rate of caesarean delivery is lower in public hospitals than private hospitals. Therefore, medical audit, quality assessment and supportive supervision should be considered to improve the quality of care in a private hospital that is likely to minimize C-section rate.

ii. The result also shows that less than 19 years and more than 25 years old of mothers age are at higher pregnancy risks for C-section. Thus, age group 20 to 24 should be safer for normal delivery. However,

future research should review maternal age when examining predictors of caesarean birth.

iii. Encouraging pregnant women to take a balanced and nutritional diet may be beneficial.

iv. Health awareness and educational programs should be given to focus on educating women, on appropriate delivery types when their health and specific status will be known.

v. Provide complete and reliable information to the mothers so that they do not opt for C-section in a state of panic or ignorance.

vi. Universities and schools who educate health team (doctors, midwives, and nurses) offer topic that directly deal with this subject.

vii. Further research at the national level with other medical procedures is highly recommended to figure out the extent of this problem in Northern region of Bangladesh.

viii. Moreover, Government should be given more attention to monitor hospital data and corresponding strategies.

Competing interests
The authors declare that they have no competing interest.

Authors' contributions
MR executed the questionnaire design, testing of interventions, analyzed data and prepared the manuscript. AAS, AS and RS participated in intervention development, editing, additional ideas and analysis activities. RMT contributed to subsequent modifications, designed and executed the overall research study. All authors contributed to the drafting of the paper and approved the final submitted version. MR, AAS and RMT are the guarantors. All authors had full access to all the data in the study, including statistical reports and tables, and can take responsibility for the integrity of the data and the accuracy of the data analysis.

Acknowledgments
We wish to thank the University of Malaya for the financial assistance in this project under UMRG grant (RG105-10AFR).

Author details
[1]University of Rajshahi, Rajshahi, Bangladesh. [2]Centre for Foundation Studies in Science, University of Malaya, Kuala Lumpur, Malaysia. [3]Department of Geography, Faculty of Arts and Social Sciences, University of Malaya, Kuala Lumpur, Malaysia. [4]Department of Obstetrics and Gynaecology, Faculty of Medicine, University of Malaya, Kuala Lumpur, Malaysia.

References
1. Kabir MA, Goh K-L, Khan MMH, Al-Amin AQ, Azam MN. Safe delivery practices: experience from cross-sectional data of Bangladeshi women. Asia Pac J Public Health. 2012 (on line published: http://aph.sagepub.com/content/early/2012/02/23/1010539512437401).
2. Bangladesh Demographic and Health Survey (BDHS). Dhaka, Bangladesh: Mitra and associates. 2011.
3. BMMS. Bangladesh maternal mortality and health care survey 2010: summary of key findings and implications. Dhaka, Bangladesh. 2010. 1–12.
4. Gomes UA, Silva AA, Bettiol H, Barbieri MA. Risk factors for the increasing caesarean section rate in Southeast Brazil: a comparison of two birth cohorts, 1978–1979 and 1994. Int J Epidemio. 1999;28:687–94.
5. Leung GM, Lam TH, Thach TQ, Wan S, Ho LM. Rates of caesarean birth in Hong Kong: 1987–1999. Birth. 2001;28:166–72.

6. Kassak KM, Ali AM, Abduallah AM. Opting for caesarean: what determines the decision? J Public Admin Manage. 2009;14(1):100–22.

7. Belizán JM, Althabe F, Barros FC, Alexander S, Showalter E, Griffin A, et al. Rates and implications of caesarean sections in Latin America: ecological study. Br Med J. 1999;319:1397–400.

8. Murray SF. Relation between private health insurance and high rates of caesarean section in Chile: qualitative and quantitative study. Br Med J. 2000;321:1501–5.

9. Martin JA, Park MM, Sutton PD. Births: preliminary data for 2001. National Vital Statistical Report. 2002;50:1–20.

10. Ravindran J. Rising caesarean section rates in public hospitals in Malaysia 2006. Med J Malaysia. 2008;63(5):434–5.

11. World Health Organization (WHO). Appropriate technology for birth. Lancet. 1985;2:436–7.

12. Savage W. The caesarean section epidemic. J Obstet Gynaecol. 2000;20:223–5.

13. Parrish KM, Holt VL, Easterling TR, Connell FA, LoGerfo JP. Effect of changes in maternal age, parity, and birth weight distribution on primary caesarean delivery rates. J Am Med Assoc. 1994;271:443–7.

14. Ecker JL, Chen KT, Cohen AP, Riley LE, Lieberman ES. Increased risk of caesarean delivery with advancing maternal age: indications and associated factors in nulliparous women. Am J Obstet Gynaecol. 2001;185:883–7.

15. Peipert JF, Bracken MB. Maternal age: an independent risk factor for caesarean delivery. Obstet Gynaecol. 1993;81:200–5.

16. Mossialos E, Allin S, Karras K, Davaki K. An investigation of caesarean section in three greek hospitals: the impact of financial incentives and convenience. Eur J Public Health. 2005;15:288–95.

17. Cnattingius R, Cnattingius S, Notzon FC. Obstacles to reducing caesarean rates in a low-caesarean setting: the effect of maternal age, height, and weight. Obstet Gynaecol. 1998;92(4 Pt 1):501–6.

18. Gould JB, Davey B, Stafford RS. Socioeconomic differences in rates of caesarean section. N Engl J Med. 1989;321:233–9.

19. Skalkidis Y, Petridou F, Papathoma E, Revinthi K, Tong D, Trichopoulos D. Are operative delivery procedures in Greece socially conditioned? Int J Qual Health Care. 1996;8:159–65.

20. Parazzini F, Pirotta N, La Vecchia C, Fedele L. Determinants of caesarean section rates in Italy. BJOG: Int J Obstet Gynaecol. 1992;99:203–6.

21. Tatar M, Gunalp S, Somunoglu S, Demirol A. Women's perceptions of caesarean section: reflections from a Turkish teaching hospital. Soc Sci Med. 2000;50:1227–33.

22. Hurst M, Sumney PS. Childbirth and social class: the case of caesarean delivery. Soc Sci Med. 1984;18:621–31.

23. Taffel SM. Caesarean delivery in the United States, 1990. Vital Health Statistics. 1994;51:1–24.

24. Spaans WA, Sluijs MB, Van Roosmalen J, Bleker O. Risk factors at caesarean section and failure of subsequent trial of labour. Eur J Obstet Gynaecol Reprod Biol. 2002;100:163–6.

25. Lynch CM, Kearney R, Turner MJ. Maternal morbidity after elective repeat caesarean section after two or more previous procedures. Eur J Obstet Gynaecol Reprod Biol. 2002;4320:1–4.

26. Signorelli C, Cattaruzza MS, Osborn JF. Risk factors for caesarean section in Italy: results of a multicentre study. Public Health. 1995;109:191–9.

27. Wilkinson C, McIlwaine G, Boulton-Jones C, Cole S. Is a rising caesarean section rate inevitable? BJOG: Int J Obstet Gynaecol. 1998;105:45–52.

28. Hall M. When a woman asks for a caesarean section. Br Med J. 1987;294:201–2.

29. Mould TA, Chong S, Spencer JAD, Gallivan S. Women's involvement with the decision preceding their caesarean section and their degree of involvement. BJOG: Int J Obstet Gynaecol. 1996;103:1074–7.

30. Shearer EL. Caesarean section: medical benefits and costs. Soc Sci Med. 1993;37:1223–31.

31. Barros FC, Vaughan JP, Victora CG, Huttly SR. Epidemic of caesarean sections in Brazil. Lancet. 1991;338:167–9.

32. Bertollini R, DiLallo D, Spadea T, Perucci C. Caesarean section rates in Italy by hospital payment mode: an analysis based on birth certificates. Am J Public Health. 1992;82:257–61.

33. Sufang G, Padmadas SS, Fengmin Z, Brown JJ, Stones RW. Delivery settings and caesarean section rates in China. Bulletin of World Health Org, Geneva. 2007;85:10.

34. Mishra US, Ramanathan M. Delivery-related complications and determinants of caesarean section rates in India. Health Policy Plan. 2002;17:90–8.

35. Therneau T, Grambsch P. Modelling survival data: extending the cox model. New York: Springer-Verlag; 2000. p. 14.

36. Green MS, Symons MJ. A comparison of the logistic risk function and the proportional hazards model in prospective epidemiological studies. J Chron Dis. 1983;36(10):715–24.

37. Khawaja M, Jurdi R, Kabakian T. Rising trends in caesarean section rates in Egypt. Birth. 2004;31(1):12–6.

38. Parkhurst JO, Rahman SA. Life saving or money wasting? Perceptions of caesarean sections among users of services in rural Bangladesh. Health Policy. 2007;80:392–401.

39. Abu-Heija AT, Jallad MF, Abukteish F. Obstetrics and prenatal outcome for pregnancies after the age of 45. J Obstet Gynaecol. 1999;19:486–8.

40. Padmadas S, Kumar S, Nair S, Kumari A. Caesarean section delivery in Kerala, India: evidence from a national family health survey. Soc Sci Med. 2000;51:511–21.

41. Nassar N, Sullivan E. Australia's Mothers and Babies, 1999, AIHW Cat. no. PER19, Perinatal Statistics Series no. 11, AIHW National Perinatal Statistics Unit, Sydney. 2001.

42. Webster L, Daling J, Mcfarlane C, Ashley D, Warren C. Prevalence and determinants of caesarean section in Jamaica. J Bio Sci. 1992;24:515–25.

43. Stanton CK, Holtz SA. Levels and trends in caesarean birth in the developing world. Stud Fam Plann J. 2006;37(1):41–8.

44. Villar J, Valladares E, Wojdyla D, Zavaleta N, Carroli G, Velazco A, et al. Caesarean delivery rates and pregnancy outcomes: the 2005 WHO global survey on maternal and prenatal health in Latin America. Lancet. 2006;367(9525):1819–29.

45. Chaudhury N, Hammer JS. Ghost doctors: absenteeism in Bangladesh health facilities, Policy Research Working Paper. Washington, D.C: World Bank; 2003. p. 3065.

High risk of malnutrition associated with depressive symptoms in older South Africans living in KwaZulu-Natal, South Africa: a cross-sectional survey

I. Naidoo[1], Karen E. Charlton[2]* (iD), TM Esterhuizen[3] and B. Cassim[1]

Abstract

Background: Malnutrition contributes to functional and cognitive decline in older adults, which results in decreased quality of life and loss of independence. This study aimed to identify determinants of nutritional risk among community-dwelling adults in KwaZulu-Natal, South Africa.

Methods: A cross-sectional survey was undertaken in 1008 subjects aged 60 years and over who were randomly selected by systematic sampling. Demographics, socioeconomic data and self-reported history of medical conditions were recorded. The Mini Nutritional Assessment-Short Form (MNA-SF) was used to screen for nutritional risk, and the Centre for Epidemiologic Studies Depression scale was administered to all subjects. Descriptive statistics and the Pearson chi-square and Kruskal-Wallis tests were used for statistical analysis. Logistic regression modelling determined predictors of nutritional risk.

Results: Of the 984 participants (mean age = 68.8 ± 7.4 years; range 60–103 years) who completed the MNA-SF, 51 % were classified as having a normal nutritional status, 43.4 % at risk for malnutrition and 5.5 % classified as malnourished. Men were more likely to be either at risk for malnutrition or be malnourished than women ($p = 0.008$), as were subjects with a monthly household income of ≤R1600 per month (~133 USD) ($p = 0.003$). In logistic regression models, depressed people were 2.803 ($p < 0.001$) times more likely to be at risk or be malnourished than those not depressed.

Conclusion: A high prevalence of risk of malnutrition was identified in older South Africans living in an urban area with poor infrastructure. Further investigations are warranted to determine whether the higher prevalence of depressive symptomatology in nutritionally at risk individuals is a determinant or a consequence of malnutrition, in order to develop targeted nutritional interventions in this age group.

Keywords: Nutrition screening, Mini Nutritional Assessment, Elderly, Urban, African

Background

Worldwide, there is a demographic transition with a rapidly increasing proportion of persons aged 60 years and over. South Africa (SA) has the highest percentage of older persons in sub-Saharan Africa, numbering 3.8 million persons or 7.6 % of the total population in this age group with a projected increase to 4.24 million (9.5 % of population) by the year 2015 [1].

In SA, as in many other developing countries undergoing the socio-demographic transition, health challenges that face the older sector of the population include an increased prevalence of non-communicable diseases, accompanied by a functional and cognitive decline, all of which are aggravated by the dynamic socioeconomic environment in the country [2]. The migration of younger members of rural households to cities in search of employment, combined with the effects of international migration

* Correspondence: karenc@uow.edu.au
[2]School of Medicine, Faculty of Science, Medicine and Health, University of Wollongong, Wollongong, Australia
Full list of author information is available at the end of the article

and the pandemic of HIV/AIDS in the context of wide-spread poverty, has resulted in a change in family structures and an erosion of traditional support systems for vulnerable older persons [1]. As a legacy of the 40 years of apartheid in the country, more than half of older Africans (58 %) have had no formal education while 13 % of elderly headed households consisting of a single room, a backyard shack or an informal structure [1]. Notably, the HIV/AIDS pandemic has resulted in a significant loss of younger persons, the consequences of which have led to a loss of principal sources of financial and material support for older persons. This has resulted in the preponderance of multigenerational households that are headed by older women, who are often primary caregivers for their grandchildren [1].

Given the socioeconomic hardships of older Africans, it is not surprising that this group may be at particular nutritional risk. Even in high-income countries, malnutrition is a frequent problem in persons aged 65 years and older [3]. Global estimates of malnutrition indicate a prevalence of 22.8 %, with considerable differences between health and residential settings (rehabilitation, 50.5 %; hospital, 38.7 %; residential aged care, 13.8 %; community, 5.8 %) [3]. In community-dwelling older adults, an additional 32 % of this group is classified as at risk of malnutrition [3]. It is well documented that socioeconomic status, physiological changes of ageing, the burden of chronic diseases and medications [4], together with a decline in functional status, and psychosocial and psychiatric factors adversely influence nutritional status [5]. In turn, malnutrition also contributes to functional [6] and cognitive decline, sarcopenia, diminished immunity, an increased susceptibility to disease as well as a decreased quality of life [7] and an overall higher mortality [8, 9].

Few studies have investigated the nutritional status of older Africans [10, 11]. Between 43 and 50 % of elderly headed South-African households have been reported to experience food poverty whereby they are unable to afford a basic subsistence diet to meet the needs of household members [12]. Rural households and those with a higher number of occupants were more likely to experience food poverty compared to those in urban areas and those comprising only one or two people.

While a number of different methods have been used to assess nutritional status, including anthropometry, biochemical indicators and dietary intake, there is no single ideal measurement for defining malnutrition in the elderly. Anthropometric measures include body mass index (BMI) and mid-upper arm circumference (MUAC). The accuracy of conventional BMI measurement may be compromised due to changes in body composition and kyphosis in older persons [13], while the MUAC is a relatively insensitive measure. Specialized laboratory services required for the biochemical and haematological biomarkers related to malnutrition are often prohibitively expensive and not practical for community-based studies, while dietary intake assessments rely on memory recall from older adults.

The Mini Nutritional Assessment (MNA) comprises four domains that include anthropometry, general assessment, a short dietary assessment and a subjective health assessment. The MNA has been validated in older persons in many countries [14] and has been shown to correlate with clinical indicators and detailed biochemistry. The MNA has a high sensitivity and specificity and is able to detect an increased risk of malnutrition, even when albumin and BMI are in the normal range. The MNA-Short Form (MNA-SF) was subsequently developed to allow a two-step process in low-risk populations, while retaining the validity of the full MNA [15]. The short form version takes 5 min to complete and has been shown to be a reliable and efficient screening tool for community-dwelling elderly patients.

KwaZulu-Natal (KZN), one of the nine provinces in SA, is home to 19.6 % of the total number of persons aged 60 years and over in the country. Most older South Africans subsist on a government old age pension [16] which was R1010 (approximately 84 USD) per month at the time of the current survey. The present study was undertaken to identify the risk of malnutrition in older persons in KZN and to determine its association with other health parameters.

Methods
Study design and sampling
A cross-sectional design was used for this study which was conducted in the Inanda, Ntuzuma and KwaMashu (INK) areas of KwaZulu-Natal, SA. According to the 2001 general census [17], 18,812 persons aged 60 years resided in the study area. Using a conservative prevalence estimate of 50 % for a chronic disease, disability or impairment, a sample size of $n = 1010$ was estimated, using a confidence level of 95 % and a precision level of 3 %. A two-staged sampling method was used. Firstly, the sample was distributed proportionately within the wards of Inanda, KwaMashu and Ntuzuma and within formal and informal dwellings in each of the three areas. Thereafter, systematic sampling was used at the level of the street/tract to identify respondents who met the inclusion criteria. The starting points were randomly selected and defined using global positioning system (GPS) coordinates for both formal and informal areas. Starting at the predefined points, skip method was used to identify households. The process continued on street or tract (for informal areas) until a maximum of 25 % of the quota for that segment of the ward was obtained, before the process was repeated on another street/tract. At

household level, eligible persons who were 60 years and older were identified, and one person was randomly selected using a Kish grid.

Inclusion criteria included age 60 years and over and the ability to speak and understand English or IsiZulu and to give informed consent. A detailed questionnaire was administered by trained fieldworkers and included demographic and socioeconomic data (educational level (classified as none, primary, secondary and tertiary) and household income), as well as information on housing structure, and household composition. The CAGE questionnaire was used to assess risk of alcohol abuse [18]. To determine the presence of chronic diseases, subjects were asked "Has a doctor or other health professional ever told you that you have any of the following?" from a list of common medical conditions.

To assess oral health, a response of very often, often, sometimes and never was recorded in response to the question "In the last six months how often did you have to avoid eating certain foods because of problems with your mouth, teeth or dentures?" The Centre for Epidemiologic Studies Depression (CESD) scale was completed for all subjects, and scores were categorized as normal (<16) or having depressive symptomatology (≥16) [19].

The MNA-SF was used to categorize subjects as having normal nutrition (score >12), being at risk of malnutrition (10–12) or being malnourished (<10) [20]. Physical activity was assessed by asking whether subjects walked outside, worked in their gardens and/or performed light or heavy household tasks. Food insecurity was assessed by a single question "How often does your household run out of food?" Responses provided as "often" and "about half the time" were classified as indicating food insecurity.

Ethical approval was obtained from the Biomedical and Research Ethics Committee of University of KwaZulu-Natal.

Data analysis

Data were encoded to ensure anonymity and were double captured and entered into a database supported by Epi-Info 2000. SPSS version 15.0 (SPSS Inc., Chicago, Illinois) was used to analyze the data. A two-tailed p value of <0.05 was considered as statistically significant. The demographic characteristics of the study population and the nutritional status are described using frequency tables, percentages and 95 % confidence intervals and displayed graphically using bar charts. Quantitative variables are summarized using summary statistics, and the Pearson chi-square and Kruskal-Wallis tests were used to determine the association between the demographic characteristics, socioeconomic status, prevalence of chronic diseases, alcohol intake, physical maintenance scales and oral health, and nutritional status. A backward stepwise logistic regression method based on likelihood ratios, with entry and removal probabilities set at 0.05 and 0.1, respectively, was used to generate models that predicted either being classified as at risk of malnutrition or being malnourished (binary variable) compared to being well nourished. Variables entered into the models were identified as being significant in bivariate analyses.

Results

Of the 1010 subjects enrolled in the study, two subjects did not meet the age criterion and were excluded. Complete details on the MNA-SF were available in 984 subjects (20 of the 24 individuals without full MNA-SF details were unable to have height and weight measurements taken because of being bedridden or unable to stand). The majority 978 (99.4 %) were African with 6 (0.6 %) being of mixed ancestry. Most (97.1 %) were in receipt of a government old age pension. The demographic and socioeconomic characteristics of the study subjects are shown in Table 1. Fifty-one percent ($n = 503$) of participants were classified as being well nourished, 43.4 % were considered to be at risk of malnutrition ($n = 427$) and 5.5 % as malnourished ($n = 54$). According to BMI categories, 18 (1.8 %) subjects were classified as

Table 1 Characteristics of the study population n (%)

	Men $n = 224$	Women $n = 760$	Total $N = 984$
Age (mean ± SD years)	68.0 (7.2)	69.0 (7.4)	68.9 ± 7.4
Range	60–91	60–94	60–94
Marital status			
Widowed	52 (23.2 %)	369 (48.9 %)	434 (44.1 %)
Never married	37 (16.5 %)	217 (28.7 %)	258 (26.2 %)
Married	106 (47.3 %)	102 (13.5 %)	211 (21.4 %)
Separated/divorced	13 (5.8 %)	55 (7.3 %)	81 (8.2 %)
Household Income			
<R1600	136 (61.3 %)	505 (66.7 %)	641 (65.5 %)
≥R1600	86 (38.7 %)	252 (33.3 %)	338 (34.5 %)
No. of persons in household			
Median	5.0	5.0	5.0
Range	1–20	1–16	1–20
Number of households with grandchildren	126 (56.3 %)	588 (77.4 %)	735 (72.9 %)
Housing type			
Formal	122 (54.7 %)	440 (58.0 %)	520 (53.6 %)
Informal	101 (45.3 %)	319 (42.0 %)	451 (46.4 %)
Level of education			
No education	51 (22.8 %)	203 (26.7 %)	254 (25.8 %)
Primary level only	95 (42.4 %)	308 (40.6 %)	403 (41.0 %)
Secondary level	77 (34.4 %)	231 (30.4 %)	308 (31.3 %)
Tertiary level	1 (0.4 %)	17 (2.2 %)	18 (1.8 %)

undernourished (BMI ≤ 18.5 kg/m^2), 196 (19.9 %) as desirable (BMI 18.5–24.9 kg/m^2), 298 (30.3 %) as overweight (BMI 25–29.9 kg/m^2) and 472 (48.0 %) as obese (BMI ≥ 30 kg/m^2). There was no significant difference in categorization of nutritional risk, according to age categories ($X^2 = 5.4$, df = 10, $p = 0.857$). Men were more likely to be either at risk for malnutrition or malnourished than women (58 % compared to 46.2 %; $X^2 = 9.76$, df = 2, $p = 0.008$), as were subjects with a monthly household income of less than or equal to R1600 (approximately 133 USD) compared to those with an income above R1600 ($X^2 = 11.714$, df = 2, $p = 0.003$), (Tables 2 and 3). Fifty-eight percent of respondents were classified as being food insecure (23.5 % reported often running out of food; 32.5 % reported about half the time); however, these participants did not have a higher prevalence of being at risk of malnutrition compared to those that were food secure. Fifty-eight percent of respondents were classified as being food insecure (23.5 % reported often running out of food; 32.5 % reported about half the time).

There was no association between nutritional status (MNA category) and having more than five persons in the household ($X^2 = 2.402$, df = 2, $p = 0.301$), whether there were grandchildren in the household or not ($X^2 = 0.602$, df = 2, $p = 0.740$), nor with level of education ($X^2 = 5.936$, df = 6, $p = 0.430$).

Of the 109 subjects (10.8 % of total sample) who reported consuming alcohol, 62 (56.9 %) had a CAGE score of <2 and 47 (43.1 %) a CAGE score of ≥ 2, but this did not differ across nutritional risk categories ($X^2 = 4.28$, df = 2, $p = 0.118$). Sixty-three percent of subjects reported attending regular social activities and meetings with a trend for those not participating in social activities being more likely to be malnourished ($X^2 = 17.880$, df = 10, $p = 0.057$). Subjects who did not walk outside were more likely to be at risk for malnutrition or malnourished compared to those who did ($X^2 = 15.5$, df = 2, $p < 0.001$). Five hundred and nine subjects (51.7 %) had poor oral health as defined by having to avoid eating certain foods (often or very often) in the past 6 months because of problems with their mouth, teeth or dentures. These participants were not more likely to be at risk for malnutrition/malnourished, compared to those subjects who did not report oral problems ($X^2 = 46.2$, df = 6, $p = 0.056$).

Based on the CESD, 487 (49.5 %) of subjects had depressive symptoms. Of those characterized as being well nourished, 189 (37.6 %) were depressed; of those at risk of malnutrition, 255 (59.7 %) were depressed; and of the malnourished, 43 (79.6 %) were depressed ($X^2 = 66.0$, df = 2, $p = <0.001$).

Two logistic regression models were identified. For model 1, variables entered into a backward stepwise model were age, gender, income, household size, poor oral health, walking outside to the shops and performing heavy household tasks. The following variables remained in the final model: gender, income, household size and walking outside to the shops. Males were 1.68 times more at risk than females, those with income below R1600 were 1.43 times more at risk, those with larger household sizes were 1.32 times more at risk and those who do not walk outside to the shops were 1.9 times more at risk than those who did. In model 2, depression was added and the adjusted odds ratio for at risk/malnutrition in depressed people was 2.8 ($p < 0.001$). In this model, household size and income were no longer associated with malnutrition (Table 4).

Table 2 Demographic and socioeconomic characteristics according to classification of nutritional risk according to MNA-SF n (% MNA-SF category)

	Nutritional categories of MNA-SF			p value[a]
	Normal	At risk of malnutrition	Malnourished	
Male	42	51.8	6.2	0.008
Female	53.8	41	5.2	
Income <R1600	313 (62.4 %)	282 (66.7 %)	46 (85.2 %)	0.003
Households with >5 persons	244 (48.8 %)	229 (53.8 %)	29 (53.7 %)	0.301
Households with grandchildren	361 (71.8 %)	315 (73.8 %)	38 (70.4 %)	0.740
Informal housing	281 (56.0 %)	257 (60.3 %)	24 (44.4 %)	0.061
Education				
No schooling	137 (27.3 %)	103 (24.1 %)	14 (25.9 %)	0.430
Primary schooling	197 (39.2 %)	189 (44.3 %)	17 (31.5 %)	
Secondary schooling	160 (31.9 %)	126 (29.5 %)	22 (40.7 %)	
Tertiary education	8 (1.6 %)	9 (2.1 %)	1 (1.9 %)	

[a]Pearson chi-square test for differences between categories of MNA-SF for variable

Table 3 Association between MNA-SF nutritional categories and behavioural and clinical indicators, expressed as percentage within each MNA-SF category

		Nutritional categories of MNA-SF, %			p value[b]
		Normal	At risk of malnutrition	Malnourished	
BMI (kg/m^2)					
Undernourished	<18.5	0	2.1	16.7	<0.001
Normal	18.5–24.9	14.7	25.1	27.8	
Overweight	25–29.9	32.4	28.8	22.2	
Obese	≥30	52.9	44.0	33.3	
Poor oral health					
Yes		22.3	27.9	16.7	0.056
Alcohol intake[a]					
CAGE score ≥2		42.6	48.0	0	0.118
Social networks					
Attended social meetings					0.057
Walked to the shops					
Yes		90.1	85.5	72.2	<0.001
Worked in the garden					
Yes		50.6	56.1	92.9	0.013
Performed light household tasks					
Yes		69.6	66.3	59.3	0.228
Performed heavy household tasks					
Yes		38.0	32.9	24.1	0.057
Depressed					
CESD score ≥16		37.6	59.7	79.6	<0.001
Diagnosed clinical conditions (n (%))					
Hypertension (n = 982)		334 (66.5 %)	269 (63.1 %)	34 (63.0 %)	0.535
Diabetes mellitus (n = 983)		96 (19.1 %)	83 (19.4 %)	14 (25.9 %)	0.485
Stroke (n = 983)		9 (0.9 %)	20 (2.0 %)	1 (1.9 %)	0.033
Arthritis (n = 983)		210 (41.8 %)	155 (36.3 %)	155 (36.3 %)	0.005
Tuberculosis (n = 983)		6 (1.2 %)	6 (1.4 %)	4 (7.4 %)	0.002

[a]n = 109 answered this question
[b]Pearson chi-square test for difference in variables according to MNA-SF categories

Discussion

To our knowledge, this is the largest study to report on the nutritional risk of community-living persons aged 60 years and over from an African country. Using the validated MNA-SF, 43.4 % of participants were considered to be at risk of malnutrition, while 5.5 % had an MNA-SF score that indicates malnutrition. The prevalence of malnutrition is considerably higher than that reported in community-dwelling older populations from higher-income countries [21–24]. In a sample of 22,007 subjects in Spain, a similar prevalence of malnutrition was identified (4.3 %), but a smaller proportion of individuals was characterized as being at risk (25.4 %) [25]. A cross-sectional study conducted in another developing country, India, in 227 participants aged 60 years and

over, found that 14 % were malnourished and 49 % were at risk using the full MNA instrument [26] while in Bangladesh, of the 625 subjects interviewed, 26 % of subjects were malnourished and 55 % were at risk [27]. In both these studies, participants had no income, incurred a high burden of disease, resided in multigenerational households and had poor or no education, all of which were reported as likely contributing factors to low MNA scores. Similarly in a Ugandan study that used BMI to assess nutritional status, 33 % of the subjects aged between 60 and 90 years were classified as malnourished [6]. Ugandan older persons also had no income or government pensions, resided in multigenerational homes and had a high burden of disease. In contrast, most of our study subjects were in receipt of a

Table 4 Logistic regression models for classification of nutritional risk. Outcome variable is "at risk of malnutrition" and "malnourished", according to MNA-SF classification

Variables		B	S.E.	Wald	df	Sig.	OR	95 % CI for OR	
								Lower	Upper
Model 1									
Step 4[a]	Gender: male vs female	.521	.157	11.018	1	.001	1.684	1.238	2.291
	Income: <R1600 vs ≥ R1600	.355	.141	6.300	1	.012	1.425	1.081	1.880
	Household (HH) size: ≥5 vs <5	.280	.134	4.396	1	.036	1.324	1.018	1.720
	Not walking outside to the shops (vs yes)	.643	.200	10.308	1	.001	1.901	1.284	2.815
	Constant	−.621	.152	16.787	1	.000	0.537		
Model 2									
Step 5[b]	Gender: male vs female	.592	.163	13.275	1	.000	1.808	1.315	2.486
	Not walking outside to the shops (vs yes)	.460	.210	4.808	1	.028	1.584	1.050	2.389
	Not performing heavy household tasks (vs yes)	.267	.145	3.417	1	.065	1.307	.984	1.735
	Depressed (vs not depressed)	1.031	.135	58.508	1	.000	2.803	2.153	3.650
	Constant	−.656	.117	31.384	1	.000	.519		

[a]Variables entered in step 1: age, gender, income, HH size, poor oral health, walking outside to the shops, performing heavy household tasks
[b]Variables entered in step 1: age, gender, income, HH size, poor oral health, walking outside to the shops, performing heavy household tasks and depression

non-contributory government-funded old age pension, which may explain, in part, the lower prevalence of nutritional risk.

Determinants of poor nutritional status are varied and numerous. Several studies have shown that older adults are more vulnerable to malnutrition than younger adults due to the presence of multiple pathologies and associated decreased oral intakes [25–27] while other studies have shown no significant association between age and nutritional status [28, 29]. The lack of an age association with nutritional risk in our sample may be related to the age distribution of our sample being mostly between 60 and 64 years and relatively few older participants.

The overall socioeconomic status of subjects was poor; most participants received a monthly pension of R1010 as their principal or only source of income. Subjects living in households with a cumulative income of <R1600 were more likely to have an MNA-SF score that indicates nutritional risk. This is consistent with findings of other studies conducted in SA [12, 30]. Other socio-demographic characteristics, including household size, living in a multigenerational household and level of education, were not associated with an MNA-SF score.

Decreased physical activity can impact on nutritional status by limiting the ability of an older person to produce, acquire and/or prepare food. In this study, subjects who reported that they did not walk to the shop were more at risk of malnutrition or malnourished, as has been reported by others [6].

The lack of an association between poor oral health and malnutrition is inconsistent with findings from other studies [28, 29, 31]. A Brazilian study found that poor oral health, defined as edentulism without denture-wearing, was more likely to be associated with unfavourable body mass, both underweight (OR = 3.94; 1.14–13.64) and overweight/obesity (OR = 2.88; 1.12–7.40), taking into account confounders of physical activity and depressive symptomatology [32]. In our sample, poor oral health was self-reported by over half of participants but was not predictive of nutritional risk, presumably because of more important overriding socioeconomic determinants. The South African Demographic and Health Survey [27] reported that 36 % of participants had oral health problems, and these were more common in older persons and those with lower educational and income levels. In a later study, while 76.3 % of South African adults aged 16+ years rated their oral health as good, only 38.1 % of those aged 65+ years rated their oral health as good [28]. In that study, participants who had no education or were unemployed were also more likely to have oral problems. The high prevalence of oral/dental problems in SA is thought to be due to poor access to dental care especially in the public sector, where it is estimated that there are approximately only 0.004 dentists per 1000 population [29].

Depression has been shown to be a major determinant of malnutrition in older adults [33]. Depressive symptomatology was strongly associated with suboptimal nutritional status in the present study, and inclusion of this variable in regression models negated the effect of socio-demographic influences. Whether this is a cause or effect is unclear.

Food insecurity was reported by over half of the study population, as has been reported in another South-African study [34]. Although these households were more likely to have a higher total monthly income, they comprised more household members and had a greater proportion of inhabitants being classified as depressed or being at risk for excessive alcohol intake.

Our study has a number of limitations. Data related to components of the MNA-SF was self-reported and may either over- or under-represent the presence of risk factors included within the screening instrument. Height and weight were measured but not available for 20 participants who were bedridden and who may have been more likely to be nutritionally compromised. Thus, the prevalence of malnutrition may have been under-reported. Lastly, food insecurity was assessed using a single question, and this may have been insensitive in a population of low socioeconomic status.

Conclusions

In this community-based study, more than half of older adults were considered to be at risk of malnutrition or malnourished. These findings highlight a need for nutritional screening to be included in primary care settings and followed up with appropriate clinical pathways and referral systems, particularly to mental health services.

Competing interests

This study was supported by a research grant from the South African Netherlands Research Programme on Alternatives in Development (SANPAD). The authors declare that they have no competing interests.

Authors' contributions

BC and KC contributed to the study design. BC was responsible for data collection and overseeing the fieldwork and data entry and analysis. KC interpreted the data and took responsibility for the manuscript. IN wrote the first draft of the manuscript. TE performed statistical analyses. All authors contributed to editing the manuscript. All authors read and approved the final manuscript.

Acknowledgements

The INK Area Based Management and INK area community members are thanked for their involvement in the study.

Author details

[1]Department of Geriatrics, University of KwaZulu-Natal, Durban, South Africa. [2]School of Medicine, Faculty of Science, Medicine and Health, University of Wollongong, Wollongong, Australia. [3]Centre for Evidence Based Health Care, Department of Interdisciplinary Health Sciences, Faculty of Medicine and Health Sciences, Stellenbosch University, Stellenbosch, South Africa.

References

1. Lombard A, Kruger E. Older persons: the case of South Africa. Ageing Int. 2009;34:119–35.
2. Ataguba JE, Akazili J, McIntyre D. Socioeconomic-related health inequality in South Africa: evidence from General Household Surveys. Int J Equity Health. 2011;10(1):48. doi:10.1186/1475-9276-10-48.
3. Kaiser M, Bauer JM, Rämsch C, Uter W, Guigoz Y, Cederholm T, et al. Frequency of malnutrition in the elderly: a multinational perspective using the Mini Nutritional Assessment (MNA®). J Am Ger Soc. 2010;58(9):1734–8.
4. Roe D. Medications and nutrition in the elderly. Prim Care. 1994;21(1):135–47.
5. BAPEN. The executive summary of the 'MUST' report [Online]. Available: http://www.bapen.org.uk/must_report.html 2003. Accessed 03/03/2015.
6. Kikafunda J, Lukwago FB. Nutritional status and functional ability of the elderly age 60–90 years in the Mpigi district of Central Uganda. Nutrition. 2005;21:59–66.
7. Millen B. Preventive nutrition services for the aging population. Springer, 1999: p. 121–132.
8. Charlton KE, Nichols C, Batterham M, Bowden S, Lambert K, Baronne L, et al. Poor nutritional status of older rehabilitation patients predicts clinical outcomes and mortality at 18 months of follow up. Eur J Clin Nutr. 2012;66:1224–8.
9. Charlton K, Batterham M, Bowden S, Ghosh A, Caldwell K, Potter J, et al. A high prevalence of malnutrition in acute geriatric patients predicts adverse clinical outcomes and mortality at 12 months. e-SPEN J. 2013;8:e120–5.
10. Charlton K, Kolbe-Alexander TL, JH N. The MNA, but not the DETERMINE, screening tool is a valid indicator of nutritional status in elderly Africans. Nutrition. 2007;23:533–42.
11. Kimokoti RW, Hamer DH. Nutrition, health, and aging in sub-Saharan Africa. Nutr Rev. 2008;66(11):611–23.
12. Charlton K, Rose D. Nutrition among older adults in Africa: the situation at the beginning of the millennium. Nutrition and Dietetics Unit, Department of Medicine, University of Capetown: Cape Town, South Africa.
13. Pieterse S, Manandhar M, Ismail S. The nutritional status of older Rwandan refugees. Pub Health Nutr. 1998;1:259–64.
14. Guigoz Y, Vellas B, Garry PJ. Assessing the nutritional status of the elderly: the Mini Nutritional Assessment as part of the geriatric evaluation. Nutr Rev. 1996;54:S59–65.
15. Kaiser M, Bauer JM, Rämsch C, Uter W, Guigoz Y, Cederholm T, et al. Validation of the Mini Nutritional Assessment® Short-Form (MNA-SF): a practical tool for identification of nutritional status. J Nutr Health & Aging. 2009;13:782–8.
16. Barrientos, A., Ferreira, M., Gorman, M., Heslop, A., Legido-Quigley, H., Lloyd-Sherlock, P. et al. Noncontributory pensions and poverty prevention: a comparative study of South Africa and Brazil. HelpAge International and Institute for Development Policy and Management, London, UK, 2003.
17. Magnusson R, Reeve B. 'Steering' private regulation? A new strategy for reducing population salt intake in Australia. Sydney Law Review. 2014;36(2):255–89.
18. Ewing A. Detecting alcoholism: the CAGE questionnaire. JAMA. 1984;252:1905–7.
19. Radloff, L., Centre for Epidemiologic Studies, N.I.o.M. Health, Editor, West Publishing Company.
20. A guide to completing the MNA-SF, Nestle Nutrition Institute. Available at: http://www.mna-elderly.com/forms/mna_guide_english_sf.pdf. Accessed 7/10/2015.
21. Winter J, Flanagan D, McNaughton SA, Nowson C. Nutrition screening of older people in a community general practice, using the MNA-SF. J Nutr Health Aging. 2013;17:322–5.
22. Nykänen I, Lönnroos E, Kautiainen H, Sulkava R, Hartikainen S. Nutritional screening in a population-based cohort of community-dwelling older people. Eur J Public Health. 2013;23:405–9.
23. Timpini A, Facchi E, Cossi S, Ghisla MK, Romanelli G, Marengoni A. Self-reported socio-economic status, social, physical and leisure activities and risk for malnutrition in late life: a cross-sectional population-based study. J Nutr Health Aging. 2011;15:233–8.
24. Ülger Z, Halil M, Kalan I, Yavuz BB, Cankurtaran M, Güngör E, et al. Comprehensive assessment of malnutrition risk and related factors in a large group of community-dwelling older adults. Clin Nutr. 2010;29:507–11.
25. Cuervo M, Garcia A, Ansorena D, Sanchez-Villegas A, Martinez-Gonzalez M, Astiasaran I, et al. Nutritional assessment interpretation on 22,007 Spanish community-dwelling elders through the Mini Nutritional Assessment test. Pub Health Nutr. 2009;1:82–90.
26. Vedantam A, Subramanian V, Rao NV, John KR. Malnutrition in free-living elderly in rural south India: prevalence and risk factors. Pub Health Nutr. 2010;9(13):1328–32.
27. Ferdous T, Kabir ZN, Wahlin A, Streatfield K, Cederholm T. The multidimensional background of malnutrition among rural older individuals in Bangladesh—a challenge for the Millennium Development Goal. Pub Health Nutr. 2009;12(12):2270–8.
28. Soini H, Routasalo P, Lagstrom H. Characteristics of MNA in elderly home care patients. Eur J Clin Nutr. 2004;58:64–70.
29. Iizaka S, Tandaka E, Sandada H. Comprehensive assessment of nutritional factors in the healthy, community dwelling elderly. Geriatric and Gerontology International. 2004;8:24–31.
30. Oldwage-Theron W, Salami L, Zotor FB. Health status of an elderly population in Sharpeville. South Africa Health SA Gesondheid. 2008;13(3):3–17.

High risk of malnutrition associated with depressive symptoms in older South Africans living...

131

31. Lamy M, Mojon P, Kalykakis G, Legrand R, Butz-Jorgensen E. Oral status and nutrition in the institutionalized elderly. J Dent. 1999;6:443–8.
32. Tôrres L, Da Silva DD, Neri AL, Hilgert JB, Hugo FN, Sousa ML. Association between underweight and overweight/obesity with oral health among independently living Brazilian elderly. Nutrition. 2013;29:152–7.
33. Feldblum I, Germa L, Castel H, Harm-Boehm I, Bilenko N. Characteristics of undernourished older medical patients and identification of predictors for an undernourished state. Nutr J. 2007;7:37.
34. Rose D, Charlton KE. Prevalence of household food poverty in South Africa: results from a large, nationally representative survey. Pub Health Nutr. 2002;5(3):383–9.

Socio-economic determinants of household food security and women's dietary diversity in rural Bangladesh: a cross-sectional study

Helen Harris-Fry[1*], Kishwar Azad[2], Abdul Kuddus[2], Sanjit Shaha[2], Badrun Nahar[2], Munir Hossen[2], Leila Younes[1], Anthony Costello[1] and Edward Fottrell[1]

Abstract

Background: There has been limited decline in undernutrition rates in South Asia compared with the rest of Asia and one reason for this may be low levels of household food security. However, the evidence base on the determinants of household food security is limited. To develop policies intended to improve household food security, improved knowledge of the determinants of household food security is required.

Methods: Household data were collected in 2011 from a randomly selected sample of 2,809 women of reproductive age. The sample was drawn from nine unions in three districts of rural Bangladesh. Multinomial logistic regression was conducted to measure the relationship between selected determinants of household food security and months of adequate household food provisioning, and a linear regression to measure the association between the same determinants and women's dietary diversity score.

Results: The analyses found that land ownership, adjusted relative risk ratio (RRR) 0.28 (CI 0.18, 0.42); relative wealth (middle tertile 0.49 (0.29, 0.84) and top tertile 0.18 (0.10, 0.33)); women's literacy 0.64 (0.46, 0.90); access to media 0.49 (0.33, 0.72); and women's freedom to access the market 0.56 (0.36, 0.85) all significantly reduced the risk of food insecurity. Larger households increased the risk of food insecurity, adjusted RRR 1.46 (CI 1.02, 2.09). Households with vegetable gardens 0.20 (0.11, 0.31), rich households 0.46 (0.24, 0.68) and literate women 0.37 (0.20, 0.54) were significantly more likely to have better dietary diversity scores.

Conclusion: Household food insecurity remains a key public health problem in Bangladesh, with households suffering food shortages for an average of one quarter of the year. Simple survey and analytical methods are able to identify numerous interlinked factors associated with household food security, but wealth and literacy were the only two determinants associated with both improved food security and dietary diversity. We cannot conclude whether improvements in all determinants are necessarily needed to improve household food security, but new and existing policies that relate to these determinants should be designed and monitored with the knowledge that they could substantially influence the food security and nutritional status of the population.

Keywords: Household food security, Nutrition assessment, Determinants, MAHFP, Dietary diversity, Bangladesh

* Correspondence: h.fry.11@ucl.ac.uk
[1]UCL Institute for Global Health, 30 Guilford Street, London, WC1N 1EH, UK
Full list of author information is available at the end of the article

Background

Undernutrition is in decline globally [1], yet, in Bangladesh, chronic undernutrition remains high with 24 % of women of reproductive age undernourished [2]. An underlying cause of undernutrition is household food insecurity [1]; Bangladesh has the lowest availability of calories per capita in South Asia [3]. With a projected increase in the incidence of erratic weather events such as flooding and drought, climate change poses particular risks to future domestic agricultural productivity and subsistence-level food production in Bangladesh [4]. To compound this problem, our understanding of the determinants of household food security remains largely theoretical and any policies aimed at improving household food insecurity will be developed from a limited evidence base.

This paper aims to improve our understanding of household food security in Bangladesh. Focussing on rural areas in the districts of Bogra, Faridpur and Moulavibazar we describe the status and socioeconomic determinants of household food security, and the relationship between these determinants, adequacy in household food provisioning and dietary diversity among women of reproductive age.

Methods

Our theoretical framework of the determinants of household food security in Fig. 1 is based on the UNICEF undernutrition framework, which illustrates how food availability, access and utilisation are the three 'pillars' of food security [1], and Pinstrup-Andersen's framework of food security linkages [5]. This framework categorises determinants and enables us to explore variables likely to affect household food security. One determinant is the complex concept of agency, for which we adopt Sen's definition as "what a person is free to do and achieve in pursuit of whatever goals or values he or she regards as important" [6].

Study setting and population

The research was conducted in nine unions of Bogra, Faridpur and Moulavibazar districts in Bangladesh, covering a sample of 2,809 women of reproductive age (15–49 years). Bogra is located to the north of Dhaka in a plain and has fertile soils. The northerly study sites in this district are widely dispersed and human resource capacity is relatively limited. Faridpur is south of Dhaka and features many large rivers that make it susceptible to flooding and make some areas difficult to access. Moulavibazar, in eastern

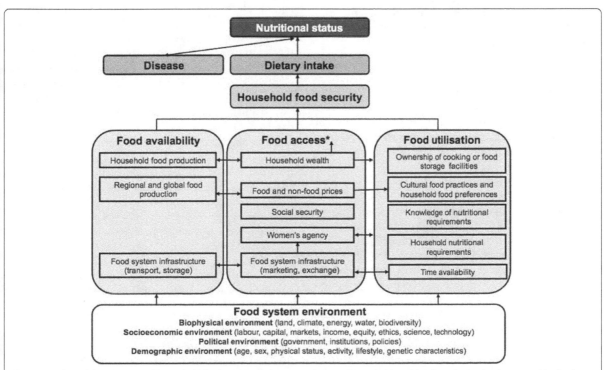

Fig. 1 Hypothetical determinants of household food security and nutritional status. *Household wealth is hypothesised to interact with all other food access determinants. For presentation purposes, the framework does not illustrate how household food security and nutritional status can reciprocally impact upon the determinants; this will need to be explored if attempting to determine causality

Bangladesh, is a hilly district, posing challenges for travel. It is characterised by tea garden estates with tea garden workers who are mostly poor and landless.

The sites were selected based on criteria for cluster randomised controlled trials that were conducted by the Diabetic Association of Bangladesh (BADAS) and University College London and are described elsewhere [7–9]. Briefly, districts were purposively sampled according to their proximity to BADAS offices and, within each district, six unions were randomly allocated to the control or intervention arm, resulting in nine intervention and nine control clusters. The sample described in this paper is women from the control arm where there was no intervention other than low intensity health system strengthening initiatives, and is likely to be more representative of the rural Bangladeshi population.

Sample size and sampling
The random sample of women included in this study represents the control arm sample of a baseline survey taken as part of a formative evaluation of an intervention to improve women's and reproductive health. The sample size of the control arm therefore relates to the intervention sample size and was powered for a quasi-experimental study to be reported elsewhere. Stratified random sampling was used to select the sample from lists of all households with women of reproductive age and children under five.

Data collection
From October to December 2011, 36 trained, local data collectors conducted a cross-sectional survey of women using a piloted structured questionnaire. Data were collected on women's socio-economic status, dietary diversity, knowledge on healthy diets, and women's autonomy and decision-making ability.

Respondents were interviewed in their homes and approximately 10 % of questions from 10 % of the questionnaires were crosschecked by supervisors who revisited the households. Questionnaires were checked for completeness in the district BADAS offices before being sent for data entry at BADAS headquarters in Dhaka. The data were also reviewed at BADAS headquarters by surveillance and data managers and inconsistencies were reported to the district offices for correction or verification. Data were entered into a Microsoft Access database and further checked.

Analysis
Indicators and proxy measures of food security determinants were categorised under food availability, access and utilisation (Fig. 1), and are listed in Table 1.

Indicators of household food security included a measure of household food shortages, Months of Adequate Food Provisioning (MAHFP), and an individual-level Women's Dietary Diversity Score (WDDS). MAHFP is the number of months per year that households reported no food shortages and was calculated according to Food and Nutrition Technical Assistance Project (FANTA) guidelines [10]. WDDS uses the following nine food group indicators: starchy staples, legumes and nuts, dairy, organ meat, eggs, flesh meat and fish, dark green leafy vegetables, other vitamin A-rich vegetables and fruits, and other fruits and vegetables [11]. Respondents reported whether or not they had eaten each food group over the last 24 h.

Socio-demographic variables measured were quality of wall, roof and floor materials in the home, ownership of homestead land and ownership of 22 assets such as electricity, bicycle or sewing machine. We used a Principal Component Analysis (PCA) to derive relative wealth groups, divided into tertiles. Some variables such as ownership of land, livestock and some assets were not included in the PCA because they were hypothesised (in Fig. 1) to be separate determinants of household food security that are independent of wealth.

MAHFP data were not normally distributed, with heaping at 0 and 12 months. Based on this, we deemed a logical categorisation of low, moderate and high food insecurity to be <9, 9–11, and 12 MAHFP respectively. Another study also used this categorisation, based on the assumption that extreme values are meaningful [12]. We used multinomial logistic regression to assess crude associations between the food security determinant variables and MAHFP. Crude associations with WDDS were assessed using linear regression. On the basis that socio-demographic characteristics and food security determinants may confound associations being tested, we controlled for these factors in multivariate regression models adjusting for age, religion and pregnancy status and all other measured food security determinants.

To test for collinearity between variables, we calculated the binary association between variables using an adjusted Wald test and the multivariate variance inflation factors (VIFs).

Analyses were conducted in Stata/IC 12.1 and we used the svyset function with weighting to account for the stratified cluster survey sampling used. Results with a p value of < = 0.05 were considered statistically significant.

Ethics
Ethical approval was obtained from the ethics committees of BADAS, Dhaka, Great Ormond Street Hospital and Institute of Child Health (GOSH-ICH), London. Women who chose to participate in the

Table 1 Indicators and proxy measures of food security determinants

Food security determinant	Indicator or proxy measure	Survey question
		• Response option
Food availability		
Household food production	Ownership of land	Does your household own any land (other than the homestead land)?
		• Yes; No; Don't know
	Ownership of livestock	Does your household own any livestock, farm animals or poultry?
		• Yes; No; Don't know
	Use of vegetable gardens	Does your household grow its own fruits and vegetables in a homestead garden or plot?
		• Yes; No; Don't know
Regional and global food production	Not available	Not available
Food system infrastructure	Not available	Not available
Food access		
Household wealth	Principal Component Analysis	Which of these do you presently have in your household?
		• Electricity; fan; mobile phone; non-mobile phone; fridge; almirah/wardrobe; table; chair/bench; cot/bed; mattress; sewing machine; watch/clock; generator; bicycle; motorcycle/scooter/tempo; animal-drawn cart; car/truck/bus/microbus; boat; rickshaw/van
		What is the main material of the floor in the house where the woman lives? (Record your observation)
		• Earth/sand; wood planks; palm/bamboo; parquet or polished wood; ceramic tiles; cement; carpet; other; don't know.
		What is the main material of the roof in the house where the woman lives? (Record your observation)
		• No roof; thatch/palm leaf; bamboo; wood planks; cardboard; tin; wood; ceramic tiles; cement; stone with lime/cement; roofing shingles; other; don't know.
		What is the main material of the exterior walls in the house where the woman lives? (Record your observation)
		• No walls; cane/palm/trunks/straw; dirt; bamboo/bamboo with mud; stone/stone with mud; plywood; cardboard; tin; cement; stone with lime/cement; bricks; wood planks/shingles; other; don't know.
		Does your household own any homestead? *If no, probe*: Does your household own homestead in any other places?
		• Yes; No; Don't know
Food and non-food prices	Not available	Not available
Social security	Not available	Not available
Women's agency	Freedom for women to always or sometimes access the market by herself	Are you allowed to go to the market/ shops without the company of another adult?
		• Always; sometimes; never allowed to go without company; never allowed to go even with company
	Involvement in decision-making relating to daily household expenditures (by herself or with her husband).	Who has the greatest say in the decision regarding how household money is spent for daily necessities, such as food?
		• Woman; woman and her husband jointly; husband; mother-in-law; father-in-law; mother; father; sister-in-law; brother-in-law; other family members; other; don't know.
Food system infrastructure	Not available	Not available
Ownership of cooking or food storage facilities	Not available	Not available

Table 1 Indicators and proxy measures of food security determinants *(Continued)*

Food utilisation		
Knowledge of nutritional requirements	Knowledge of malnutrition prevention (number of methods named)	What can women do to stay well nourished? What else? Do not prompt. (Multiple answer)
		• Eat adequate amount of nourishing/vitamin rich food every day; eat plenty of vegetables; eat eggs/milk/dairy products; prevent childhood (and early) marriage; prevent adolescent pregnancy; eat more food during pregnancy; adequate rest during pregnancy; prevent frequent pregnancy/space births by more than 2 ½ years; increase food quantity during lactation; maintain hygiene and cleanliness/look after one's health; other (specify); don't know.
	Women's literacy	Can you read this passage for me please?
		(Interviewer to decide the ability level)
		• Easily; with difficulty; cannot read.
	Access to media (ownership of radio or television) Taken from asset score, which is partially used in the PCA.	Which of these do you presently have in your household?
		• Radio/tape recorder; television with cable; television without cable.
Household size	Not available	Not available
Larger household	Number of women of reproductive age in the household	How many women aged 15–49 live in your household?
		• Number of women
Intra-household food distribution and food control	Not available	Not available
Cultural practices and individual practices	Not available	Not available

study gave verbal consent and were free to stop the interview at any time.

Results

We obtained responses from 93 % of the target sample. Reasons for not successfully interviewing the women were because the respondents were not at home, the woman had divorced, or the respondent had died. We were unable to check for response bias due to the lack of data on non-responders. 6.6 % (n 189) of women were excluded from the WDDS analysis because they had celebrated or feasted within the previous 24 h. Reporting of a feast day was not associated with any household characteristics or variables used in the analysis, except households with more than one woman of reproductive age were less likely to report a feast ($\chi^2 = 5.25$, $p = 0.04$). We expect that this is a spurious finding because we cannot identify any rationale for bigger households feasting less, since wealth is not associated. Nevertheless, interpretation of results must be done with the usual caution applied to sample surveys with incomplete response.

Study population characteristics

The study population characteristics are summarised in Table 2. All respondents were women of reproductive age, with a mean age of 30.8 years (SD 8.0; range 15, 49). 90 % of respondents were Muslim; the remaining 10 %

were Hindu. Approximately two thirds of respondents were literate.

Household food security

The percentage of respondents reporting adequate household food provisioning in 2010–11 is displayed by Gregorian months in Fig. 2. The month with the highest proportion (almost one third) of households facing food shortages was Kartik (October to November); in Agrahaiyan (November to December) food shortages fell sharply to 16 %. Over half of respondents reported no food shortages over the year. Of those that did, respondents faced shortages for an average of half of the year and 54.7, 19.1, and 26.2 % of households had 12, 9–11 and <9 months of adequate food provisioning respectively.

Respondents had a mean WDDS of 3.8 (range 1, 9). Consumption of food groups by all women is shown in Fig. 3. There was no significant difference in WDDS or consumption of food groups depending on pregnancy status of women (results not shown).

Food availability determinants

The determinants of food availability are listed in Table 1. Five percent of respondents reported that they owned land. Of those who owned land, respondents owned an average of 0.7 acres (range 0.05, 22.1). Eighty percent of respondents reported owning livestock; farm animals, or

Table 2 Summary of respondent characteristics

Characteristic	Bogra	Faridpur	Moulavibazar	Total % (n)
Total	$n = 818$	$n = 1,163$	$n = 828$	100 $n = 2,809$
Age (years)	$n = 818$	$n = 1,163$	$n = 827$	$n = 2,808$
Mean	30.6 (SD = 8.1)	30.2 (SD = 7.7)	32.8 (SD = 8.2)	30.8 (SD = 8.0)
≤19	7.5 (61)	4.0 (47)	3.0 (25)	5.3 (133)
20–24	18.0 (147)	21.7 (252)	14.1 (117)	18.5 (516)
25–29	24.1 (197)	26.6 (309)	21.6 (179)	24.5 (685)
30–34	18.3 (150)	19.2 (223)	22.1 (183)	19.5 (556)
≥35	32.2 (263)	28.6 (332)	39.1 (324)	32.4 (918)
Religion	$n = 818$	$n = 1,163$	$n = 828$	$n = 2,809$
Islam	93.9 (768)	93.1 (1083)	78.4 (649)	90.3 (2500)
Hindu	6.1 (50)	6.9 (80)	21.6 (179)	9.7 (309)
Pregnancy status	$n = 818$	$n = 1,163$	$n = 828$	$n = 2,809$
Pregnant	5.1 (42)	5.7 (66)	5.0 (41)	5.3 (149)
Not pregnant	94.9 (776)	94.3 (1097)	95.1 (787)	94.7 (2660)
PCA wealth score[a]	$n = 814$	$n = 1,160$	$n = 824$	$n = 2,798$
Lowest tertile	26.3 (214)	34.2 (397)	39.0 (321)	31.9 (932)
Middle tertile	39.7 (323)	28.5 (331)	26.2 (216)	32.8 (870)
Top tertile	34.0 (277)	37.2 (432)	34.8 (287)	35.4 (996)
Mean number of assets owned	7.0 (2.6)	7.0 (3.0)	6.7 (SD = 3.0)	6.9 (SD = 2.8)
Educational status	$n = 818$	$n = 1,163$	$n = 828$	$n = 2,809$
None or less than 1 year	51.3 (420)	56.8 (660)	55.2 (457)	54.1 (1,537)
Primary (any level)	23.5 (192)	18.5 (215)	21.3 (176)	21.2 (583)
Secondary and higher	25.2 (206)	24.8 (288)	23.6 (195)	24.7 (689)
Literacy	$n = 818$	$n = 1,163$	$n = 828$	$n = 2,809$
Cannot read	37.5 (307)	33.6 (391)	36.2 (300)	35.5 (998)
Can read (easily or with difficulty)	62.5 (511)	66.4 (772)	63.8 (528)	64.5 (1,811)

[a]0.04 % missing data for PCA wealth score

poultry and they owned on average 9 animals (range 1, 106). Just over half of respondents reported use of a homestead garden.

Food access determinants

Respondents reported owning an average of 7 (range 0, 16) out of 22 assets, such as electricity or a table.

Women's freedom to shop alone was limited; almost half of respondents were never allowed to shop without company, and 6 % were never allowed to shop, with or without the company of another adult. Sixty three percent of respondents reported that they (alone or with their husband) were the main decision-makers for purchasing daily necessities such as food.

Food utilisation determinants

Respondents could name an average of 2 (range 0, 9) ways for women to stay well-nourished. The commonest methods listed were to eat plenty of vegetables; to eat eggs, milk or dairy products; and to eat an adequate amount of nourishing, vitamin-rich food every day. Most respondents (86 %) thought that women should eat more than usual during pregnancy, and 5 % thought women should eat less. Over one third of respondents reported ownership of a radio or a television.

Analysis of the determinants of MAHFP and WDDS

Testing for collinearity between determinants, we found an expected positive and significant association between relative wealth (PCA score) and land ownership ($F_{1,6} = 132.71$, $p = <0.000$), ownership of livestock ($F_{1,6} = 21.37$, $p = 0.004$) and access to media ($F_{1,6} = 474.80$, $p = <0.000$). However, VIFs were sufficiently low, ranging between 1.03 and 2.16, indicating that the inclusion of the separate determinants in the model is statistically valid.

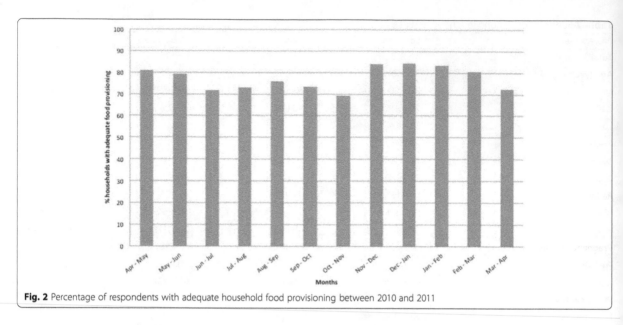

Fig. 2 Percentage of respondents with adequate household food provisioning between 2010 and 2011

Table 3 shows results from crude and adjusted multinomial logistic regression analysis of the associations between measures of food security determinants and MAHFP. Determinants of food availability, access and utilisation were associated with food insecurity. Wealth and land ownership were the strongest protective factors against food insecurity; both factors reduced the risk of low food security by more than 70 % and 80 % respectively. Literacy and access to media also significantly reduced the risk of food insecurity, with the likelihood of low food security being up to a third lower amongst the literate and 50 % lower where households had access to media. The ownership of livestock and the women's freedom to go to the market alone were protective against severe food insecurity but there was no evidence of an association with mild food insecurity. Having more than one woman of reproductive age living in the same

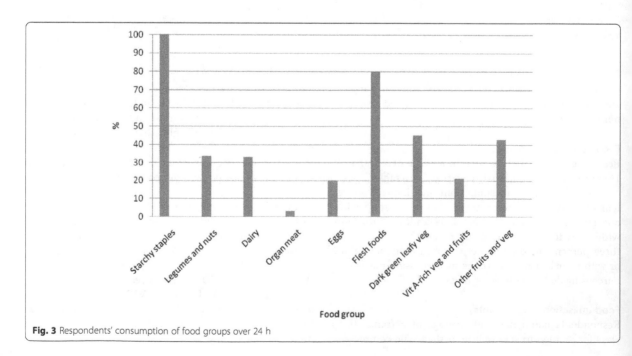

Fig. 3 Respondents' consumption of food groups over 24 h

Table 3 Associations between possible food security determinants and months of adequate household food provisioning

| Possible determinants of MAHFP | Total | MAHFP | Crude[a] | | | | Adjusted[b] | | | |
| | | | Moderate food security | | Low food security | | Moderate food security | | Low food security | |
	Weighted % (n)	mean (95 %CI)	RRR (95 % CI)	p value	RRR (95 % CI)	p value	RRR (95 % CI)	p value	RRR (95 % CI)	p value
Total	(2808)	9.3 (range 0, 12)								
Respondent characteristics										
Age	(2808)		1.03 (1.01, 1.04)	0.007	1.04 (1.03, 1.04)	0.000	1.02 (1.01, 1.04)	0.005	1.04 (1.03, 1.05)	0.000
Religion										
Islam[c]	90.3 (2499)	9.3 (8.2, 10.4)								
Hindu	9.7 (309)	8.9 (7.6, 10.2)	1.16 (0.44, 3.04)	0.715	1.16 (0.57, 2.37)	0.632	1.47 (0.60, 3.65)	0.335	1.31 (0.55, 3.12)	0.481
Pregnancy status										
Not pregnant[c]	94.7 (2659)	9.3 (8.2, 10.3)	0.64 (0.32, 0.74)	0.176	1.01 (0.74, 1.39)	0.932	0.76 (0.43, 1.35)	0.289	1.12 (0.78, 1.61)	0.464
Pregnant	5.3 (149)	9.2 (7.6, 10.7)								
Food availability determinants										
Ownership of land										
Does not own land[c]	53.7 (1534)	8.0 (6.2, 8.9)								
Owns land	46.3 (1271)	10.7 (10.1, 11.3)	0.35 (0.28, 0.44)	0.000	0.19 (0.14, 0.28)	0.000	0.47 (0.39, 0.57)	0.000	0.28 (0.18, 0.42)	0.000
Ownership of livestock										
Does not own livestock[c]	19.9 (598)	7.8 (6.3, 7.3)								
Owns livestock	80.1 (2210)	9.6 (8.6, 10.6)	0.87 (0.58, 1.32)	0.453	0.46 (0.37, 0.57)	0.000	1.13 (0.71, 1.81)	0.543	0.65 (0.51, 0.82)	0.004
Use of vegetable gardens										
Do not use gardens[c]	48.3 (1293)	9.1 (7.8, 10.4)								
Use gardens	51.8 (1515)	9.4 (8.3, 10.5)	0.54 (0.28, 1.04)	0.062	0.79 (0.41, 1.54)	0.427	0.65 (0.40, 1.07)	0.081	1.05 (0.57, 1.94)	0.853
Food access determinants										
Wealth (PCA)										
Lowest tertile[c]	31.9 (931)	7.2 (5.5, 8.8)								
Middle tertile	32.8 (870)	9.5 (8.3, 10.6)	0.61 (0.42, 0.90)	0.020	0.34 (0.22, 0.51)	0.001	0.81 (0.56, 1.19)	0.230	0.49 (0.29, 0.84)	0.018
Top tertile	35.4 (996)	11.0 (10.7, 11.3)	0.20 (0.10, 0.37)	0.001	0.08 (0.05, 0.14)	0.000	0.36 (0.18, 0.70)	0.010	0.18 (0.10, 0.33)	0.000
Woman's freedom travel to market alone										
Never[c]	62.9 (1835)	8.9 (7.8, 10.1)								
Always or sometimes	37.1 (973)	9.8 (8.9, 10.8)	1.19 (0.50, 2.86)	0.639	0.61 (0.39, 0.96)	0.037	1.12 (0.48, 2.61)	0.759	0.56 (0.36, 0.85)	0.015
Woman's participation in decision-making relating to daily expenditures										
No[c]	63.2 (1794)	9.2 (7.9, 10.5)								
Yes	36.8 (1014)	9.4 (8.5, 10.3)	1.42 (0.99, 2.02)	0.053	1.04 (0.58, 1.86)	0.886	1.35 (0.88, 2.08)	0.139	1.07 (0.66, 1.71)	0.751
Food utilisation determinants										
Knowledge of undernutrition prevention methods (number of methods known)										
0–2[c]	76.2 (2101)	9.2 (7.9, 10.4)								
≥3	23.8 (707)	9.6 (8.9, 10.3)	0.85 (0.39, 1.86)	0.631	0.86 (0.46, 1.58)	0.560	1.10 (0.57, 2.14)	0.728	1.05 (0.58, 1.90)	0.854
Women's literacy										
Cannot read[c]	35.9 (998)	7.9 (6.5, 9.4)								
Can read	64.2 (1810)	10.0 (9.2, 10.9)	0.36 (0.27, 0.49)	0.000	0.27 (0.19, 0.39)	0.000	0.64 (0.44, 0.95)	0.031	0.64 (0.46, 0.90)	0.019
Access to media										
No radio or television[c]	63.9 (1815)	8.5 (7.2, 9.8)								
Own radio or television	36.1 (993)	10.7 (10.0, 11.3)	0.34 (0.24, 0.50)	0.000	0.22 (0.15, 0.33)	0.000	0.56 (0.35, 0.90)	0.024	0.49 (0.33, 0.72)	0.004

Table 3 Associations between possible food security determinants and months of adequate household food provisioning *(Continued)*

Number of women of reproductive age in the household									
1 woman[c]	76.9 (2115)	9.2 (8.1, 10.3)							
>1 woman	23.1 (693)	9.4 (8.5, 10.4)	0.90 (0.64, 1.28)	0.505	0.95 (0.82, 1.10)	0.427	1.30 (0.82, 2.08)	0.214	1.46 (1.02, 2.09)	0.041

We have a maximum of 0.04 % missing data on background information and food utilization determinants, a maximum of 0.14 % missing data on food availability determinants, and a maximum of 0.43 % missing data on food access determinants

[a]Adjusted for clustering and stratification only

[b]Adjusted for socio-demographic characteristics (age and religion), pregnancy status and the other determinants of food security

[c]Reference group

household was associated with an increased risk of severe food insecurity in the adjusted analysis and age was associated with a slight increase in all categories of food insecurity.

Table 4 shows results from linear regression analysis of associations between possible food security determinants and WDDS. The adjusted analysis found that use of vegetable gardens, increasing wealth, literacy and increasing household size were significantly associated with increases in dietary diversity scores of between 0.21 and 0.5.

Discussion and conclusion

Our data show that populations in Bogra, Faridpur and Moulavibazar had sufficient food in the household (MAHFP) for only 9.3 (range 0, 12) months over a year, between 2010 and 2011. The highest prevalence of food shortages corresponds with the main harvest; after this there was a sharp fall in food shortages. Women in the household also reported consumption of an average of 3.8 (range 1, 9) food groups over one day. Another study found a comparable WDDS of 4.3 in Bangladesh [13], but what the WDDS means in public health terms is unclear because there are no cut-off points; new guidelines, developed after our survey, propose five out of ten different food groups as 'adequate' [14].

After adjusting for confounders, the food security determinants associated with a reduced risk of mild household food insecurity were household food production (measured by ownership of land), household wealth (highest tertile), and knowledge of nutritional requirements (women's literacy and access to media). The determinants associated with reduced risk of high food insecurity were the same as above, as well as ownership of livestock, both middle and highest wealth tertiles, women's agency (freedom to travel to the market), and household size (fewer women of reproductive age in the household). Determinants associated with increased WDDS were household food production (use of vegetable gardens), wealth (top tercile), ownership of cooking or food storage facilities (refrigerator ownership), knowledge of nutritional requirements (women's literacy) and household size.

Strengths and limitations of the research

The large sample, geographical representation of the sample and simple metrics used provide a useful snapshot household food security and its proximate determinants, and this study contributes to the scarce literature on measures of household food security [12, 15]. The very high response rate is also a notable strength of our study, although being cross-sectional we were unable to assess any bias that from nonresponders. The cross-sectional design also prevents an analysis of temporal associations and causality. Since nutritional outcomes could reciprocally affect food security determinants, reverse causality is possible. Prospective monitoring of food security and its determinants is required to elucidate the direction of causation. Also, the measures used do not quantify all hypothetical determinants; this limits the study in the comprehensiveness of the analysis and possibility of missing confounders.

MAHFP is limited in its representation of 'household food security' because it captures the respondents' perceptions of whether they had enough food; MAHFP might only measure calorie, but not micronutrient, security. Therefore, WDDS was used as a measure of household access to a micronutrient-rich diet. Although WDDS is a measure of individual dietary intake, intra-household food distribution in Bangladesh tends to be biased against women, so WDDS is likely to be a conservative estimate of household nutritional security [16, 17]. Future studies could use a Household Dietary Diversity Score, [18] or the Household Food Insecurity Access Scale [19].

Determinants of household food availability

The strong, significant association between ownership of land and reduced risk of food insecurity is consistent with publications from other parts of the world [20] but is also of particular concern in Bangladesh, given the population growth and decreasing land available per capita. This indicates a continued importance of the promotion of equitable land tenure laws and employment schemes for the landless poor.

The use of vegetable gardens is interesting because it had no association with MAHFP but did show a weak

Table 4 Associations between possible food security determinants and women's dietary diversity score

Possible determinants of WDDS	Total	WDDS	Crude[a]		Adjusted[b]	
	% (n)	Mean (95 % CI)	Coeff. (95 % CI)	p value	Coeff. (95 % CI)	p value
Total	100 (n = 2620)	3.8 (range 1,9)				
Respondent characteristics						
Age	2620		−0.01 (−0.01, 0.00)	0.036	0.00 (−0.01, 0.01)	0.973
Religion						
Islam[c]	90.2 (2328)	3.7 (3.6, 3.9)				
Hindu	9.8 (292)	4.2 (3.7, 4.6)	0.42 (−0.06, 0.90)	0.075	0.32 (0.00, 0.65)	0.052
Pregnancy status						
Not pregnant[c]	94.7 (2480)	3.8 (3.7, 3.9)				
Pregnant	5.3 (140)	4.0 (3.6, 4.5)	0.26 (−0.13, 0.65)	0.154	0.21 (−0.07, 0.48)	0.118
Food availability determinants						
Ownership of land						
Does not own land[c]	54.2 (1443)	3.6 (3.5, 3.7)				
Owns land	45.8 (1174)	4.0 (3.9, 4.1)	0.39 (0.30, 0.48)	0.000	0.10 (−0.01, 0.21)	0.070
Ownership of livestock						
Do not own livestock[c]	19.6 (552)	3.7 (3.6, 3.9)	0.06 (−0.10, 0.23)	0.369	−0.06 (−0.21, 0.08)	0.327
Own livestock	80.4 (2068)	3.8 (3.7, 3.9)				
Use of vegetable gardens						
Do not use gardens[c]	48.3 (1199)	3.6 (3.5, 3.8)				
Use gardens	51.7 (1421)	3.9 (3.8, 4.1)	0.32 (0.19, 0.46)	0.001	0.20 (0.11, 0.31)	0.003
Food access determinants						
Wealth (PCA)						
Lowest tertile[c]	32.2 (876)	3.4 (3.3, 3.5)				
Middle tertile	32.8 (815)	3.7 (3.5, 3.9)	0.33 (0.11, 0.55)	0.011	0.17 (−0.03, 0.37)	0.083
Top tertile	35.0 (918)	4.2 (4.0, 4.3)	0.85 (0.59, 1.12)	0.000	0.46 (0.24, 0.68)	0.002
Freedom travel to market alone						
Never[c]	63.0 (1718)	3.8 (3.6, 4.0)				
Always or sometimes	37.0 (902)	3.8 (3.5, 4.0)	−0.05 (−0.47, 0.36)	0.763	−0.04 (−0.40, 0.33)	0.810
Women's involvement in decision-making relating to household food expenditure						
No	63.2 (1668)	3.8 (3.7, 3.9)				
Yes	36.8 (952)	3.8 (3.6, 4.0)	0.02 (−0.20, 0.23)	0.849	0.03 (−0.16, 0.21)	0.731
Food utilisation determinants						
Knowledge of undernutrition prevention methods (number of methods known)						
0-2	76.3 (1963)	3.7 (3.6, 3.9)				
≥3	23.7 (657)	4.0 (3.7, 4.4)	0.30 (−0.09, 0.68)	0.112	0.14 (−0.16, 0.45)	0.296
Women's literacy						
Cannot read[c]	36.2 (940)	3.4 (3.3, 3.5)				
Can read	63.8 (1680)	4.0 (3.9, 4.1)	0.59 (0.46, 0.72)	0.000	0.37 (0.20, 0.54)	0.002
Access to media						
Do not own radio or television	64.1 (1698)	3.6 (3.5, 3.7)				
Own radio or television	35.9 (922)	4.2 (3.9, 4.4)	0.58 (0.27, 0.88)	0.004	0.24 (−0.01, 0.50)	0.056

Table 4 Associations between possible food security determinants and women's dietary diversity score *(Continued)*

Number of women of reproductive age in the household						
1 woman[c]	77.4 (1985)	3.7 (3.6, 3.8)				
>1 woman	22.6 (635)	4.0 (3.8, 4.2)	0.33 (0.22, 0.43)	0.000	0.17 (0.05, 0.29)	0.012

We have a maximum of 6.73 % missing data on background information and food utilization determinants, a maximum of 6.84 % missing data on food availability determinants, and a maximum of 7.12 % missing data on food access determinants
[a]Adjusted for clustering and stratification only
[b]Adjusted for socio-demographic characteristics (age and religion), pregnancy status and the other determinants of food security
[c]Reference group

association with WDDS. It is possible that gardens only improve household food intake in seasons when crop yields are high, food prices are lower, and households are already food secure. The latter association with WDDS is consistent with findings that a vegetable garden programme in Bangladesh improved macronutrient and micronutrient consumption [21].

Determinants of household food access
Respondents in the highest wealth tertile were significantly less likely to experience food shortages. An international review supports this [22], as does a study that found Bangladeshi cash-for-work programmes increased food consumption and nutritional status [23]. We also found an association between wealth and WDDS, reflecting findings from a comparative study from Kenya, the Philippines and Bangladesh [24].

Given control over food purchasing, women tend to prioritise expenditure of household resources on food [25, 26]. Our results showed risks of food insecurity were lower if women could access the market, but no effect was found for involvement in budgetary decisions—maybe because the measures used are crude representations of complex concepts of decision-making and empowerment.

Determinants of household food utilisation
We hypothesised that access to media and literacy would improve food security by increasing access to and comprehension of health-promoting mass media campaigns. Although access to media and literacy were associated with a reduced risk of food shortages, and literacy was associated with higher dietary diversity, women's nutritional knowledge was not associated with MAHFP or WDDS. This is surprising since we expect literacy and access to media to have an impact through its effect upon women's nutrition knowledge [27] and it would appear that literacy and media access affect food security through alternative pathways.

Policy implications
This research provides a starting point for further quantification of the largely assumed, hypothetical determinants of household food security. To be comprehensive, exploration of other determinants in the framework is

required. Research to validate the use of MAHFP would add to early discussions on its appropriateness as a new measure of household food security [28, 29].

Our cross-sectional research identifies numerous possible food security determinants relating to land tenure, use of vegetable gardens, income generation and women's empowerment. Although we cannot conclude whether improvements in all determinants are required to improve household food security, we have shown the multi-dimensionality of the determinants of household food security. Therefore, policies relating to these determinants, irrespective of their primary objectives, should be designed with the knowledge that they could influence the food security and nutritional status of the population.

Competing interests
The authors declare that they have no competing interests.

Authors' contributions
HHF and EF prepared the first draft of the manuscript and conducted data analysis. LY and EF devised the sampling strategy and designed survey tools. KA and AK are the project director and project manger, respectively, in Bangladesh, and were responsible for day to day oversight and coordination of data collection. AC is the principal investigator of the project. SS and MH provided and monitored data capture and management. All authors participated in the interpretation of results and revisions of the manuscript. All authors read and approved the final manuscript.

Acknowledgements
This research is funded by a Big Lottery Fund International Strategic Grant. We would like to thank Dr. Malay Kanti Mridha for his helpful input into our analysis and conclusions.

Funding
This research was funded by the Big Lottery Fund. The funding body had no involvement in any part of the study design, implementation or analysis.

Author details
[1]UCL Institute for Global Health, 30 Guilford Street, London, WC1N 1EH, UK. [2]Perinatal Care Project, Diabetic Association of Bangladesh, 122 Kazi Nazrul Islam Avenue, Dhaka 1000, Bangladesh.

References
1. Black RE, Allen LH, Bhutta ZA, Caulfield LE, De Onis M, Ezzati M, et al. Maternal and child undernutrition: global and regional exposures and health consequences. Lancet. 2008;371(9608):243–60.
2. BDHS. Bangladesh Demographic and Health Survey. National Institute of Population Research and Training (NIPORT), Mitra and Associates, and ICF International. 2011.

3. Ericksen P, Thornton P, Notenbaert A, Cramer L, Jones P, Herrero M. Mapping hotspots of climate change and food insecurity in the global tropics. 2011.

4. Ruane AC, Major DC, Winston HY, Alam M, Hussain SG, Khan AS, et al. Multi-factor impact analysis of agricultural production in Bangladesh with climate change. Glob Environ Chang. 2013;23(1):338–50.

5. Pinstrup-Andersen P, Watson II DD. Food Policy for Developing Countries: The Role of Government in Global, National, and Local Food Systems: Cornell University Press. 2011.

6. Sen A. Well-being, agency and freedom: the Dewey lectures. J Philos. 1984;1985:169–221.

7. Azad K, Barnett S, Banerjee B, Shaha S, Khan K, Rego AR, et al. Effect of scaling up women's groups on birth outcomes in three rural districts in Bangladesh: a cluster-randomised controlled trial. Lancet. 2010;375(9721):1193–202.

8. Houweling T, Azad K, Younes L, Kuddus A, Shaha S, Haq B, et al. The effect of participatory women's groups on birth outcomes in Bangladesh: does coverage matter? Study protocol for a randomized controlled trial. Trials. 2011;12(1):208.

9. Fottrell E, Azad K, Kuddus A, Younes L, Shaha S, Nahar T, et al. The Effect of Increased Coverage of Participatory Women's Groups on Neonatal Mortality in Bangladesh: A Cluster Randomized Trial. JAMA Pediatrics. 2013;167(9):816–25.

10. Bilinsky P, Swindale A. Months of adequate household food provisioning (MAHFP) for measurement of household food access: indicator guide: Food and Nutritional Technical Assistance Project, Academy for Educational Development. 2007.

11. Kennedy G, Ballard T, Dop MC. Guidelines for measuring household and individual dietary diversity. Food and Agriculture Organization of the United Nations. 2011.

12. Leah J, Pradel W, Cole DC, Prain G, Creed-Kanashiro H, Carrasco MV. Determinants of household food access among small farmers in the Andes: examining the path. Public Health Nutr. 2013;16(01):136–45.

13. Arsenault JE, Yakes EA, Islam MM, Hossain MB, Ahmed T, Hotz C, et al. Very low adequacy of micronutrient intakes by young children and women in rural Bangladesh is primarily explained by low food intake and limited diversity. J Nutr. 2013;143(2):197–203. doi:10.3945/jn.112.169524.

14. FAO. Introducing the Minimum Dietary Diversity—Women (MDD W) Global Dietary Diversity Indicator for Women, http://www.fantaproject.org/monitoring-and-evaluation/minimum-dietary-diversity-women-indicator-mddw. FANTA project. 2014.

15. De Cock N, D'Haese M, Vink N, Van Rooyen CJ, Staelens L, Schönfeldt HC, et al. Food security in rural areas of Limpopo province, South Africa. Food Security. 2013;5(2):269–82.

16. Pitt MM, Rosenzweig MR, Hassan MNH. Productivity, Health and Inequality in the Intrahousehold Distribution of Food in Low-Income Countries. Am Econ Rev. 1990;80(5):1139–56.

17. Bouis H, Peña C, Haddad L, Hoddinott J, Alderman H. Inequality in the intrafamily distribution of food: the dilemma of defining an individual's"fair share". Intrahousehold resource allocation in developing countries: models, methods, and policy. 1997. p. 179–93.

18. Ruel MT. Is dietary diversity an indicator of food security or dietary quality? International Food Policy Research Institute (IFPRI). 2002.

19. Coates J, Swindale A, Bilinsky P. Household Food Insecurity Access Scale (HFIAS) for measurement of food access: indicator guide. Washington: Food and Nutrition Technical Assistance Project, Academy for Educational Development; 2007.

20. Tschirley DL, Weber MT. Food security strategies under extremely adverse conditions: The determinants of household income and consumption in rural Mozambique. World Dev. 1994;22(2):159–73.

21. Campbell AA, Akhter N, Sun K, de Pee S, Kraemer K, Moench-Pfanner R, et al. Relationship of homestead food production with night blindness among children below 5 years of age in Bangladesh. Public Health Nutr. 2011;14(09):1627–31.

22. Arimond M, Hawkes C, Ruel M, Sifri Z, Berti P, Leroy J, et al. In: Thompson B, Amoroso L, editors. Agricultural interventions and nutrition: lessons from the past and new evidence. 2011. p. 41–75.

23. Mascie-Taylor C, Marks M, Goto R, Islam R. Impact of a cash-for-work programme on food consumption and nutrition among women and children facing food insecurity in rural Bangladesh. Bull World Health Organ. 2010;88(11):854–60.

24. Bouis HE, Eozenou P, Rahman A. Food prices, household income, and resource allocation: socioeconomic perspectives on their effects on dietary quality and nutritional status. Food Nutr Bull. 2011;32(Supplement 1):14S–23S.

25. Kennedy E, Peters P. Household food security and child nutrition: the interaction of income and gender of household head. World Dev. 1992;20(8):1077–85.

26. Quisumbing AR, Brown LR, Feldstein HS, Haddad L, Peña C. Women: The key to food security: International Food Policy Research Institute Washington, DC. 1995.

27. Hussain A, Aarø L, Kvåle G. Impact of a health education program to promote consumption of vitamin A rich foods in Bangladesh. Health Promot Int. 1997;12(2):103–9.

28. Webb P, Coates J, Frongillo EA, Rogers BL, Swindale A, Bilinsky P. Measuring household food insecurity: why it's so important and yet so difficult to do. J Nutr. 2006;136(5):1404S–8S.

29. Coates J, Wilde PE, Webb P, Rogers BL, Houser RF. Comparison of a qualitative and a quantitative approach to developing a household food insecurity scale for Bangladesh. J Nutr. 2006;136(5):1420S–30S.

High prevalence of typhoidal *Salmonella enterica* serovars excreting food handlers in Karachi-Pakistan: a probable factor for regional typhoid endemicity

Taranum Ruba Siddiqui[1*], Safia Bibi[1], Muhammad Ayaz Mustufa[2], Sobiya Mohiuddin Ayaz[1] and Adnan Khan[3]

Abstract

Background: Typhoid fever is the persistent cause of morbidity worldwide. *Salmonella enterica* serovar's carriers among food handlers have the potential to disseminate this infection on large scale in the community. The purpose of this study was to determine the prevalence of typhoidal *S. enterica serovars* among food handlers of Karachi.

Methods: This cross-sectional study was conducted in Karachi metropolis. A total of 220 food handlers were recruited on the basis of inclusion criteria from famous food streets of randomly selected five towns of Karachi. Three consecutive stool samples were collected from each food handler in Carry Blair transport media. Culture, biochemical identification, serotyping, and antimicrobial susceptibility tests for *S. enterica* serovars were done.

Results: Out of 220 food handlers, 209 consented to participate, and among them, 19 (9.1 %) were positive for *S. enterica* serovars. Serotyping of these isolates showed that 9 (4.3 %) were typhoidal *S.* serovars while 10 (4.7 %) were non-typhoidal *S.* serovars. Of the typhoidal *S.* serovars, 7 were *S. enterica* serovar Typhi and 1 each of *S. enterica* serovar Paratyphi A and B. The resistance pattern of these isolates showed that 77.7 % were resistant to ampicillin and 11.1 % to cotrimoxazole. All typhoidal *S. enterica* serovar isolates were sensitive to chloramphenicol, ceftriaxone, cefixime, nalidixic acid, and ofloxacin.

Conclusions: Carrier rate of typhoidal *S. enterica* serovars in food handlers working in different food streets of Karachi is very high. These food handlers might be contributing to the high endemicity of typhoid fever in Karachi, Pakistan.

Keywords: Typhoid fever, Diarrhea, Endemics, *Salmonella enterica* serovars, Carriers

Background

Typhoid fever remains a public health problem worldwide. It is caused by *Salmonella enterica* serovar Typhi and *S. enterica* serovar Paratyphi A, Paratyphi B, and Paratyphi C. A recent study on global burden of typhoid fever reported 26.9 million illnesses and 200,000 to 600,000 deaths annually due to typhoid fever [1]. Typhoid is endemic in most of the developing countries like Pakistan. A prospective population-based surveillance conducted in five Asian countries including Pakistan revealed that the annual typhoid incidence is the second highest, i.e., 412.9 (per 100,000 person years), in Pakistan [2]. A study conducted in Pakistan in pediatric population also reported 170/100,000 incidence of typhoid fever annually [3]. This high incidence of typhoid fever in Pakistan is mainly contributed by persistent poverty, poor personal hygiene, and sanitary condition [4].

Typhoid fever can be cured with appropriate antimicrobial treatment still 3–5 % of patients become lifelong carriers [5]. Since the organism is transmitted

---

* Correspondence: elegy_tt@hotmail.com
[1]Gastroenterology and Hepatology unit, Pakistan Medical Research Council, Research Center, Jinnah Postgraduate Medical Center, Refiquee Shaheed Road, Karachi 75510, Pakistan
Full list of author information is available at the end of the article

through fecal oral route, hence, these carriers serve as a main source for the transmission of infection as they continue to harbor and excrete the organism in their feces. Carriers of these pathogens among food handlers may be another reason for endemicity in these areas as they transmit the infection on a large scale in the community. Worldwide it is recommended that in case of food handlers, microbiological clearance of cases, carriers, and contact cases should be performed. At least five consecutive negative sets of cultures should be done to ensure safe food handling [6].

Although many studies have been previously conducted in Pakistan on typhoid incidence, antimicrobial resistance in *Salmonella* and its serovars, we could not find any data regarding prevalence of *Salmonella* carrier in our population particularly in food handlers [3, 7–9]. Taking into account the poor condition of sanitation, hygiene, and no guidelines for safe food handling in this highly endemic area, estimation of *Salmonella* carrier state particularly in food handlers is of the utmost importance. The aim of this paper is to describe the estimate of *Salmonella* carrier state in food handlers working in different regions of Karachi. Evidence from this paper is useful to do intervention-based study which leads to the formulation of guidelines for safe food handling in our setup. Keeping in view the high resistance rate in *S. enterica* serovars and emerging multiple drug resistance from previous study [2], the antimicrobial susceptibility pattern of *Salmonella* isolated from food handlers' stool samples is also assessed in this study.

Methods
Study setting
It was a cross-sectional study in which from eighteen towns of Karachi, five towns, named as Gulberg Town, Jamsheed Town, Sardar Town, North Nazimabad Town, and Korangi Town, were randomly selected. From each selected towns, four food streets were recruited for the study (Figs. 1, 2, 3, 4, 5, and 6). These selected food streets were visited to approach food handlers for interview and stool samples.

Sample size
On the basis of previous study [10] with 7 % precision and the design effect (D_{eff}) of 2 at the 95 % confidence level, the sample size for this study was calculated as 220 food handlers (with 5 % extra due to noncompliance).

Study population
Food handler was defined as "A person involved in the preparation, cooking, serving or transportation of food in any part of the institute or hotel or restaurant" [11].

Apparently, healthy food handlers were recruited. Those who have recalled past 3 months illness with high-grade fever (>38 °C) and diarrhea or recently confirm typhoid cases in food handlers were excluded from the study.

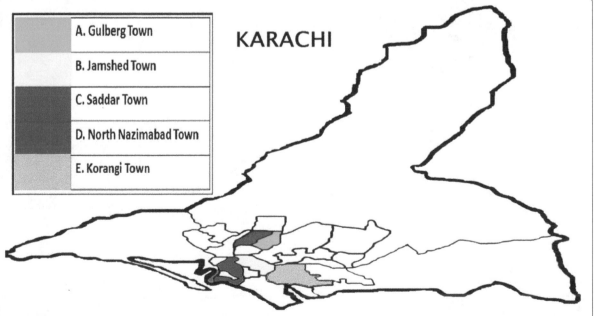

Fig. 1 Map of Karachi Metropolis, Sindh, Pakistan, showing towns distribution. Study towns are colored (Karachi and towns maps are adopted from the official website of Metropolis Karachi) http://www.kmc.gos.pk/

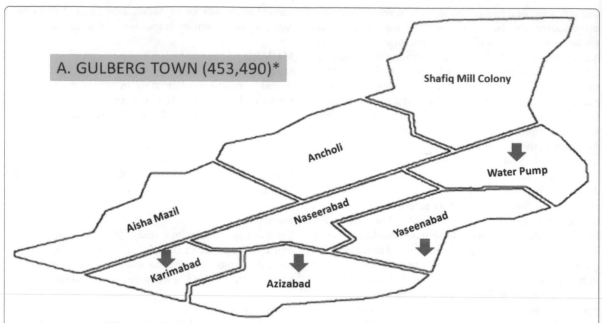

Fig. 2 Gulberg Town showing with arrow signs pointing to food streets area visited in this study for data collection. Asterisk showing population of this town according to the last census 1998. (Karachi and towns map is adopted from the official website of Metropolis Karachi) http://www.kmc.gos.pk/

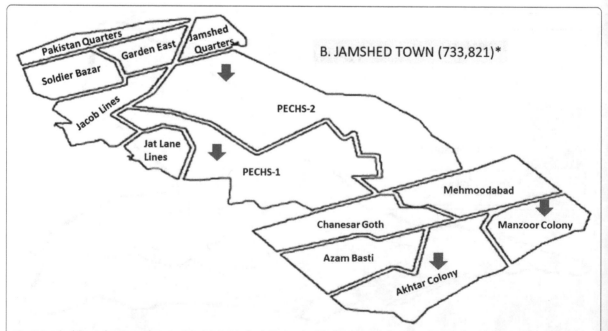

Fig. 3 Jamshed Town showing with *arrow signs* pointing to food streets area visited in this study for data collection. *Asterisk* showing population of this town according to the last census 1998. (Karachi and towns map is adopted from the official website of Metropolis Karachi) http://www.kmc.gos.pk/

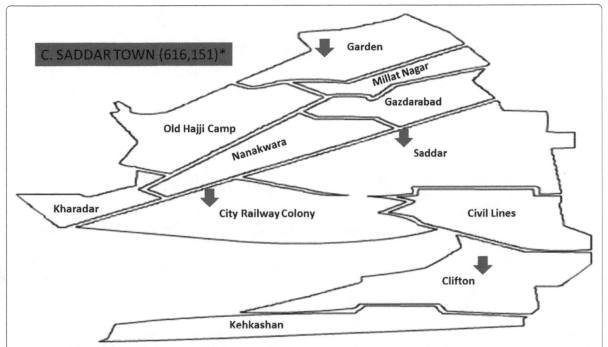

Fig. 4 Saddar Town showing with arrow signs pointing to food streets area visited in this study for data collection. *Asterisk* showing population of this town according to the last census 1998. (Karachi and towns map is adopted from the official website of Metropolis Karachi) http://www.kmc.gos.pk/

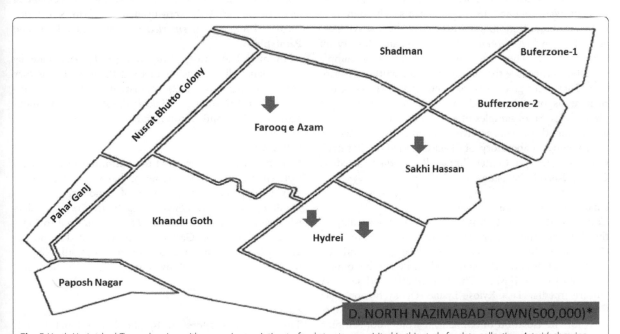

Fig. 5 North Nazimabad Town showing with arrow signs pointing to food streets area visited in this study for data collection. *Asterisk* showing population of this town according to the last census 1998. (Karachi and towns map is adopted from the official website of Metropolis Karachi) http://www.kmc.gos.pk/

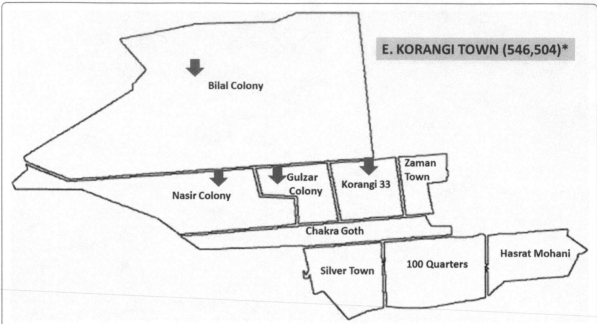

Fig. 6 Korangi Town showing with arrow signs pointing to food streets area visited in this study for data collection. *Asterisk* showing population of this town according to the last census 1998. (Karachi and towns map is adopted from the official website of Metropolis Karachi) http://www.kmc.gos.pk/

Sampling

Food handlers from selected food street were approached for demographic information and stool samples. The purpose of the study was explained, and written informed consent was obtained from participants. Through pretested structured questionnaire, food handlers were interviewed regarding typhoid risk factors and history of typhoid fever. They were briefed about stool sample collection procedure through verbal and a written description. They were given a sterile stool container and Cary-Blair transport media with a cotton swab in air-tight plastic bags. Stool samples of each food handler were collected for three consecutive days and transported to Microbiology Laboratory of "Pakistan Medical Research Council, Research Center; Jinnah Postgraduate Medical Center," Karachi Pakistan.

Laboratory procedure

Culture and sensitivity test was performed according to the Clinical and Laboratory Standards Institute 2012 (CLSI) guidelines in Microbiology Diagnostic and Research laboratory of "Pakistan Medical Research Council, Research Center, JPMC." Three differential and selective culture media, i.e., Xylose-Lysine Deoxycholate agar, Cysteine F broth and Salmonella Shigella Agar, were used for the isolation of Salmonella from stool samples. Biochemical identification of pathogens was performed on the bases of oxidase test, sulfide production, motility test, indole test, urea test, and reaction on triple sugar iron (TSI). For further identification of Salmonella serovars, serotyping was done by slide agglutination test (as per kit recommendation for each antigen). Polyvalent "O," Salmonella Factor 2, 4, and 9, and Vi Salmonella antisera (Remel, UK) were used to confirm S. enterica serovar Typhi and S. enterica serovar Paratyphi A and Paratyphi B.

Antimicrobial susceptibility test (AST) was done by Kirby-Bauer disk diffusion method (Clinical Laboratory Standards Institute 2012) against ampicillin, chloramphenicol, ceftriaxone, nalidixic acid, ofloxacin, cotrimoxazole, cefixime, and ciprofloxacin.

Follow-up

Food handlers were revisited to communicate their stool test reports, information about proper hygienic practices emphasizing on the importance of hand hygiene while handling foods were conveyed to them. Food handlers who were positive for Salmonella were referred to "Specialized Centre of Gastroenterology and Hepatology unit, PMRC, JPMC" for treatment and counseling in order to maintain strict hygienic practices while handling food.

Ethics

The study was approved by the Institutional Review board (IRB) of Jinnah Postgraduate Medical Center. Written informed consents were taken from all the study participants prior to the data collection.

Statistical analysis

Data analysis was done on computer software SPSS version 17.0 and Microscoft Excel. The chi-square test is used to check the possible association of typhoidal *Salmonella* isolates with risk factors. p value <0.05 was consider significant.

Results

Out of 220 food handlers, 209 consented to participate and gave three consecutive stool samples. Their ages ranged from 13–70 years (Mean ± SD 30 ± 10.9). Only four food handlers were females. Of the total, 88 (42.1 %) were working as cook, 54 (25.8 %) as helper (those who helps in kitchen and serving food), and 67 (32 %) as steward.

Piped water for household and drinking was available to 171 (82 %) of food handlers while 61 (29 %) were treating their drinking water prior to use. Carrier cases and source of drinking water showed no significant association with carrier state.

Salmonella carrier rate was higher in food handler who belonged to middle socioeconomic group (p value 0.029). Hand washing before taking meal was practiced by 181 (86.6 %) of food handlers. Hand washing was infrequently practiced in *Salmonella* carriers as compared to noncarrier food handlers (p value 0.005). No significant association was observed between eating habit and carrier state. Among food handlers, 121 (58 %) food handlers used soap for hand washing.

Consumption of fruits and vegetable without washing with carrier state in food handlers showed a significant association (p value 0.002).

A total of 38 (18 %) food handlers had the history of typhoid fever, and 15 (39.4 %) of them were hospitalized due to typhoid fever. In food handlers who were carriers of *Salmonella*, only 5 (55.5 %) had history of typhoid fever due to which 2 (22.2 %) were hospitalized. Significant association was observed between carrier state and history of typhoid fever in food handlers (p value 0.011). Family members of *Salmonella* carriers 3 (33.3 %) had history of typhoid fever. The detailed finding regarding hygienic practices and history of typhoid fever is given in Tables 1 and 2.

Total of 19 (9.1 %) food handlers were positive for *S. enterica* serovars while 9 (4.3 %) isolates were typhoidal *S. enterica* serovars. Seven (3.3 %) isolates were *S. enterica* serovar Typhi, 1 each (0.47 %) was *S. enterica* serovar Paratyphi A and B. Out of 19 isolates, 10 (4.7 %) isolates were non-typhoidal *S. enterica* serovars.

Susceptibility pattern of typhoidal *S. enterica* serovars showed that 77.7 % were resistant to ampicillin and 11.1 % to cotrimoxazole. All typhoidal *S. enterica* serovar isolates were sensitive to chloramphenicol, ceftriaxone, cefixime, nalidixic acid, and ofloxacin. Non-typhoidal *S. enterica* serovar was 100 % resistance to ampicillin, 40 % to cotrimoxazole, 30 % to nalidixic acid, and 10 % each to chloramphenicol, ceftrixone, and cefixime. All isolates were sensitive to ofloxacin (Fig. 7).

Table 1 Risk factors in *Salmonella* carriers

	Risk factors	Salmonella carrier (Typhoidal + non-typhoidal)		p value
		Yes ($n = 19$)	No ($n = 190$)	
1	Socioeconomic status			
	Low	4 (21 %)	90 (47.4 %)	0.029
	Middle	15 (78.9 %)	90 (47.4 %)	
	High	0	10 (5.3 %)	
2	Washing of hands before taking meal			
	Always	12 (63.15 %)	169 (88.9 %)	0.005
	Never	7 (36.8 %)	21 (11 %)	
3	Eating habit			
	Always eat food cooked at home	9 (47.4 %)	79 (41.6 %)	0.400
	Eat from small restaurant (Thelas/Chapra hotels)	10 (52.6 %)	111 (58.4 %)	
4	Use of soap for washing			
	Always	13 (68.4 %)	108 (56.8 %)	0.234
	Sometime	6 (31.6 %)	82 (43.1 %)	
5	Washing of fruits and vegetables before consumption			
	Always	4 (21 %)	108 (56.8 %)	0.002
	Sometimes/never	15 (78.9 %)	82 (43 %)	

Table 2 Typhoid history in typhoidal *Salmonella* carriers

History of typhoid fever		Typhoidal (n = 09)	Non-typhoidal and not carrier (n = 200{10 + 190})	p value
1	History of typhoid fever in food handlers			0.011
	Yes	5 (55.5 %)	33 (16.5 %)	
	No	4'(44.4)	167 (83.5 %)	
2	Typhoid treatment taken by food handler			0.104
	Yes	3 (15.8 %)	25 (13.2 %)	
	No	6 (66.6 %)	175 (87.5 %)	
3	Hospital admission for typhoid fever			0.129
	Yes	2 (22.2 %)	13 (6.5 %)	
	No	7 (77.7 %)	187 (93.5 %)	
4	Family member had typhoid fever			0.056
	Yes	3 (15.8 %)	19 (10.0 %)	
	No	6 (66.6 %)	181 (90.0 %)	

Out of 19 food handlers who carried *Salmonella*, 9 had typhoidal serovars; of them, 3 were cooks, 2 were stewards, and 4 were helpers, while 10 food handlers were positive for non-typhoidal serovars were 4 cooks, 4 stewards, and 2 helpers.

Discussion

Present study showed that 4.3 % healthy food handlers were carriers of typhoidal *S. enterica* serovars which is much higher than the study reported from Iran, i.e., 1.88 % [12]. Another study conducted in India showed 16.6 % carriers' rate which is comparably very high [13]. We may correlate this dissimilarity in carrier rate with a population based surveillance data, showing higher incidence rate of typhoid, i.e., 493.5/100,000 in India followed by 412.9/100,000 in Pakistan [2].

The overall carrier rate of *Salmonella* serovars was 9 %. This is similar to studies from China [14] and UK [15] where 9.5 and 12.3 % were carriers of *S. enterica* serovars. However, this rate is much higher as compared to the studies carried out in Ethiopia and Ghana [16, 17]. Fecal carriage of non-typhoidal *Salmonella* in asymptomatic food handlers is 4.7 % which is higher as compared to study from Ghana which reported 1.1 % carriers of non-typhoidal *Salmonella* among food handlers [17].

Previous study showed that multidrug resistance (MDR) *S. enterica* is increasing [18] and varying geographically [2]. In present study, 77.7 % isolates showed resistance to ampicillin and 11 % showed resistance to cotrimoxazole; it is observed that none of the isolates was resistant against chloramphenicol, cephalosporins,

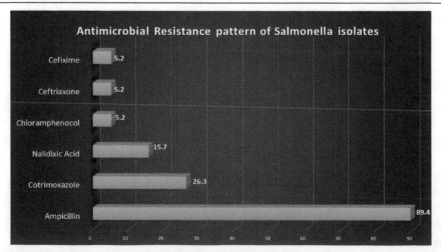

Fig. 7 Figure showing Antimicrobial Resistance pattern of *Salmonella* isolates

and quinolone group. No typhoidal *Salmonella* MDR strain was isolated in the study which is comparable with the study from Nepal showing no MDR isolates [19], but contrast to the local hospital-based study which showed 30.5 % resistance to all three first line drugs in typhoidal *Salmonella* serovars isolated from typhoid cases [20]. Another local study [21] also stated 30 % resistance strains against nalidixic acid which is used as a marker to detect intermediate/reduced susceptibility of cipro-floxacin against *S. enterica* serovars Typhi [22]. In the present study, none of the typhoidal *Salmonella* isolate showed resistance against nalidixic acid.

Out of 4.7 % non-typhoidal *Salmonella* carriers, 10 % MDR strains were isolated. Since salmonellosis (non-typhoidal) is a food-borne disease caused by consumption of contaminated foods and also contracted through fecal-oral route. In the existence of poor hygienic condition, this high rate of MDR is an alarming situation for public health concerns.

Though the treatment for *Salmonella* carrier is chole-cystectomy, as gall bladder is the reservoir for this disease, but being an invasive procedure gall bladder removal is not feasible. Present study showed that fluoroquinolone (ofloxacin/ciprofloxacin) can be the drug of choice for the treatment of these carriers. A previous study from neighboring country also stated ofloxacin as a better option in presence of MDR *S. enterica* [23].

Assessment of living behavior and life style in relation to typhoid carrier state of food handlers revealed that most of the *Salmonella* carriers were not practicing hand washing before taking meal. World Health Organization (WHO) recommends safe water access and hygienic food handling to prevent typhoid (www.who.int/water_sanitation_health/diseases/typhoid/en/). In Karachi, thousands of food handlers are working in different restaurants/hotels. Many of these restaurants are small and located in insanitary areas. Besides that a large number of street food vendors are also working in approximately all localities of Karachi, there is almost no provision of sink and toilet in case of street food vendors. Hand washing is an established way to prevent disease transmission, but this basic step which breaks the infection chain is not routinely performed by most of the food handlers of Karachi. Other factors like eating outside from restaurants or stalls, washing of vegetables and fruits before consumptions, and history of typhoid fever in food handlers or within their families showed contributing factors which might lead to *Salmonella* infection/carrying *Salmonella* in their feces. Present study showed significant association between *Salmonella* carrier state and hygienic practices like hand washing and washing of raw food before consumption. In present study, the prevalence of *Salmonella* carrier was significantly higher in lower and middle socioeconomic classes; it was found that none of the food handlers belonging to higher class were

Salmonella carrier. Findings of food handlers' behavior towards hygiene are comparable with the study conducted in Indonesia; these findings confirm that poor hygienic practices of lower and middle socioeconomic classes are risk factors of acquiring this disease [24].

Conclusions

It may be concluded from the present study that the carrier rate of typhoidal *Salmonella* serovars in food handlers is quite high. In an environment of poor sanitation and hygiene, this high rate signifies wide dissemination of typhoid pathogen through food handlers and indicates one of the probable reasons of typhoid endemicity in Karachi.

Recommendation

It is recommended that local food regularity authority should establish pre-employment screening and medical clearance of food handlers; food handlers should also be screened periodically for *Salmonella* carrier state. In order to evaluate food handlers' practices and contamination level, it is suggested that level of personal hygiene practices during their work should also be assessed (hand swabbing and microbiological analysis can be the assessing tool). Food handlers need to be aware of the importance of personal health and hygiene for the safety of food. It is recommended that awareness program should be organized for food handlers to encourage and motivate them about good practices. These efforts might play an important role in reducing the burden of typhoid endemicity in Karachi Metropolis.

Competing interests
The authors declare that they have no competing interests.

Authors' contributions
TRS conceived and designed the study. TRS, SB, and MAM supervised the data collection. TRS, SB, SMA, and AK analyzed the data. TRS wrote the first draft. All authors critically revised the draft for intellectual content. All authors read and approved the final manuscript.

Acknowledgements
This research project is funded by Pakistan Medical Research Council; grant was awarded to Taranum Ruba Siddiqui. We would like to acknowledge Professor Dr. Saleem Hafiz from the Department of Clinical Pathology, Sindh Institute of Urology and transplantation (SIUT), for helping in the critical review of the final manuscript.

Author details
[1]Gastroenterology and Hepatology unit, Pakistan Medical Research Council, Research Center, Jinnah Postgraduate Medical Center, Refiquee Shaheed Road, Karachi 75510, Pakistan. [2]Pakistan Medical Research Council, Research Center, National Institute of Child Health, Karachi, Pakistan. [3]Microbiology Department, University of Karachi, Karachi, Pakistan.

References
1.　Buckle GC, Fischer Walker CL, Black RE. Typhoid fever and paratyphoid fever: systematic review to estimate global morbidity and mortality for 2010. J glob health. 2012;2(1).

2.   Ochiai RL, Acosta CJ, Danovaro-Holliday M, Baiqing D, Bhattacharya SK, Agtini MD, et al. A study of typhoid fever in five Asian countries: disease burden and implications for controls. Bull World Health Organ. 2008;86:260–8.

3.   Siddiqui FJ, Rabbani F, Hasan R, Nizami SQ, Bhutta ZA. Typhoid fever in children: some epidemiological considerations from Karachi, Pakistan. Int J infectious dis. 2006;10–3:215–22.

4.   Arif A, Naheed R. Socio-economic determinants of diarrhoea morbidity in Pakistan. Academic Research International 2.1 (2012): 23-9944.

5.   Brooks GF, Carroll KC. Enteric gram- negative rods (Enterobacteriaceae), chap. 16. In: Brooks GF, Carroll KC, Butel JS, Morse SA, editors. Jawetz, Melnick & Adelberg's medical microbiology, 24th Edition. US: McGraw-Hill; 2004.

6.   Braddick MR, Crump BJ, Yee ML. How long should patients with *Salmonella* typhi or *Salmonella* paratyphi be followed-up? A comparison of published guidelines. J Public Health. 1991;13–2:101–7.

7.   Mirza SH, Khan MA. Low level quinolone resistance in multidrug resistant typhoid. J Coll Physicians Surg Pak. 2008;18–1:13–6.

8.   Butt T, Ahmed RN, Salman M, Kazmi SY. Changing trends in drug resistance among typhoid *Salmonella* in Rawalpindi. Pakistan East Mediter Health J. 2005;11(5–6):1038–44.

9.   Wain J, House D, Zafar A, Baker S, Nair S, Kidgell C, et al. Vi antigen expression in *Salmonella enterica* serovar Typhi clinical isolates from Pakistan. J Clin Microbiol. 2005;43–3:1158–65.

10. Senthilkumar B, Prabakaran G. Multidrug resistant *Salmonella* typhi in asymptomatic typhoid carriers among food handlers in namakkal district, Tamil Nadu. Indian J Med Microbiol. 2005;23(2):92–4.

11. Food handlers health policy. Available at: www.occmed.oxfordjournals.org/content/suppl/2005/05/31/kqi094.DC1/kqi094suppl.pdf. Accessed 27 April, 2010

12. Yousefi-Mashouf R, Rangbar M, Mossavi MJ, Ahmady M. Prevalence of *Salmonella* carriers among food handlers and detection of drug resistance of isolates in Hamadan. J Res Health Sci. 2011;3–2:25–8.

13. Senthilkumar B, Prabakaran G. Multidrug resistant *Salmonella* typhi in asymptomatic typhoid carriers among food handlers in Namakkal district. Tamil Nadu Ind J Med Microbiol. 2005;23–2:92–4.

14. Luo Y, Li J, Ma Y, Hu C, Jin S, Cui S. Isolation and characterization of nontyphoid *Salmonella* from hospital food handlers in Beijing, China. J Food Safety. 2009;29–3:414–23.

15. Dryden MS, Keyworth N, Gabb R, Stein K. Asymptomatic foodhandlers as the source of nosocomial salmonellosis. J Hosp Infect. 1994;28–3:195–208.

16. Abera B, Biadegelgen F, Bezabih B. Prevalence of *Salmonella enterica* serovar Typhi and intestinal parasites among food handlers in Bahir Dar Town. Northwest Ethiopia Ethiop J Health Dev. 2010;24–1:46–50.

17. Feglo PK, Frimpong EH, Essel-Ahun M. Salmonellae carrier status of food vendors in Kumasi, Ghana. East Afr Med J. 2004;81–7:358–36.

18. Crump JA, Mintz ED. Global trends in typhoid and paratyphoid fever. Clin Infect Dis. 2010;50–2:241–6.

19. Dongol S, Thompson CN, Clare S, Nga TVT, Duy PT, Karkey A, et al. The Microbiological and Clinical Characteristics of Invasive Salmonella in Gallbladders from Cholecystectomy Patients in Kathmandu, Nepal. PLoS ONE. 2012;7(10):e47342. doi:10.1371/journal.pone.0047342.

20. Qaiser S, Irfan S, Khan E, Ahsan T, Zafar A. In vitro susceptibility of typhoidal salmonellae against newer antimicrobial agents: a search for alternate treatment options. J Pak Med Assoc. 2011;61–5:462.

21. Afzal A, Sarwar Y, Ali A, Haque A. Current status of fluoroquinolone and cephalosporin resistance in *Salmonella enterica* serovar Typhi isolates from Faisalabad. Pakistan Pak J Med Sci. 2012;28(4):602–7.

22. Mandal S, DebMandal M, Pal NK. Nalidixic acid resistance predicting reduced ciprofloxacin susceptibility of *Salmonella enterica* serovar Typhi. Asian Pacific J of Trop Dis. 2012;2:S585–7.

23. Kumar S, Rizvi M, Berry N. Rising prevalence of *enterica* fever due to multidrug-resistant Salmonella: an epidemiological study. J Med Microbiol. 2008;57–10:1247–50.

24. Gasem MH, Dolmans WMV, Keuter MM, Djokomoeljanto R. Poor food hygiene and housing as risk factors for typhoid fever in Semarang, Indonesia. Trop Med Int Health. 2001;6–6:484–90.

Women's participation in household decision-making and higher dietary diversity: findings from nationally representative data from Ghana

Dickson A. Amugsi[1*], Anna Lartey[2], Elizabeth Kimani[1] and Blessing U. Mberu[1]

Abstract

Background: Low-quality monotonous diet is a major problem confronting resource-constrained settings across the world. Starchy staple foods dominate the diets in these settings. This places the population, especially women of reproductive age, at a risk of micronutrients deficiencies. This study seeks to examine the association between women's decision-making autonomy and women's achievement of higher dietary diversity (DD) and determine the socio-demographic factors that can independently predict women's attainment of higher DD.

Methods: The study used data from the 2008 Ghana Demographic and Health Survey. The participants comprised of 2262 women aged 15–49 years and who have complete dietary data. The DD score was derived from a 24-h recall of intake of foods from nine groups. The score was dichotomized into lower DD (DD $\leq$4) and higher (DD $\geq$5). Logistic regression was used to assess the association between women decision-making autonomy (final say on how to spend money, making household purchases, own health care, opinions on wife-beating, and sexual intercourse with husband) and the achievement of higher DD. The logistic regression models were adjusted for covariates at the individual and household levels.

Results: The analysis showed that women participation in decision-making regarding household purchases was significantly associated with higher DD, after adjusting for individual and household level covariates. The odds of achieving higher DD were higher among women who had a say in deciding household purchases, compared to women who did not have a say (OR = 1.74, 95 % CI = 1.24, 2.42). Women who had more than primary education were 1.6 times more likely to achieve higher DD, compared to those with no education (95 % CI = 1.12, 2.20). Compared to women who lived in polygamous households, those who lived in monogamous households had higher odds of achieving higher DD (OR = 1.42, 95 % CI = 1.04, 1.93).

Conclusions: Net other covariates, women who have a say in making household purchases are more likely to achieve higher DD compare to those who do not have a say. This may indicate autonomy to buy nutritious foods, suggesting that improving women decision-making autonomy could have a positive impact on women dietary intake.

Keywords: Women, Higher, Dietary diversity, Ghana

* Correspondence: damugsi@aphrc.org
[1]African Population and Health Research Centre, APHRC Campus, P.O. Box 10787-00100, Nairobi, Kenya
Full list of author information is available at the end of the article

Background

Low-quality monotonous diet is the bane of resource constrained settings across the world [1]. Starchy staple foods dominate the diets in these settings, with fruits, vegetables, and animal source foods scarcely consumed. This places the population at high risk of micronutrient deficiencies, and women of reproductive age are particularly vulnerable [1–4]. This is the case because of increased nutrient needs for women during pregnancy and lactation, and when these needs are not met, mothers may experience wasting and fatigue that may limit their ability to fully satisfy infant needs [3]. This may result in infants who are small for gestational age and children with stunted growth and slowed cognitive development, which may persist into adulthood and transmit to the next generation [3]. Thus, the consequences of micronutrient malnutrition do not only affect the health and survival of women, but also their offspring. It is estimated that 2 billion people around the world suffer from micronutrient deficiency, and 19 million pregnant women are vitamin A deficient [2, 5]. The vast majority of these people live in the developing countries. There is a growing consensus that increasing the dietary diversity (more food groups) can help improve diet quality, especially among women [2, 3, 6]. A new dietary diversity indicator, called minimum dietary diversity-women (MDD-W) has recently been developed as a proxy indicator of the micronutrient adequacy of the diet of women [6–8]. The proponents of this indicator posit that women consuming foods from five or more food groups out of ten have a greater likelihood of meeting their micronutrient needs than women consuming foods from fewer food groups [8].

There is evidence that women's participation in household decision-making and ability to purchase food (an aspect of empowerment) is significantly associated with availability of diverse diet in the household [9]. This enforces the idea that women's decision-making autonomy is an important aspect of women empowerment, as it relates to women's dietary diversity and subsequently, better nutritional status. Various elements of women empowerment and disempowerment for that matter have been linked to lower or higher nutritional risks respectively. For instance, domestic abuse and sexual coercion have an impact on women's nutrition. A study in South India observed that mothers who had endured domestic abuse and sexual coercion were at higher risk of poor nutrition, so did their children [10]. Also, a positive association between increases in women's empowerment and improved nutrition outcomes has been documented and, that any actions leading to women's disempowerment can result in adverse nutritional impacts for women [11–13]. A study in Bangladesh and Vietnam observed a positive association between maternal education and maternal

dietary diversity [14]. Women who have greater education tend to have higher dietary diversity (DD). Murakami and colleagues [15] investigated the association between maternal education and individual food consumption among Japanese women. They observed that higher education is associated with a higher intake of vegetables, fish and shellfish, and potatoes, but not with bread, noodles, confectioneries and sugars, fats and oils, pulses and nuts, meat, eggs, dairy products, or fruits [15]. Mirmiran and colleagues [16] also found significant positive association between educational level and improvement in women's dietary intake.

A number of studies have found a significant association between Socio-economic status (SES) and women's dietary diversity [16, 17]. A study in Nepal concludes that higher SES is associated significantly with more frequent consumption of most food groups, including in-season fruits and vegetables [17]. Other factors such as place of residence, presence of co-wives in the household and sex of household head have been found to associate importantly with women eating patterns [18–20]. For example, systematic review of studies on dietary patterns in low- and middle-income countries reveals that living in urban areas is associated with overall healthier dietary patterns [18].

The literature reviewed above helps one appreciate the significance of women's decision-making autonomy in promoting women's DD. However, the challenge with the foregoing literature is the glaring lack of evidence on African countries. In Ghana for instance, studies on how women participation in decision-making at the household level impacts on their dietary diversity is almost non-existent. This highlights the need to examine data from Ghana on the subject of decision-making and DD. The present study was therefore set out to (1) examine the association between women's decision-making autonomy and women's achievement of higher dietary diversity (DD); (2) determine the socio-demographic factors that can independently predict women's attainment of higher DD.

Methods
Data sources and study population
This analysis used data from the Ghana Demographic and Health Surveys (GDHS) [21]. The surveys were conducted in Ghana in 2008 (September to November) by the Ghana Statistical Service and the Ghana Health Service, with technical support from ICF Macro through the MEASURE DHS programme. The surveys were designed to be representative at the national, regional and rural-urban levels. The Ghana DHS employed a two-stage sampling design. The first stage involved selection of clusters from a master sampling frame constructed from the 2000 national population and housing

census. The second stage involved the selection of households from these clusters. All women and men aged 15–49 and 15–59, respectively, in the selected households were eligible to participate in the survey. Three questionnaires were used for the data collection: the Household Questionnaire, the Women's Questionnaire, and the Men's Questionnaire. The household response rate was 98.9 %. In this analysis, we used data of 2262 women aged 15–49 years and who have complete dietary data. Ethical clearance was sought from Ghana Health Service ethics review committee (GHS-ERC) before the surveys were conducted. Individual written informed consent was obtained from study participants before they were allowed to participate in the study. The data were completely anonymous; therefore, the authors of the present study did not have to seek further ethical clearance.

Measures
Women's dietary diversity
The women's DD score was constructed based on the 24-h recall of food consumption. The DD score is a count of the number of food groups consumed by the woman during the 24 h prior to the in-home survey. Fourteen (14) types of foods contained in the data were regrouped into nine (9) main food groups [3]: (1) grain, tubers, roots; (2) flesh meat (beef, pork, chicken, fish etc.); (3) dairy products (milk, cheese, yogurt etc.); (4) legumes (food made from beans, peas, lentils, nuts); (5) eggs; (6) organ meat (liver, heart, kidney etc.); (7) dark green vitamin A rich leafy vegetables; (8) vitamin A rich fruits and other vitamin A vegetables; (9) other fruits. The women reported whether or not they have consumed any of the above mentioned food groups. A "yes" response was scored "1" and "no" response scored "0". The scores were then summed up to create the women DD score, which ranged from 0 to 9. This score was dichotomised into consumption of four or less food groups (DD ≤4)—lower DD, and consumption of five or more food groups (DD ≥5)—higher DD, and used in the subsequent analysis. The selection of higher DD threshold of five (5) food groups was informed by the new recommended dietary diversity indicator for women, called minimum dietary diversity-women (MDD-W), for assessing micronutrient adequacy for women's diets [6]. This indicator reflects consumption of at least five of ten food groups. However, because the food groups used in this paper were not the actual representation of the MDD-W indicator, the use of the term MDD-W had been avoided.

Women's decision-making autonomy (empowerment) variables
Women empowerment variables used in this analysis included, final say on how to spend money, final say in making household purchases, final say on own health care, opinion on wife-beating, and ability to refuse husband sex on justifiable grounds. Some of the variables were recoded. Final say on making large household purchases and final say on making purchases for daily needs were recoded into "final say on making household purchases". Also, final say on deciding what to do with money husband earns and who decides how to spend money in the household were recoded into "final say on how to spend money". In addition, two indices on women autonomy were created [22]: the number of reasons that justify wife-beating in the respondent's opinion and the respondent's opinion on the number of circumstances under which a wife is justified in refusing to have sexual intercourse with her husband. Details on the construction of these indices have been published elsewhere [23].

Socio-demographic factors
These factors were collected both at the woman and household levels. The woman level factors included but are not limited to age, education, parity, occupation, ethnicity, and religion. The household level factors included sex of household head, place of residence, household wealth index, presence of co-wives, number of children under 5 years, and number of household members. Ethnicity and religion were recoded into "Akan" and other ethnicities" and "Christian and other religions", respectively. The occupation variable was also recoded into "white collar and agriculture/labour".

Statistical analysis
The data were analysed using IBM SPSS version 21. Descriptive analysis was conducted to examine the background characteristics of the study samples. Bivariate analysis was carried out to assess the association between the predictor variables and higher women's DD. Only significant predictors in bivariate analysis were used in the multivariate analysis. Logistic regression was used to assess the association between women decision-making autonomy (final say on how to spend money, making household purchases, own health care, opinions on wife-beating, and sexual intercourse with husband), and the achievement of higher DD. The logistic regression models were adjusted for covariates at the individual level (age, parity, education, occupation, ethnicity and religion), and household level (sex of household head, place of residence, wealth index, co-wives, number of children under 5 years and number of household members). Results were considered statistically significant when $P < .05$.

Results
Descriptive analysis results
Table 1 presents descriptive statistics of the sample. The average age of the study participants was 30 years (SD =

Table 1 Descriptive analysis of the study sample ($n = 2262$): categorical and continuous variables

Variables	Means ± SD/%
Women dietary diversity (DD)	
Women DD ≤4	56.9
Women DD ≥5	43.1
Food groups used in creating women DD	
Grains-tubers-roots (yes)	97.9
Flesh food (beef, pork, fish etc.) (yes)	82.2
Dairy products (milk, cheese, yogurt etc.)(yes)	58.1
Legumes (food made from beans, peas, lentils, nuts) (yes)	28.4
Eggs (yes)	19.2
Organ meat (yes)	10.2
Dark green vitamin A rich leafy vegetables (yes)	55.6
Vitamin A rich fruits and other vitamin A vegetables (yes)	16.1
Other fruits (yes)	63.0
Socio-demographic factors	
Maternal occupation	
Agriculture/labour	54.2
White collar	45.8
Maternal education	
No education	37.8
Primary	24.1
Secondary+	38.0
Final say on own health care	
Has a say	65.2
Final say in making household purchases	
Has a say in taking final decision	79.2
Presence of co-wives in household	
There are co-wives	21.0
There are no co-wives	79.0
Continuous variables	
Maternal age	30.10 ± 7.02
Maternal parity	3.70 ± 2.24
Number of children under 5 years	1.78 ± 0.99
Number of household members	5.88 ± 2.76

7.02). Twenty-one percent (21 %) of the study sample lived in polygamous households, and each household in the sample had approximately six members. Expectedly, almost all the women (98 %) in this sample consumed starchy food (grains, tubers, roots). The second highest consumed food group was flesh meat (82 %). The least consumed food groups were organ meat (10 %) and vitamin A rich fruits and other vitamin A vegetables (16 %). Additionally, 63 % of the women consumed non-vitamin A rich fruits (other fruits) while a total of 43 % consumed foods from five or more food groups.

Bivariate analysis results

In the bivariate analysis, the following decision-making autonomy variables were positively and significantly associated with higher DD among women: final say on household purchases ($\beta = 0.56$, $P = .001$), final say on how to spend money ($\beta = 0.51$, $P = .026$), women opinion on wife-beating ($\beta = 0.07$, $P = .022$), and ability to refuse husband sex on justifiable grounds ($\beta = 0.11$, $P = .043$). Additionally, socio-demographic variables such as woman age, parity, education, occupation, ethnicity, religion, sex of household head, household wealth index, presence of co-wives, and number of household members were also significantly associated with higher women's DD.

Multivariate analysis results

Table 2 presents the results of the multiple logistic regression analysis. In this analysis, women decision-making autonomy regarding household purchases was significantly associated with higher DD (consumption of five or more food groups), after adjusting for individual and household level covariates. Compared with women who have no say in deciding household purchases, women who had a say were almost twice as likely to achieve higher DD (OR = 1.74, 95 % CI = 1.24, 2.42). The other decision-making variables (final say on how to spend money, women's opinion on wife-beating, ability to refuse husband sex on justifiable grounds) did not reach statistical significance in the multivariate analysis. Women educational level was also associated with higher DD—women who had higher than primary education were 1.6 times more likely to achieve higher DD than those with no education (95 % CI = 1.12, 2.20). Compared to women in the poorest wealth quintile, women in the richer and richest quintiles were 1.7 (95 % CI = 1.07, 2.64) and 1.8 (95 % CI = 1.05, 3.14) times respectively, more likely to achieve higher DD. Women who live in non-polygamous households had higher odds of achieving higher DD than those who lived in polygamous households (OR = 1.42, 95 % CI = 1.04, 1.93). There were significant negative associations between Christian religion and Akan ethnic group, and higher DD respectively.

Discussion

The results of our analyses show a strong positive association between women's participation in decision-making (indication of empowerment) regarding household purchases and higher DD. Women who participate in final decision-making are almost two times more likely to achieve higher DD compared to those who do not participate in household decision-making. This association remains after adjusting for other important socio-demographic determinants of women's dietary diversity at the individual and household levels. These

Table 2 Multivariate logistic regression analysis of the association between women's decision-making autonomy, socio-demographic factors, and women's dietary diversity (DD)[a] (n = 2262)

Variables	Coefficients	SE	OR	95 % CI for OR	Wald F	P
Women decision-making autonomy						
Final say on how to spend money						
Has no say in making final decision	Ref	Ref	Ref	Ref	Ref	Ref
Has a say in making final decision	0.32	0.25	1.38	0.84, 2.25	1.63	0.200
Final say on making Household purchases						
Has no say in making final decision	Ref	Ref	Ref	Ref	Ref	Ref
Has a say in making final decision	0.55	0.17	1.74	1.24, 2.42	10.53	.001
Final say on own health care						
Has no say in making final decision	Ref	Ref	Ref	Ref	Ref	Ref
Has a say in making final decision	−0.25	0.13	0.78	0.60, 1.01	3.63	.057
Wife-beating not justified score	−0.01	0.04	0.99	0.92, 1.07	0.02	.900
Refused husband sex score	0.07	0.07	1.07	0.94, 1.23	1.03	.310
Woman level factors[b]						
Maternal age	0.01	0.01	1.01	0.98, 1.04	0.40	.530
Maternal parity	−0.04	0.05	0.96	0.88, 1.05	0.87	.350
Maternal education						
No education	Ref	Ref	Ref	Ref	Ref	Ref
Primary	0.17	0.16	1.18	0.86, 1.62	1.06	.300
Secondary or higher	0.45	0.17	1.57	1.12, 2.20	6.87	.009
Maternal occupation						
Agriculture/labour	Ref	Ref	Ref	Ref	Ref	Ref
White collar	−0.11	0.14	0.90	0.69, 1.17	0.66	.420
Maternal ethnicity						
Other ethnicities	Ref	Ref	Ref	Ref	Ref	Ref
Akan	−0.36	0.14	0.70	0.53, 0.91	7.11	.008
Maternal religion						
Other religions	Ref	Ref	Ref	Ref	Ref	Ref
Christian religion	−0.30	0.14	0.75	0.56, 0.99	4.18	.041
Household level factors[b]						
Sex of household head						
Male	Ref	Ref	Ref	Ref	Ref	Ref
Female	−0.18	0.14	0.84	0.63, 1.11	1.59	.210
Place of residence						
Rural	Ref	Ref	Ref	Ref	Ref	Ref
Urban	0.10	0.17	1.11	0.80, 1.55	0.38	.540
Household wealth index						
Poorest	Ref	Ref	Ref	Ref	Ref	Ref
Poor	−0.34	0.18	0.71	0.51, 1.01	3.71	.054
Middle	−0.31	0.21	0.73	0.48, 1.10	2.23	.140
Richer	0.52	0.23	1.68	1.07, 2.64	4.98	.026
Richest	0.60	0.28	1.81	1.05, 3.14	4.49	.034

Table 2 Multivariate logistic regression analysis of the association between women's decision-making autonomy, socio-demographic factors, and women's dietary diversity (DD)[a] (n = 2262) (Continued)

Present of co-wives in household						
There are co-wives	Ref	Ref	Ref	Ref	Ref	Ref
There are no co-wives	0.35	0.16	1.42	1.04, 1.93	4.86	.028
Number of under five children	0.03	0.08	1.03	0.89, 1.19	0.13	.720
Number of household members	0.04	0.03	1.04	0.98, 1.11	1.92	.170

[a]Dietary diversity (DD) is the number of food groups consumed over 24-h period
[b]Women and household levels factors were adjusted for in the multivariate analysis

results suggest that women's decision-making autonomy at the household level is crucial for the consumption of diverse diet. The findings of the present study are consistent with previous studies. In India and Bangladesh, women's participation in household decision-making and ability to purchase food, have positive impact on the availability of diverse diet in the household, and consequently adequate dietary diversity intake among women and children [9, 24]. This suggests that programmes to improve women's nutrition could focus on increasing women's decision-making power. Similarly, several other studies report positive associations between women's empowerment and dietary diversity [11, 13, 25]. These studies conclude that any actions that lead to women disempowerment can result in adverse nutritional impact for women as well as for their children. Hence, it stands to reason that investment in women empowerment would have a beneficial effect on women and their children [13, 26, 27]. It is evident from the foregoing that women's participation in decision-making (an indicator of empowerment) associates importantly with women dietary intake, although the underlying mechanisms may be complex.

Our analysis also reveals a number of socio-demographic factors that are associated significantly with women's DD. One of such factors is women's education. The results show that high level of women's education increases the likelihood of achieving higher DD. This is probably because women who have high education are likely to earn their own income, thereby becoming financially autonomous. Indeed, it is a documented fact that financial autonomy has a positive influence on women's nutrition [28]. This is so, because higher financial autonomy gives women more negotiation powers with regards to food purchases [1, 13, 28]. Our findings are comparable with previous studies. In Vietnam and Bangladesh, positive and significant association was observed between maternal education and maternal dietary diversity [14]. Nevertheless, in Japan, the effect of education on the intake of individual foods is mixed. While higher education was associated with a higher intake of vegetables, fish and shellfish, and potatoes, there was no association between education and intake of bread, noodles, confectioneries

and sugars, fats and oils, pulses and nuts, meat, eggs, dairy products, or fruit [15]. This implies that when dietary diversity is disaggregated, the influence of education may not be across all food groups. Further analysis could focus on both dietary diversity and the individual food groups.

Furthermore, household wealth (an indicator of socio-economic status) was found in this analysis to associate significantly with women's DD. Women in the richest wealth quintile have higher odds of achieving higher DD compared to those in the poorest wealth quintiles. The probable explanation is that women in the richest quintile in Ghana are likely to have available to them, a disposable income and other resources. This may increase the ability of women in these households to make household purchases [9]. The importance of food purchasing ability on the availability of dietary diversity in households has been documented [9].The findings of the present study are in line with previous studies that examined the relationship between socio-economic status (SES) and women dietary intake. Mirmiran and colleagues [16] observed a positive and significant association between SES and women dietary diversity. Additionally, two other studies concluded that higher SES is associated importantly with more frequent consumption of most food groups including seasonal fruits and vegetables, diet quality, and diversity [17, 18]. Our analysis confirms the findings from previous studies that SES is an important determinant of women's dietary intake. Interventions targeted at increasing women's SES could increase their dietary diversity.

Similarly, this study shows that compared to women who live in polygamous households, women in non-polygamous (monogamous) households are more likely to achieve a higher DD. This suggests that non-existent of co-wives reduces competition on the limited resources in the household, thereby making women in the monogamous households to have access to a diverse diet. As there is an evidence that polygamy forces women to live in poverty by forcing them to share resources in the household and thus exacerbates the impoverishment of women by limiting their access to financial and other resources in the marriage [19]. Another plausible explanation is the relationship between monogamy and women's autonomy, and the effect it has on women's dietary diversity. Nigatu and colleagues [29] observed a positive association between monogamous marriage and women's autonomy—women in monogamous marriages were more than three times likely to be autonomous compared to those in polygamous marriages'. A related study observes that women in monogamous households have considerable decision-making power, including what the household will consume, while women in polygamous households have noticeable smaller decision-making power [30].

There are a number of strengths and weakness associated with this study. One of the key strengths is the representative nature of the data used in the analysis. This means that the findings of the study can be generalised to all women in Ghana. To the best of the authors' knowledge, this is the first study in Ghana to have used nationally representative data to investigate the relationship between women's decision-making autonomy, socio-demographic factors, and women's DD.

A limitation of this study is the fact that the data are from a cross sectional study, and a causal relationship between socio-demographic factors, decision-making autonomy, and higher DD cannot be established. Therefore, the conclusions contained in this paper are based on associations between the explanatory and outcome variables, rather than causal relationships. Due to data limitation, the present study used 9-point food group instead of the newly recommended 10-point food group. Secondly, the present study included organ meat in the computation of the DD score, while the newly recommended MDD-W did not. However, since the DD use in this study is not intended to be an exact representation of the new MDD-W, and for the fact that the use of the term MDD-W had been avoided in the paper, the inclusion of organ meat might not affect the findings contained in this paper.

Conclusions

The results show that women who participate in taking household decisions making regarding household purchases are more likely to achieve higher DD compared to those who do not participate. This suggests that improving women decision-making autonomy could have a positive impact on women's dietary intake. Interventions in Ghana should target at promoting women's decision-making power at the households level. Household wealth index, education, and the absence of co-wives in the household are also positively and significantly associated with higher women's DD. Improving household wealth, promoting female education, and encouraging monogamous marriages could have a significant impact on women dietary intake in Ghana.

Acknowledgements
The authors thank MEASURE DHS for releasing the data for this study. We also wish to thank the Ghana Statistical Service and Ghana Health Service who were responsible for collecting the data, and the study participants.

Funding
This study did not receive funding from any source.

Authors' contribution
DAA conceived and designed the study, performed the data analysis, interpreted the results, and drafted the manuscript. AL, EK, and BUM contributed to the study design, data analysis and interpretation, and critical revision of the manuscript. All authors read and approved the final version. All authors take responsibility of any issues that might arise from the publication of this manuscript.

Competing interests
The authors declare that they have no competing interests.

Author details
[1]African Population and Health Research Centre, APHRC Campus, P.O. Box 10787-00100, Nairobi, Kenya. [2]Nutrition Division, Economic and Social Department, Food and Agriculture Organization, Rome, Italy.

References
1. Arimond M, Torheim LE, Wiesmann D, Joseph M, Carriquiry A. Dietary diversity as a measure of women's diet quality in resource-poor areas: results from rural Bangladesh site. Washington: Food and Nutrition Technical Assistance (FANTA); 2008.
2. Biodiversity International. Recommending dietary diversity for women. 2014. [cited 2015 02.02]. Available from: http://www.bioversityinternational.org/news/detail/recommending-dietary-diversity-for-women/.
3. USAID. Maternal dietary diversity and the implications for children's diets in the context of food security. Washington: USAID; 2012.
4. Arimond M, Wiesmann D, Becquey E, Carriquiry A, Daniels MC, Deitchler M, et al. Simple food group diversity indicators predict micronutrient adequacy of women's diets in 5 diverse, resource-poor settings. J Nutr. 2010;140(11):2059S–69S.
5. Torheim LE, Ferguson EL, Penrose K, Arimond M. Women in resource-poor settings are at risk of inadequate intakes of multiple micronutrients. J Nutr. 2010;140(11):2051S–8S.
6. Martin-Prével Y. A new indicator for global assessment of dietary diversity among women: global nutrition report; 2014. [cited 2015 02.02]. Available from: http://globalnutritionreport.org/2014/10/20/a-new-indicator-for-global-assessment-of-dietary-diversity-among-women/.
7. Food and Nutrition Technical Assistance (FANTA). New global indicator to measure women's dietary diversity. 2014. [cited 2015 2.02]. Available from: http://www.fantaproject.org/monitoring-and-evaluation/minimum-dietary-diversity-women-indicator-mddw.
8. Introducing the Minimum Dietary Diversity – Women (MDD-W). Global dietary diversity indicator for women. Washington: 2014. [cited 2015 02.02]. Available from: http://www.fantaproject.org/sites/default/files/resources/Introduce-MDD-W-indicator-brief-Sep2014.pdf.
9. Bhagowalia P, Menon P, Quisumbing AR, Soundararajan V. Unpacking the links between women's empowerment and child nutrition: evidence using nationally representative data from Bangladesh. Selected paper prepared for presentation at the 2010 Agricultural & Applied Economics Association. Denver: Agricultural & Applied Economics Association; 2010.
10. Sethuraman K, Lansdown R, Sullivan K. Women's empowerment and domestic violence: the role of sociocultural determinants in maternal and child undernutrition in tribal and rural communities in South India. Food Nutr. 2006;27(2):128–43.
11. Bhagowalia P, Menon P, Quisumbing AR, Sundararaja V. What dimensions of women's empowerment matter most for child nutrition? evidence using nationally representative data from Bangladesh. Washington: International Food Policy Research Institute; 2012.

12. Smith LC, Haddad L. Explaining child malnutrition in developing countries: a cross-country analysis. Washington: International Food Policy Research Institute; 2000.

13. Smith LC, Ramakrishnan U, Ndiaye A, Haddad L, Martorell R. The importance of women's status for child nutrition in developing countries. Washington: International Food Policy Research Institute; 2003.

14. Nguyen PH, Avula R, Ruel MT, Saha KK, Ali D, Tran LM, et al. Maternal and child dietary diversity are associated in Bangladesh, Vietnam, and Ethiopia. J Nutr. 2013;143(7):1176–83.

15. Murakami K, Miyake Y, Sasaki S, Tanaka K, Ohya Y, Hirota Y, Osaka Maternal and Child Health Study Group. Education, but not occupation or household income, is positively related to favorable dietary intake patterns in pregnant Japanese women: the Osaka Maternal and Child Health Study. Nutr Res. 2009;29(3):164–72.

16. Mirmiran P, Mohammadi F, Allahverdian S, Azizi F. Association of educational level and marital status with dietary intake and cardiovascular risk factors in Tehranian adults: Tehran lipid and glucose study (TLGS). Nutr Res. 2002;22(12):1365–75.

17. Campbell RK, Talegawkar SA, Christian P, LeClerq SC, Khatry SK, Wu LS, et al. Seasonal dietary intakes and socioeconomic status among women in the Terai of Nepal. J Health Popul Nutr. 2014;32(2):198–216.

18. Mayén AL, Marques-Vidal P, Paccaud F, Bovet P, Stringhini S. Socioeconomic determinants of dietary patterns in low- and middle-income countries: a systematic review. Am J Clin Nutr. 2014;100(6):1520–31.

19. von Struensee V. The Contribution of polygamy to women's oppression and impoverishment: an argument for its prohibition. 2005. [cited 2015 02.02]. Available from: http://www.austlii.edu.au/au/journals/MurUEJL/2005/2.html.

20. Haidar J, Kogi-Makau W. Gender differences in the household-headship and nutritional status of pre-school children. East Afr Med J. 2009;86(2):69–73.

21. MEASURE DHS. [cited 2014 28.2]. Available from: http://www.measuredhs.com/data/available-datasets.cfm.

22. Ghana, Statistical, Service (GSS), Ghana, Health, Service (GHS) et al. Demographic and health survey 2008. Accra: GSS, GHS, and ICF Macro; 2009.

23. Amugsi DA, Mittelmark MB, Lartey A, Matanda DJ, Urke HB. Influence of childcare practices on nutritional status of Ghanaian children: a regression analysis of the Ghana Demographic and Health Surveys. BMJ Open. 2014;4(11):e005340.

24. Menendez KP, Mondal SK, McQuestion MJ, Pappu K, Dreyfuss ML. Women's decision-making autonomy and dietary intake in Jharkhand State, India. 2006. [cited 2015 02.02]. Available from: https://apha.confex.com/apha/134am/techprogram/paper_140244.htm.

25. Smith L, Haddad LJ. Explaining malnutrition in developing countries: a cross country analysis. Washington: International Food Policy Research Institute; 2000.

26. Quisumbing AR. Household decisions, gender, and development. A synthesis of recent research. Food policy. Washington: International Food Policy Research Institute; 2003.

27. Yoong J, Rabinovich L, Diepeveen S. The impact of economic resource transfers to women versus men, A systematic review. Technical report. London: London EPPI-Centre, Social Science Research Unit, Institute of Education, University of London; 2012.

28. Shroff M, Griffiths P, Adair L, Suchindran C, Bentley M. Maternal autonomy is inversely related to child stunting in Andhra Pradesh, India. Matern Child Nutr. 2009;5(1):64–74.

29. Nigatu D, Gebremariam A, Abera M, Setegn T, Deribe K. Factors associated with women's autonomy regarding maternal and child health care utilization in Bale Zone: a community based cross-sectional study. BMC Womens Health. 2014;14:79.

30. Santos F, Fletschner D, Savath V. An intrahousehold analysis of access to and control over land in the Northern province, Rwanda: World Bank conference on land and poverty. The World Bank - Washington DC,: Rural development institute; 2014. [cited 2015 02.02]. Available from: http://www.landesa.org/wp-content/uploads/An-Intrahousehold-Analysis-of-Access-to-and-Control-Over-Land-Santos-Savath-Fletschner-March-2014.pdf.

Water Quality Index for measuring drinking water quality in rural Bangladesh: a cross-sectional study

Tahera Akter[1], Fatema Tuz Jhohura[1], Fahmida Akter[1], Tridib Roy Chowdhury[1], Sabuj Kanti Mistry[1], Digbijoy Dey[3], Milan Kanti Barua[3], Md Akramul Islam[2,3] and Mahfuzar Rahman[1*]

Abstract

Background: Public health is at risk due to chemical contaminants in drinking water which may have immediate health consequences. Drinking water sources are susceptible to pollutants depending on geological conditions and agricultural, industrial, and other man-made activities. Ensuring the safety of drinking water is, therefore, a growing problem. To assess drinking water quality, we measured multiple chemical parameters in drinking water samples from across Bangladesh with the aim of improving public health interventions.

Methods: In this cross-sectional study conducted in 24 randomly selected *upazilas*, arsenic was measured in drinking water in the field using an arsenic testing kit and a sub-sample was validated in the laboratory. Water samples were collected to test water pH in the laboratory as well as a sub-sample of collected drinking water was tested for water pH using a portable pH meter. For laboratory testing of other chemical parameters, iron, manganese, and salinity, drinking water samples were collected from 12 out of 24 *upazilas*.

Results: Drinking water at sample sites was slightly alkaline (pH 7.4 ± 0.4) but within acceptable limits. Manganese concentrations varied from 0.1 to 5.5 mg/L with a median value of 0.2 mg/L. The median iron concentrations in water exceeded WHO standards (0.3 mg/L) at most of the sample sites and exceeded Bangladesh standards (1.0 mg/L) at a few sample sites. Salinity was relatively higher in coastal districts. After laboratory confirmation, arsenic concentrations were found higher in Shibchar (Madaripur) and Alfadanga (Faridpur) compared to other sample sites exceeding WHO standard (0.01 mg/L). Of the total sampling sites, 33 % had good-quality water for drinking based on the Water Quality Index (WQI). However, the majority of the households (67 %) used poor-quality drinking water.

Conclusions: Higher values of iron, manganese, and arsenic reduced drinking water quality. Awareness raising on chemical contents in drinking water at household level is required to improve public health.

Keywords: Water quality index, Chemical parameters, WASH program, BRAC, Bangladesh

Background

Quality of drinking water indicates water acceptability for human consumption. Water quality depends on water composition influenced by natural process and human activities. Water quality is characterized on the basis of water parameters (physical, chemical, and microbiological), and human health is at risk if values exceed acceptable limits [1–3]. Various agencies such as the World Health Organization (WHO) and Centers for Disease Control (CDC) set exposure standards or safe limits of chemical contaminants in drinking water. A common perception about water is that clean water is good-quality water indicating knowledge gap about the presence of these substances in water. Ensuring availability and sustainable management of good-quality water is set as one of the Sustainable Development Goals (SDGs) and is a challenge for policy makers and Water, Sanitation and Hygiene (WASH) practitioners, particularly in the face of changing climatic conditions, increasing populations, poverty, and the negative effects of human development.

* Correspondence: mahfuzar.rahman@brac.net
[1]BRAC Research and Evaluation Division, BRAC Centre, 75 Mohakhali, Dhaka 1212, Bangladesh
Full list of author information is available at the end of the article

Water Quality Index (WQI) is considered as the most effective method of measuring water quality. A number of water quality parameters are included in a mathematical equation to rate water quality, determining the suitability of water for drinking [4]. The index was first developed by Horton in 1965 to measure water quality by using 10 most regularly used water parameters. The method was subsequently modified by different experts. These indices used water quality parameters which vary by number and types. The weights in each parameter are based on its respective standards, and the assigned weight indicates the parameter's significance and impacts on the index. A usual WQI method follows three steps which include (1) selection of parameters, (2) determination of quality function for each parameter, and (3) aggregation through mathematical equation [5]. The index provides a single number that represents overall water quality at a certain location and time based on some water parameters. The index enables comparison between different sampling sites. WQI simplifies a complex dataset into easily understandable and usable information. The water quality classification system used in the WQI denotes how suitable water is for drinking. The single-value output of this index, derived from several parameters, provides important information about water quality that is easily interpretable, even by lay people [6]. In a resource-poor country like Bangladesh where ensuring availability and sustainable management of water is one of the challenging areas towards development. The present study embraced weighted arithmetic WQI method to deliver water quality information to WASH practitioners. One of the merits of this method is that a less number of parameters are required to compare water quality for certain use [5].

The WASH program of the Bangladesh Rural Advancement Committee (BRAC) has provided interventions in 250 *upazilas* in Bangladesh since 2006 with the aim of improving the health of the rural poor. The BRAC WASH program selects intervention areas on the basis of some criteria such as high poverty rate, poor sanitation coverage, and lack of access to safe water due to high arsenic, salinity, and other contaminants [7]. The program has adopted a holistic approach integrating water, sanitation, and hygiene components. The water component promotes use of safe water through a number of activities: (1) deep tubewell installation in arsenic-affected areas; (2) loan to construct tubewell platform in order to protect groundwater from pollutions; and (3) water quality testing [8]. Besides, awareness building and behavioral change remain at the core of the WASH program [9] to improve health and hygiene of the rural poor. The types of interventions vary according to households' economic status.

Earlier, we conducted a number of studies on water- and hygiene-related issues in intervention areas, such as use of tubewell water and water safety practices [8], women in water hygiene [10], and knowledge gap on hygiene and safe water [7]. Some impeding factors towards access to safe drinking are poverty, unhygienic sanitation practices, low groundwater levels, and impacts of natural hazards (e.g., arsenic, salinity, extreme weather events) [11]. The program assessed water safety in a crude way by some proxy indicators such as awareness on brick-built tubewell platform, its cleanliness, and no waterlogging at the bottom of the tubewell. To our knowledge, the present study on water quality assessment based on some water parameters has been the first study conducted for the BRAC WASH program. We aimed through this research to understand households' exposure to these water parameters according to their background characteristics which might have programmatic implications in the future. The present study measures drinking water quality with the application of weighted arithmetic WQI method based on some chemical parameters. These parameters used for drinking water quality assessment were selected as the requirement of BRAC WASH program. The relevance of the present study lies in programmatic implications by providing evidence-based and useful information on drinking water quality in a simple way. We expect that the findings will help in designing program interventions to ensure safe drinking water either by raising awareness about chemical contamination of water or by improving water quality through provision of hardware supply.

Methods

Study design and area

This study was part of our research on "The status of household WASH behaviors in rural Bangladesh," conducted in 24 randomly selected *upazilas* (5 % of total). The current study on the assessment of drinking water quality used a cross-sectional study design and was conducted in 12 out of 24 *upazilas* across the country: Alfadanga (Faridpur), Kendua (Netrokona), Shibchar (Madaripur), Rupsha (Khulna), Debhata (Satkhira), Patharghata (Barguna), Rangabali (Patuakhali), Anwara (Chittagong), Bijoynagar (Brahmanbaria), Shajahanpur (Bogra), Kamalganj (Moulvibazar), and Kurigram Sadar (Kurigram) (Fig. 1).

Study procedure

A total of 960 households from 24 *upazilas* (40 households in each *upazila*) were randomly selected for socioeconomic survey and arsenic test on the spot using test kit at household level. Twelve out of 24 *upazilas* were considered to collect water samples from drinking water sources and to test chemical parameters in the laboratory. A total of 542 water samples were collected from 293 randomly selected households. In each *upazila*, 20 out of 40 households were

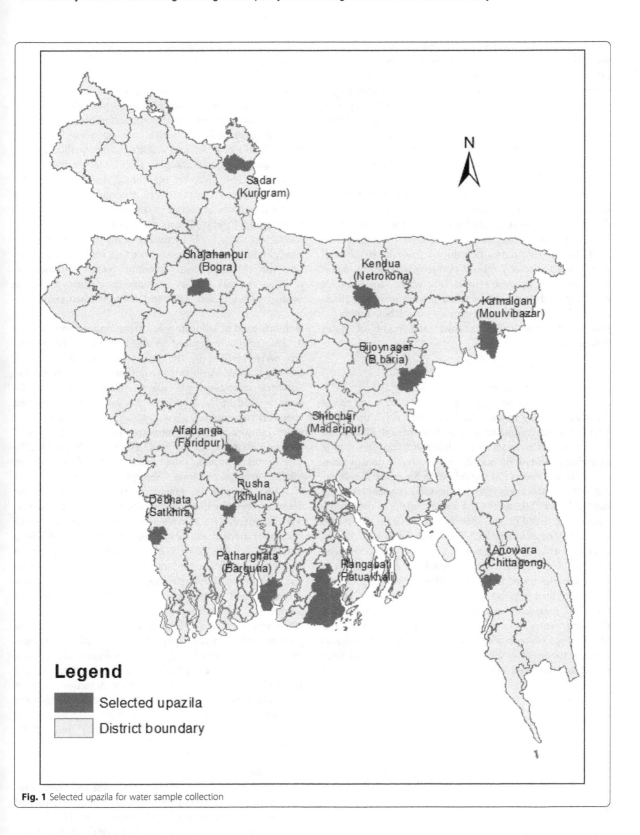

Fig. 1 Selected upazila for water sample collection

initially selected for water samples collection. However, the total number of samples varied due to some reasons: (1) samples collected from shared tubewells increased the number of households; and (2) a few water samples were discarded due to label numbers being washed away, rendering them unidentifiable. Of the total water samples collected, same samples (293 samples) were used to test both iron and manganese levels in water. Similarly, the remaining 249 water samples were used to test both pH and salinity (Table 1).

A total of 36 research assistants were recruited and grouped into 12 to collect water samples from selected *upazilas*. They were trained intensively for 3 days and a field test was conducted nearby Dhaka prior to actual field survey. Groundwater samples from each tubewell were collected after 2 min of pumping in order to obtain deep water as the test sample. The water samples were collected in 100-mL pre-washed bottles with watertight seals. The collected water samples were labeled with the household identification number and name of water parameters.

Arsenic test on the spot

A total of 960 households from 24 *upazilas* were visited for arsenic testing in the field. Simultaneously, a pre-tested structured questionnaire was used to obtain household-level information on socioeconomic condition. Of the total households visited, 66 and 31 % households used shallow (<300 ft) and deep (≥300 ft) tubewells for collecting drinking water, respectively. Out of the total households using tubewells, 645 tubewells (424 shallow and 221 deep tubewells) were tested on the spot for arsenic using the "econo quick (EQ) arsenic test kit." The nature of EQ kit reading is quantitative. A color chart in a scale of values between 0.0 and 1.0 mg/L was used to record the arsenic status of water samples tested in the field. The EQ kit was preferred to use in field test because of its high accuracy (about 90 %) of measuring arsenic status of the tubewells [12]. Drinking water sources of the remaining households (33 %) were not considered for arsenic testing for various reasons: tubewells of 29 % of households had already been tested and declared arsenic free (0.0 mg/L) in the recent

past, and 4 % used pond water for drinking and were excluded from arsenic testing.

Testing of water samples using pH meter

Acid-base balance is assessed by the pH value of water [13]. A controlled water pH is suggested in WHO guidelines to reduce adverse health consequences. According to the WHO guidelines of drinking water quality, exposure to both high and low pH values causes irritation the eyes, skin, and mucous membrane for humans [14]. Here, 123 water samples were randomly selected from the total samples collected to test the pH. A portable pH meter (model PHS-25) was used in the BRAC head office to test the pH. pH meter operating instructions were carefully followed: the meter was first calibrated by putting the electrode into standard buffer solutions of pH 6.86 and pH 4.00 at set temperature prior to being washed with distilled water and sample measurement.

Methods used at laboratory for measuring parameters

Arsenic results measured in the field using the testing kits were verified in the laboratory. About 10 % of collected water samples were picked at random for laboratory validation. pH meter values were similarly crosschecked in the laboratory for validation. The other chemical contents (e.g., iron, manganese, and salinity) in water samples were also measured in the Water Quality Testing Laboratory of the NGO Forum for Public Health. The water samples were analyzed by flow-injection hydride generation atomic absorption spectrometry (FI-HG-AAS) method for arsenic detection. The minimum detection level for this method was 3 (μg/L). Total arsenic was measured. The efficiency of field kits used by NGO Forum for arsenic testing was reported to have low failure rate (11 % for Merck kit, 6.2 % for NIPSOM), supporting high kit's performance in arsenic testing [15]. Manganese was analyzed in Flame (air-acetylene) AAS. The minimum detection limit of this method was 0.01 ppm. For both arsenic and manganese, AAS of Shimadzu (model: AA-6300) was used at the laboratory. Iron was analyzed by phenanthroline method using UV-visible spectrophotometer where iron was brought into a solution, reduce to a ferrous state by treating with acid and hydroxylamine and 1, 10-phenanthroline. The minimum detection limit of this method was 0.05 ppm. UV-visible spectrophotometer of Shimadzu (model: UV-1601) was used at the laboratory. Salinity was measured at the laboratory by conductivity method using an appropriate electrode.

Data analysis

Descriptive statistics were used to analyze the mean, median, standard deviation, interquartile range (IQR), and frequency distribution of each parameter. The households' wealth index was developed based on ownership

Table 1 Sample distribution

Chemical parameter	Spot test	Laboratory test				
	Arsenic (As)	Arsenic (As)	Manganese (Mn)	Iron (Fe)	pH	Salinity (NaCl)
Households visited	960	293				
Sample tested	645	64	293	293	249	249
Total sample	645	542				

of valued items. Bangladesh and WHO guideline standards were considered in the evaluation of the number of household members exceeding acceptable drinking water limits. The exposure level of household members was analyzed by their background characteristics which included age, sex, education, economic status, and media access at home, NGO membership, wealth index, and type of water sources used. The households were classified as ultra-poor, poor, and non-poor as per the following criteria of the BRAC WASH program: households that owned less than 404.7 m^2 of land, had no fixed source of income, or were headed by a female were classified as "ultra-poor"; households with land holdings between 404.7 and 4047 m^2 and/or sold manual labor for a living were classified as "poor"; and households that did not fall into either of the above categories were classified as "non-poor." Wealth index was developed based on the ownership of valued items at household level.

Weighted arithmetic Water Quality Index (WQI) method

The weighted arithmetic WQI method [16, 17] was applied to assess water suitability for drinking purposes. In this method, water quality rating scale, relative weight, and overall WQI were calculated by the following formulae:

$$q_i = (C_i/S_i) \times 100$$

where q_i, C_i, and S_i indicated quality rating scale, concentration of i parameter, and standard value of i parameter, respectively.

Relative weight was calculated by

$$w_i = 1/S_i$$

where the standard value of the i parameter is inversely proportional to the relative weight.

Finally, overall WQI was calculated according to the following expression:

$$\mathrm{WQI} = \sum q_i w_i / \sum w_i$$

Ethics statement

The research protocol was approved by the ethical review committee of James P Grant School of Public Health, BRAC University.

Results

Demographic and socioeconomic profile of households

The background characteristics of households from whom water samples were collected for laboratory testing are shown in Table 2. A total of 293 households comprising 1491 members were included in the analysis. The proportions of male and female household members were 51 and 49 %, respectively. Over half of members

had higher secondary education and above followed by secondary (22 %), primary (20 %), and no schooling (8 %). Members belonged to poor (37 %), ultra-poor (30 %), and non-poor (32 %) economic groups. The study participants represented six divisions (highest administrative boundary of Bangladesh) including Dhaka and Khulna (8 % in each), Chittagong and Barisal (about 28 % in each), Rajshahi (11 %), and Sylhet (18 %). The majority had access to media (radio and/or television) at home (51 %), and 55 % of the members had no NGO membership.

pH levels in the drinking water

The median of pH value was 7.4, while IQR values at different sample sites varied between 0.2 and 0.4, respectively. The highest frequency value was pH 7.4 (34 %) followed by pH 7.2 (13 %) and pH 7.6 (9 %). pH values at selected sites ranged between 6.6 and 8.4 (Table 3), within acceptable limits (6.5–8.5). The mean pH values in both shallow (7.5 ± 0.4) and deep tubewells (7.4 ± 0.3) varied, but median value was found the same in both types (7.4 mg/L).

Manganese concentrations in drinking water

In our samples, manganese concentrations varied between 0.1 and 5.5 mg/L with a median value of 0.2 mg/L (Table 3). At most sample sites, the median value exceeded the Bangladesh standard of 0.1 mg/L, except Rangabali (Patuakhali) and Bijoynagar (B.Baria). The highest median value (0.9 mg/L) was observed in Shibchar (Madaripur), which exceeded the WHO standard of 0.4 mg/L. Exposure to manganese in drinking water according to the household member characteristics is shown in Table 4. High exposure levels exceeding standards (0.1 mg/L) were found in Chittagong (27 %), Barisal (23 %), and Sylhet (19 %). Those belonging to the lowest wealth group (26 %) had higher exposure to manganese (>0.1 mg/L) than those in the highest wealth group (16 %). When the WHO standard of 0.4 mg/L was considered, the majority of households (82 %) were within acceptable limits. According to Bangladesh standards, about half (51 %) of the households exceeded acceptable limits (>0.1 mg/L).

Iron (Fe) in drinking water

The median iron concentration values in water exceeded WHO standards (0.3 mg/L) at all sample sites except Bijoynagar. The median iron values at a few sites exceeded Bangladesh limits (1.0 mg/L) (Table 3). The highest median iron concentration value was in Kamalganj (Moulvibazar) (2.3 mg/L) followed by Anwara (Chittagong) (2.0 mg/L), Shibchar (Madaripur) (2.0 mg/L), and Rupsha (Khulna) (1.4 mg/L). The lowest median value was observed in Bijoynagar (B.Baria) (0.3 mg/L).

Table 2 Demographic and socioeconomic characteristics of households

Characteristics	Frequency (HH[a] members)	Percentage (%)
Sex		
Male	757	50.8
Female	734	49.2
Age(years)		
≤4	106	7.2
5–20	516	34.9
21–40	455	30.8
41–60	300	20.3
≥61	102	6.9
Educational level		
No schooling	62	7.6
Primary	166	20.3
Secondary	177	21.6
Higher secondary and above	414	50.5
Division		
Dhaka	115	7.7
Chittagong	414	27.8
Rajshahi	160	10.7
Khulna	121	8.1
Barisal	411	27.6
Sylhet	270	18.1
Occupation		
Agriculture	123	9.0
Laborer (skilled/unskilled)	123	9.0
Housewife/homestead task	408	29.9
Service/professional	87	6.4
Business	88	6.5
Student	427	31.3
Unemployed/disabled	70	5.1
Others	38	2.8
Household economic status		
Ultra-poor	452	30.3
Poor	557	37.4
Non-poor	482	32.3
Marital status		
Unmarried	692	46.4
Married	728	48.8
Widow/separated/divorced	71	4.8
Access to media at home		
No access to media	730	49.0
Access to media	761	51.0
NGO membership		
No membership	816	54.7

Table 2 Demographic and socioeconomic characteristics of households (Continued)

Member of any NGO	675	45.3
Wealth index		
Lowest	342	23.1
Second	301	20.3
Middle	265	17.9
Fourth	262	17.7
Highest	313	21.1
Total	1491	100

[a]Household

About 7 % of young children (≤4 years) were exposed to iron levels in drinking water that exceeded WHO and Bangladesh standards. The highest exposure levels, exceeding the WHO's acceptable limit of 0.3 mg/L, were in Barisal (29 %) followed by Chittagong (23 %) and Sylhet (20 %) (Table 4). In Dhaka, only 7 % of household members were exposed to greater than 0.3 mg/L iron in drinking water. Only 18 % households met WHO standards (≤0.3 mg/L), while a large proportion (82 %) were exposed to high concentrations of iron in drinking water (>0.3 mg/L). The median iron concentration in deep tubewells was slightly higher (0.8 mg/L)than in shallow tubewells (0.7 mg/L), although median values in both cases exceeded WHO and lower limit of Bangladesh standards.

Salinity (NaCl) levels
Division-wise variations in sodium chloride levels in drinking water are shown in Table 4. The highest proportion of household members exposed to more than 600 mg/L sodium chloride was found in Dhaka (40 %) followed by Barisal (35 %) and Khulna (26 %). Considering Bangladesh standards (upper limit 600 mg/L), more females than males exceeded their exposure limits (54 % vs. 46 %) (Table 4). As shown in Table 3, excess sodium chloride was detected in Rupsha (Khulna) (1050 mg/L) when the upper limit of Bangladesh standard (600 mg/L) was considered.

Arsenic (As) concentrations in drinking water
Arsenic testing in the field revealed high arsenic concentrations exceeding Bangladesh standards in Shibchar (Madaripur), Biswanath (Sylhet), and Dhaka. A random sub-sample (over 10 %) was selected for laboratory validation, which showed that water samples collected from Shibchar (Madaripur) (median 0.05 mg/L) and Alfadanga (Faridpur) (median 0.03 mg/L) showed higher arsenic concentrations compared to other sample sites exceeding WHO standard (Table 3). About 68 and 77 %

Table 3 Regional variation in the values of chemical parameters of drinking water

Sample site		Chemical parameter				
		pH	Manganese (Mn) (mg/L)	Iron (Fe) (mg/L)	Salinity (NaCl) (mg/L)	Arsenic (As) (mg/L)
Alfadanga (Faridpur)	Median	7.4	0.3	0.6	400	0.033
	IQR	0.3	0.4	2.5	150	0.063
	Mean ± SD	7.4 ± 0.4	0.3 ± 0.2	2.0 ± 2.9	478.6 ± 210.0	0.047 ± 0.034
Kendua (Netrokona)	Median	7.4	0.2	0.5	200	0.007
	IQR	0.4	0.4	1.4	100	0.01
	Mean ± SD	7.6 ± 0.4	0.3 ± 0.3	1.1 ± 1.7	197.0 ± 243.0	0.031 ± 0.053
Shibchar	Median	7.4	0.9	2	450	0.045
	IQR	0.4	0.9	3.9	500	0.028
	Mean ± SD	7.4 ± 0.3	0.9 ± 0.6	2.0 ± 2.8	584.4 ± 352.1	0.057 ± 0.037
Rupsha (Khulna)	Median	7.4	0.2	1.4	1050	0.008
	IQR	0.3	0.1	2.4	1050	0.013
	Mean ± SD	7.4 ± 0.2	0.2 ± 0.1	2.3 ± 2.0	1180 ± 723.0	0.009 ± 0.006
Debhata (Satkhira)	Median	7.4	0.2	0.8	400	0.003
	IQR	0.2	0.2	0.5	150	0.001
	Mean ± SD	7.5 ± 0.4	0.3 ± 0.3	1.4 ± 1.6	391.7 ± 79.3	0.006 ± 0.006
Patharghata (Barguna)	Median	7.4	0.2	0.6	100	0.004
	IQR	0.4	0.2	0.4	400	0.000
	Mean ± SD	7.4 ± 0.3	0.2 ± 0.1	0.9 ± 0.7	717.5 ± 1133.2	0.004
Rangabali (Patuakhali)	Median	7.4	0.1	0.4	500	0.005
	IQR	0.2	0.1	0.2	100	0.002
	Mean ± SD	7.5 ± 0.3	0.1 ± 0.1	0.4 ± 0.3	557.5 ± 84.4	0.004 ± 0.001
Anwara (Chittagong)	Median	-	0.2	2.0	-	0.006
	IQR	-	1.5	3.2	-	0.008
	Mean ± SD	-	0.7 ± 0.8	2.8 ± 3.2	-	0.009 ± 0.008
Bijoynagar (B.Baria)	Median	7.3	0.1	0.3	100	-
	IQR	0.0	0.2	0.9	0	-
	Mean ± SD	-	0.3 ± 0.4	0.6 ± 0.8	-	-
Shajahanpur (Bogra)	Median	7.4	0.3	0.7	100	-
	IQR	0.5	0.4	0.9	0	-
	Mean ± SD	7.4 ± 0.3	0.4 ± 0.4	1.2 ± 1.4	-	-
Kamlganj (Moulvibazar)	Median	-	0.3	2.3	-	0.075
	IQR	-	0.5	6.2	-	0.000
	Mean ± SD	-	0.4 ± 0.3	5.0 ± 6.2	-	-
Sadar (Kurigram)	Median	7.4	-	-	100	-
	IQR	0.5	-	-	100	-
	Mean ± SD	7.5 ± 0.4	-	-	135.0 ± 62.2	-
Bangladesh standard		6.5-8.5	0.1	0.3-1.0	150-600	0.05
WHO standard		6.5-8.5	0.4	0.3	250	0.01

Water pH in shallow tubewell: median (7.4), IQR (0.5), mean (7.5), SD (0.38). Water pH in deep tubewell: median (7.4), IQR (0.4), mean (7.4), SD (0.32).

of household members in the Dhaka division were exposed to higher levels of arsenic with respect to WHO (0.01 mg/L) and Bangladesh standards (0.05 mg/L), respectively (Table 4).

Water Quality Index (WQI)

Drinking water was considered excellent in Kurigram Sadar and Rangabali (Patuakhali) (WQI value < 50) (Table 5). Of the total sample sites, 33 % (4 out of 12 sites)

Table 4 Status of chemical parameters by WHO and Bangladesh drinking water standard (%)

Characteristics	WHO drinking water standard (mg/L)								Bangladesh drinking water standard (mg/L)							
	Mn		Fe		NaCl		As		Mn		Fe		NaCl		As	
	≤0.4	>0.4	≤0.3	>0.3	≤250	>250	≤0.01	>0.01	≤0.1	>0.1	≤1.0	>1.0	≤600	>600	≤0.05	>0.05
Sex																
Male	50.3	52.8	50.8	50.8	51.7	50.3	50.0	52.3	50.3	51.2	51.8	48.9	51.9	46.1	50.2	56.7
Female	49.7	47.2	49.2	49.2	48.3	49.7	50.0	47.7	49.7	48.8	48.2	51.1	48.1	53.9	49.8	43.3
p value	0.462		0.995		0.643		0.691		0.709		0.290		0.109		0.495	
Age(years)																
≤4	7.1	8.3	8.7	7.0	7.2	7.1	7.1	6.5	6.5	7.8	4.6	6.9	7.2	7.0	7.0	6.7
5-20	35.6	30.9	37.0	34.3	35.0	35.7	35.6	39.3	37.4	32.5	34.5	34.5	35.5	34.9	35.1	53.3
21–40	30.4	32.8	28.7	31.3	32.0	32.1	31.8	23.4	29.2	32.3	30.3	32.2	31.9	32.8	30.1	20.0
41–60	20.0	21.5	18.9	20.5	20.2	17.9	17.2	24.3	20.4	20.2	20.9	18.9	19.0	17.9	19.3	20.0
≥61	7.0	6.4	6.8	6.9	5.6	7.2	8.4	6.5	6.5	7.2	6.7	7.5	6.4	7.4	8.5	90.0
p value	0.6623		0.720		0.707		0.358		0.318		0.805		0.975		0.199	
Educational level																
No education	7.1	9.8	8.8	7.3	9.5	6.8	7.5	5.0	5.7	9.4	8.0	7.1	8.0	7.1	6.9	5.0
Primary	20.0	21.2	19.2	20.4	25.9	22.2	15.0	28.3	19.9	20.7	20.9	18.9	26.3	12.7	17.9	30.0
Secondary	20.6	26.5	14.4	22.8	17.2	21.2	21.1	20.0	19.4	23.8	19.5	24.2	19.2	21.4	20.8	20.0
Higher secondary and above	52.2	42.4	57.6	49.4	47.5	49.8	56.4	46.7	55.1	46.2	51.7	49.8	46.5	58.7	54.3	45.0
p value	0.166		0.152		0.257		0.175		0.032**		0.443		0.010**		0.623	
Household economic status																
Ultra-poor	30.1	32.2	24.4	31.8	21.3	19.1	26.4	27.5	27.7	32.8	30.2	30.4	20.3	18.5	25.9	36.7
Poor	36.1	42.7	36.1	37.5	42.3	38.6	33.5	42.2	39.0	35.8	36.0	38.3	41.9	31.9	33.6	63.3
Non-poor	33.8	25.1	39.5	30.7	36.4	42.3	40.1	30.3	33.3	31.4	33.8	31.3	37.7	49.6	40.5	0.0
p value	0.018**		0.010**		0.107		0.168		0.097*		0.551		0.003***		0.000***	
Access to media at home																
No access to media	48.4	50.9	35.7	51.7	82.6	58.3	65.3	35.8	46.6	51.2	52.7	40.8	66.2	76.7	56.1	56.7
Access to media	51.6	49.1	64.3	48.3	17.4	41.7	34.7	64.2	53.4	48.8	47.3	59.2	33.8	23.3	43.9	43.3
p value	0.447		0.000***		0.000***		0.000***		0.070*		0.000***		0.002***		0.950	
NGO membership																
No membership	54.0	57.3	56.4	54.2	60.7	59.3	58.7	61.5	54.0	55.4	52.2	59.2	58.6	65.5	60.4	50.0
Member of any NGO	46.0	42.7	43.6	45.8	39.3	40.7	41.3	38.5	46.0	44.6	47.8	40.8	41.4	34.5	39.6	50.0
p value	0.324		0.513		0.622		0.622		0.579		0.009**		0.051**		0.265	
Wealth index																
Lowest	22.1	27.0	28.9	21.7	22.6	21.1	38.4	0.0	20.1	25.9	25.0	20.9	22.0	20.4	28.8	0.0
Second	20.2	21.7	17.3	21.2	18.3	19.1	12.2	9.2	15.6	24.8	21.5	18.2	17.2	25.8	11.1	13.3
Middle	19.0	12.4	19.2	17.5	31.2	24.3	28.3	20.2	21.2	14.7	20.9	13.2	26.6	29.4	26.9	13.3
Fourth	17.0	20.6	16.9	17.8	20.2	17.2	5.5	48.6	17.1	18.2	16.4	19.8	20.0	11.3	15.2	60.0
Highest	21.6	18.4	17.7	21.8	7.7	18.3	15.6	22.0	26.0	16.4	16.2	28.0	14.2	13.1	18.0	13.3
p value	0.031**		0.066*		0.000***		0.000***		0.000***		0.000***		0.004***		0.000***	
Water sources by type																
Shallow tubewell	38.2	78.3	72.9	39.4	74.2	28.4	31.0	70.6	43.0	47.8	42.9	47.2	52.8	21.1	40.2	76.7
Deep tubewell	50.0	21.7	27.1	48.8	1.8	68.6	69.0	29.4	49.4	40.4	42.2	50.9	33.1	78.9	59.8	23.3
Others	11.8	0.0	0.0	11.8	24.1	2.9	0.0	0.0	7.6	11.8	14.9	1.9	14.1	0.0	0.0	0.0
p value	0.000***		0.000***		0.000***		0.000***		0.000***		0.000***		0.000***		0.000***	

Table 4 Status of chemical parameters by WHO and Bangladesh drinking water standard (%) *(Continued)*

Division																
Dhaka	6.6	12.7	11.7	6.8	36.0	40.1	9.1	67.9	6.5	8.9	7.4	8.5	38.1	39.7	22.7	76.7
Chittagong	25.4	39.7	50.8	23.0	1.6	0.0	16.5	9.2	28.7	26.9	27.2	28.4	0.8	0.0	15.6	0.0
Rajshahi	9.3	17.2	10.2	10.8	2.7	0.0	-	-	8.3	13.1	10.8	9.0	1.4	0.0	-	-
Khulna	9.5	1.5	0.0	9.8	1.0	19.8	20.2	16.5	6.5	9.7	7.1	9.5	9.0	25.9	20.9	0.0
Barisal	32.3	5.2	20.3	29.0	24.1	38.5	54.1	0.0	32.9	22.5	41.2	6.9	32.2	34.5	40.8	0.0
Sylhet	16.9	23.6	7.1	20.4	34.6	1.7	0.0	6.4	17.2	19.0	6.3	37.6	18.5	0.0	0.0	23.3
p value	0.000***		0.000***		0.000***		0.000***		0.000***		0.000***		0.000***		0.000***	
HH[a] member (%)	82	18	17.8	82.2	40.6	59.4	68.9	31.1	48.7	51.3	61.4	38.6	81.6	18.4	91.5	8.5
HH (%)	82	18	18	82	41	59	69	31	49	51	61	39	82	18	91.5	8.5

*p < 0.10; **p < 0.05; ***p < 0.01
[a]Household

had good-quality drinking water (WQI value < 100) and the majority (67 %) had poor-quality drinking water (WQI value > 100). Quality of drinking water was found very poor in Anwara (Chittagong) and Kamalganj (Moulvivazar), while water was categorized as unsuitable for drinking only in Shibchar (Madaripur).

Discussion

Assessment of drinking water quality is a timely requirement amid emerging public health problems in this context where availability of safe water is at risk due to natural and man-made activities. This cross-sectional study conducted across the country aimed at measuring drinking water quality using WQI which delivered messages on the composite effect of chemical parameters on water. The present study is a fact finding or exploratory

Table 5 Computed water quality values for sample sites

Sample site *upazila* name (district name)	WQI value	Water quality classification based on computed WQI values in sample sites
		<50 = excellent; 50–100 = good water; 101–200 = poor water; 201–300 = very poor water, >300 = water unsuitable for drinking
Rangabali (Patuakhali)	40.05	Excellent water
Sadar (Kurigram)	11.79	Excellent water
Rupsha (Khulna)	92.14	Good water
Patharghata (Barguna)	75.35	Good water
Alfadanga (Faridpur)	169.44	Poor water
Kendua (Netrokona)	142.51	Poor water
Debhata (Satkhira)	113.18	Poor water
Shajahanpur (Bogra)	135.67	Poor water
Bijoynagar (B.baria)	111.83	Poor water
Anwara (Chittagong)	253.29	Very poor water
Kamalganj (Moulvibazar)	258.36	Very poor water
Shibchar (Madaripur)	371.50	Water unsuitable for drinking

study contributing to designing and improving program interventions which cover a larger population including high arsenic, high saline prone coastal areas. There is duality about spatial and temporal variations of some chemical parameters. A periodic assessment on arsenic concentration depicts no association with seasonal variations, while repeated assessment of arsenic contents in water based on seasons is assumed to bring little value in health surveillance [18]. In contrast, seasonal and spatial variations of arsenic concentrations in groundwater have been reported by Shrestha et al. [19].

The study findings revealed that drinking water was slightly alkaline, although the ideal pH for human consumption is stated to be 7.4 [20]. A controlled pH of water is suggested in WHO guideline to reduce the corrosion and contamination of drinking water having health consequences. Water pH is influenced by a number of factors including rock and soil composition and the presence of organic materials or other chemicals. Napacho and Manyele [21] found that pH values in shallow tubewells varied between 6.7 and 8.3 due to dissolved minerals from the soil and rocks. They further explained higher alkalinity by the presence of two common minerals, calcium and magnesium, affecting the hardness of the water. On the other hand, water with low pH values is meant to be acidic, soft, and corrosive.

The median value of manganese concentrations exceeded Bangladesh standard at most of the study sites. Other Bengali studies have reported higher manganese levels in drinking water in terms of WHO standards [22]. For example, Islam et al. [23] reported that 52 % of pond-sand filter and 45 % of pond water exceeded Bangladesh drinking water standards. The median value at our sample sites was relatively lower than some previous findings (about 0.8 and 0.9 mg/L) [24, 25] but higher than the 0.1 mg/L reported by Bouchard [26].

Children are reported to be particularly vulnerable to higher manganese concentrations due to their low protective mechanisms. Approximately 8 % of children were exposed to excess manganese concentrations that exceeded both WHO and Bangladesh standards (>0.4 and >0.1 mg/L, respectively). We found higher exposure to manganese in lowest wealth group. This finding has similarity with the other study conducted in Araihazar, Bangladesh [27]. Less exposure among the infants was reported by mothers who had access to TV. Besides, participants living in poor-quality housing type (mud vs. concrete) were more likely to report exposure among the infants. Several studies have reported that exposure to high manganese concentrations threatens children's cognitive [28], behavioral, and neuropsychological health [25]. However, the potential impact of lower exposure and interactions with other metals are less well characterized. Infants and children are reported to be more susceptible to manganese toxicity than adults [27], and a number of Bangladesh studies have shown that children's intellectual function, and consequently their academic achievement, was adversely affected by manganese exposure in drinking water [22, 25, 27]. Contradictory to these findings, a higher manganese level in drinking water was shown to be protective against fetal loss during pregnancy of undernourished women in Bangladesh [29].

In most of the sample sites (9 out of 12 sites), iron content in drinking water exceeded upper acceptable limit (1.0 mg/L) of Bangladesh standard. A previous study in rural Bangladesh revealed 50 times higher iron concentrations (mean value 16.7 mg/L) in ground water than WHO's limit (0.3 mg/L) and reported that 47 % of women consumed above the daily limit of iron (45 mg), likely to increase the risk of health problems [30]. Consumption of >30 mg of iron per day in drinking water was associated with a reduced risk of anemia in individuals without thalassemia [31]. In Gaibandha, half of female respondents consuming >42 mg of iron from drinking water stayed within tolerable limits. If this limit were exceeded, however, the populations would be likely to experience health-related problems including gastrointestinal distress, zinc absorption, and others [32].

Approximately 2 % of women in developed countries but 50 % in developing countries are anemic, contributing to high rates of maternal mortality in developing countries [33]. Iron-deficiency anemia is one of the top ten contributing factors to the global burden of diseases and is considered a public health problem with a high risk of morbidity and mortality in pregnant women and young children [34]. In our study, about half of the female participants were exposed to higher iron concentrations in drinking water which exceeded both WHO and Bangladesh standard. The health impacts of exceeding recommended WHO levels of chemical substances such as iron are often not well documented [32]. There

is a duality to iron concentrations: on the one hand, iron deficiency can cause anemia and fatigue, while on the other, excess iron can cause multiple organ dysfunction (e.g., liver fibrosis and diabetes) [35]. In a 10-year period of study in Bangladesh, the prevalence of anemia in women of reproductive age ranged between 23 and 95 % depending on age, pregnancy status, and residency. However, more recent studies have reported iron deficiency as the most important determinant of 7 to 60 % of anemia cases in Bangladesh [36].

Salinity in drinking water was found higher (>600 mg/L) only in Rupsha (Khulna) and Patharghata (Barguna). Geographically, these two *upazilas* are coastal areas. Salinity problems in coastal regions are assumed to be the effects of climate change [37], although industrial and domestic wastes [38] and geological and soil characteristics [21] are also thought to contribute. Bangladesh is at the forefront of the negative effects of climate change and has faced dramatic rises in sea level over the last three decades. Approximately 20 million people living in coastal Bangladesh [24] are dependent on tubewells, rivers, and ponds for drinking water, and these sources are increasingly becoming saline due to rising sea levels [39]. Salinity has intruded over 100 km inland from the Bay of Bengal with consequent health impacts: in a 2008 survey, higher rates of preeclampsia and hypertension were reported in the coastal than non-coastal population [40]. Consistent with this, Khan et al. [41] reported that hypertensive disorders were associated with salinity in drinking water. Furthermore, reducing salt consumption from the global estimated levels of 9–12 g/day [42] to an acceptable limit of 5 g/day [43] would be predicted to reduce blood pressure and stroke/cardiovascular disease by 23 and 17 %, respectively [44].

Most households in Dohar, Shibchar, and Sonargaon used shallow tubewells for drinking, which were affected by high levels of arsenic. In Shibchar (West Kakor village), most tubewells were affected by arsenic, and the villagers were unaware of which tubewell was arsenic free; therefore, they collected drinking water from any tubewell. In some cases (e.g., Sonargaon), people used arsenic-affected drinking water sources even though they knew that the water was contaminated and damaging to health. Bladder cancer risk is increased 2.7 and 4.2 times by arsenic exposure of 10 and 50 μg/L in water, respectively. In this study, there was an 83 % chance of developing bladder cancer and a 74 % probability of mortality at a 50 μg/L exposure level. Mortality rates are 30 % higher at 150 than 10 μg/L [45]. According to a national survey conducted in 2009 by UNICEF/BBS (2011), 53 and 22 million people were exposed to arsenic according to WHO and BDWS standards, respectively. Arsenic has been detected in the groundwater of 322 *upazilas* (subdistricts) and 61 districts in Bangladesh [46]. The health effects of prolonged and excessive inorganic arsenic exposure include arsenicosis, skin diseases, skin cancers, internal cancers (bladder, kidney, and lung), diabetes, raised blood pressure, and reproductive disorders [47].

The overall suitability of drinking water was assessed using a combined measure of water quality parameters: the WQI. The chemical parameters (pH, iron, manganese, salinity, and arsenic) of water samples were used to calculate the WQI value at each site. We applied the weighted arithmetic WQI method to calculate WQI values. In this method, the permissible WQI value for drinking is considered to be 100, the water quality being considered poor if the value exceeded this acceptable limit. Water quality was found excellent only in Rangabali (Patuakhali) and Kurigram Sadar. The water was considered excellent at these sites mainly due to low chemical parameter values contributing to lower composite effect on drinking water quality. In Shibchar (Madaripur), water was categorized as unsuitable for drinking, mainly due to high manganese and arsenic levels found in water at these sites. At most sample sites (e.g., Alfadanga, Kendua, Debhata, Shajahanpur, and Bijoynagar), water was classified as "poor" for drinking due to high manganese values. Moreover, arsenic was also found to be high in Alfadanga (Faridpur) and Kendua (Netrokona). However, in Anwara (Chittagong) and Kamalganj (Moulvibazar), the chemical parameter values in the water samples were very high and contributed to very poor-quality drinking water.

Most respondents at the sample sites used shallow tubewells to obtain drinking water due to lower installation costs. In some areas, such water from shallow tubewells was reported to have high iron and arsenic levels. In coastal districts such as Barguna, Satkhira, and Khulna, water from both shallow and deep tubewells were salty, as reported by the respondents. Yisa and Jimoh [16] reported higher levels of iron and manganese that contributed to poor-quality drinking water. These characteristics are consistent with unplanned waste disposal, agricultural run-off including pesticide or fertilizer, and other environmentally hazardous activities polluting surface water [48].

The study had some limitations. This study embraced cross-sectional study design. However, it would have been better to collect samples throughout the year addressing seasonality and depth of wells. We could not collect data on other WHO-recommended parameters which was beyond our scope of work. Therefore, the analysis has been limited to few water parameters as the requirement of BRAC WASH program and due to resource constraints. Measuring other WHO-recommended chemical parameters might have been a future concern for the program. In addition, water pH would have been tested on the spot using pH meter which was not possible for this study due to limited resources. The limitations observed in this study highlight the insights of future scope of work for research divisions and WASH program.

Conclusions

Here, we report that drinking water in Bangladesh was mainly alkaline with pH values within acceptable limits. According to WHO standards, a greater proportion of household members are exposed to excessive amounts of iron compared to manganese (82 % vs. 18 %). About half of households exceeded acceptable limits of manganese exposure when considering Bangladeshi standards. Majority of the households used poor quality of drinking water according to WQI values. Higher values of iron, manganese, and arsenic reduced drinking water quality. Awareness raising on chemical contents in drinking water at household level is required to improve public health.

Abbreviations
As: arsenic; BRAC: Bangladesh Rural Advancement Committee; CDC: Centers for Disease Control; EQ: econo quick; Fe: iron; IQR: interquartile range; MDG: Millennium Development Goals; Mn: manganese; NaCl: sodium chloride; NGO: non-government organization; UNICEF: United Nations International Children's Emergency Fund; WASH: Water, Sanitation and Hygiene; WHO: World Health Organization; WQI: Water Quality Index.

Competing interests
The authors declare that they have no competing interests.

Authors' contributions
TA, MR, FTJ, and FA conceived and designed the study. SKM, TRC, and DD contributed to the data collection. TA, FTJ, and MR conducted the data analysis and participated in the result interpretation. TA and FTJ wrote the manuscript. MR, MAi, and MKB commented on the manuscript draft. All authors read and approved the final manuscript.

Acknowledgements
We would like to thank the respondents who provided valuable information and time for this study. We thank all the interviewers involved in the data collection and the field staff of the BRAC WASH program for their assistance in conducting this study. We acknowledge the Data Management Unit of RED for their support in data entry and cleaning. Finally, we acknowledge the Government of the Netherlands for funding the study. We thank the Nextgenediting Global Initiative (www.nextgenediting.com) for editorial assistance.

Author details
[1]BRAC Research and Evaluation Division, BRAC Centre, 75 Mohakhali, Dhaka 1212, Bangladesh. [2]BRAC Tuberculosis Programme, BRAC Centre, 75 Mohakhali, Dhaka 1212, Bangladesh. [3]BRAC Water, Sanitation and Hygiene Programme, BRAC Centre, 75 Mohakhali, Dhaka 1212, Bangladesh.

References
1. Bureau of Indian Standards (BIS). Specification for drinking water. New Delhi, India: Food and Agricultural Division Council; 2012.
2. Central Pollution Control Board (CPCB). Guide manual: water and waste water. New Delhi, India: Central Pollution Control Board; 2013. Available: http://www.cpcb.nic.in/upload/Latest/Latest_67_guidemanualw&wwanalysis.pdf.
3. World Health Organization (WHO). Guideline for drinking water quality. 2012.
4. Ochuko U, Thaddeus O, Oghenero OA, John EE. A comparative assessment of water quality index (WQI) and suitability of river Ase for domestic water supply in urban and rural communities in Southern Nigeria. Int J Human Soc Sci. 2014;4(1):234–45.

5.   Tyagi S, Sharma B, Singh P, Dobhal R. Water quality assessment in terms of Water Quality Index. Am J Water Resour. 2013;1(3):34–8.

6.   Chowdhury RM, Muntasir SY, Hossain MM. Water Quality Index of water bodies along Faridpur-Barisal Road in Bangladesh. Glob Eng Tech Rev. 2012;2:1–8.

7.   Akter T, Ali ARMM. Factors influencing knowledge and practice of hygiene in Water, Sanitation and Hygiene (WASH) programme areas of Bangladesh Rural Advancement Committee. Rural Remote Health. 2014;14:2628. Online.

8.   Dey NC, Rabbi SE. Studies on the impact of BRAC WASH-1 interventions: an overview. In: achievements of BRAC Water, Sanitation and Hygiene programme towards Millennium Development Goals and beyond. Dhaka: BRAC; 2013.

9.   Rabbi SE, Dey NC. Exploring the gap between hand washing knowledge and practices in Bangladesh: a cross-sectional comparative study. BMC Public Health. 2013;13:89.

10. Dey NC, Akter T. Women in water-hygiene and sanitation management at households in rural Bangladesh: changes from baseline to end line survey. In: achievements of BRAC Water, Sanitation and Hygiene programme towards Millennium Development Goals and beyond. Dhaka: BRAC; 2013.

11. UNICEF. First annual high level meeting for sanitation and water for all aims to be a watershed for reaching the MDG targets. 2010. Available: http://www.unicef.org/bangladesh/media_6193.htm

12. George CM, Zheng Y, Graziano JH, Rasul SB, Hossain Z, Mey JL, et al. Evaluation of an arsenic test kit for rapid well screening in Bangladesh. Environ Sci Technol. 2012;46(20):11213–9.

13. World Health Organization (WHO). pH in drinking water. Guidelines for drinking water quality. Geneva: World Health Organization; 1996. Available: http://www.who.int/water_sanitation_health/dwq/chemicals/en/ph.pdf.

14. Ambica A. Groundwater quality characteristics study by using water quality index in Tambaram area, Chennai, Tamil Nadu. Middle East J Sci Res. 2014;20(11):1396–401.

15. Rahman MM, Mukherjee D, Sengupta MK, Chowdhury UK, Lodh D, Ranjan C, et al. Effectiveness and reliability of arsenic field testing kits: are the million dollar screening projects effective or not. Environ Sci Technol. 2002;36(24):5385–94.

16. Yisa J, Jimoh T. Analytical studies on water quality index of river Landzu. Am J Appl Sci. 2010;7:453–8.

17. Tyagi S, Singh P, Sharma B, Singh R. Assessment of water quality for drinking purpose in District Pauri of Uttarkhand India. Appl Ecol Environ Sci. 2014;2(4):94–9.

18. Thundiyil JG, Yuan Y, Smith AH, Steinmaus C. Seasonal variation of arsenic concentration in wells in Nevada. Environ Res. 2007;104(3):367–73.

19. Shrestha SM, Rijal K, Pokhrel MR. Spatial distribution and seasonal variation of arsenic in groundwater of the Kathmandu Valley Nepal. J Inst Sci Technol. 2014;19(2):7–13.

20. Parker KT. What are the benefits of drinking alkaline water? 2013. Available: http://www.livestrong.com/article/498701-what-are-the-benefits-of-drinking-alkaline-water/.

21. Napacho ZA, Manyele SV. Quality assessment of drinking water in Temeke district (part II): characterization of chemical parameters. Afr J Environ Sci Technol. 2010;4:775–89.

22. Khan K, Wasserman GA, Liu X, Ahmed E, Parvez F, et al. Manganese exposure from drinking water and children's academic achievement. Neurotoxicology. 2012;33:91–7.

23. Islam MA, Karim MR, Higuchi T, Sakakibara H, Sekine M. Comparison of the trace metal concentration of drinking water supply options in southwest coastal areas of Bangladesh. Appl Water Sci. 2014;4:183–91.

24. Khan AE, Ireson A, Kovats S, Mojumder SK, Khusru A, et al. Drinking water salinity and maternal health in coastal Bangladesh: implications of climate change. Environ Health Perspect. 2011;119:1328–32.

25. Wasserman GA, Liu X, Parvez F, Ahsan H, Levy D, et al. Water manganese exposure and children's intellectual function in Araihazar Bangladesh. Environ Health Perspect. 2006;114:124–9.

26. Bouchard MF, Sauve S, Barbeau B, Legrand M, Brodeur M-E, et al. Intellectual impairment in school-age children exposed to manganese from drinking water. Environ Health Perspect. 2011;119:138–43.

27. Hafeman D, Factor-Litvak P, Cheng Z, van Geen A, Ahsan H. Association between manganese exposure through drinking water and infant mortality in Bangladesh. Environ Health Perspect. 2007;115:1107–12.

28. Roels HA, Bowler RM, Kim Y, Henn BC, Mergler D, et al. Manganese exposure and cognitive deficits: a growing concern for manganese neurotoxicity. Neurotoxicology. 2012;33:1–19.

29. Rahman SM, Åkesson A, Kippler M, Grandér M, Hamadani JD, et al. Elevated manganese concentrations in drinking water may be beneficial for fetal survival. PLoS ONE. 2013;8:e74119.

30. Merrill RD. Dietary iron may flow from tubewells in rural Bangladesh, 2012. Available: http://water.jhu.edu/magazine/dietary-iron-may-flow-from-tubewells-in-rural-bangladesh/.

31. Merrill RD, Shamim AA, Ali H, Labrique AB, Schulz K, et al. High prevalence of anemia with lack of iron deficiency among women in rural Bangladesh: a role for thalassemia and iron in groundwater. Asia Pac J Clin Nutr. 2012;21:416–24.

32. Merrill RD, Shamim AA, Ali H, Jahan N, Labrique AB, et al. Iron status of women is associated with the iron concentration of potable groundwater in rural Bangladesh. J Nutr. 2011;141:944–9.

33. Baby A, Venugopal J, D'silva R, Chacko S, Vineesha P, et al. Knowledge on management of anemia during pregnancy: a descriptive study. Med Health Sci. 2014;2:140–4.

34. Kraft S. What is nutritional deficiency anemia? What causes nutritional deficiency anemia? 2014.

35. Heming N, Montravers P, Lasocki S. Iron deficiency in critically ill patients: highlighting the role of hepcidin. Crit Care. 2011;15:210.

36. Lindstrom E, Hossain MB, Lonnerdal B, Raqib R, Arifeen SE, et al. Prevalence of anemia and micronutrient deficiencies in early pregnancy in rural Bangladesh. Acta Obstet Gynecol Scand. 2011;90:47–56.

37. Haque M, Budi A, Azam Malik A, Suzanne Yamamoto S, Louis V, et al. Health coping strategies of the people vulnerable to climate change in a resource-poor rural setting in Bangladesh. BMC Public Health. 2013;13:565.

38. Egereonu UU, Nwachukwu UL. Evaluation of the surface and groundwater resources of Efuru river catchment, Mbano, South Eastern Nigeria. Modelling, Measurement and Control. 2005. 66

39. Rahman AA, Ravenscroft P. Groundwater resources and development in Bangladesh: background to the arsenic crisis, agricultural potential and the environment. Dhaka: The University Press Limited; 2003. 466 p.

40. Rasheed S, Jahan S, Sharmin T, Hoque S, Khanam MA, et al. How much salt do adults consume in climate vulnerable coastal Bangladesh? BMC Public Health. 2014;14.

41. Khan AE, Scheelbeek PFD, Shilpi AB, Chan Q, Mojumder SK, et al. Salinity in drinking water and the risk of (pre)eclampsia and gestational hypertension in coastal Bangladesh: a case-control study. PLoS ONE. 2014;9:e108715.

42. Brown IJ, Tzoulaki I, Candeias V, Elliott P. Salt intakes around the world: implications for public health. Int J Epidemiol. 2009;38:791–813.

43. World Health Organization (WHO). Population salt reduction strategies for the prevention and control of non-communicable diseases in South-East Asia region. New Delhi: World Health Organization; 2013. p. 48.

44. He FJ, Li J, MacGregor GA. Effect of longer term modest salt reduction on blood pressure: Cochrane systematic review and meta-analysis of randomized trials. BMJ. 2013;346.

45. Saint-Jacques N, Parker L, Brown P, Dummer T. Arsenic in drinking water and urinary tract cancers: a systematic review of 30 years of epidemiological evidence. Environ Health. 2014;13:44.

46. Hossain M, Rahman SN, Bhattacharya P, Jacks G, Saha R, et al. Sustainability of arsenic mitigation interventions—an evaluation of different alternative safe drinking water options provided in MATLAB, an arsenic hot spot in Bangladesh. Front Environ Sci. 2015;3.

47. Santra SC, Samal AC, Bhattacharya P, Banerjee S, Biswas A, et al. Arsenic in food chain and community health risk: a study in gangetic west Bengal. Procedia Environ Sci. 2013;18:2–13.

48. Chapman D. Water quality assessment—a guide to use biota, sediment and water in environmental monitoring. Report No. 041921590. London: E&FN Spon, an imprint of Chapman & Hall; 1996. 626 p.

20

What does quality of care mean for maternal health providers from two vulnerable states of India? Case study of Bihar and Jharkhand

Shilpa Karvande, Devendra Sonawane, Sandeep Chavan and Nerges Mistry[*]

Abstract

Background: Quality instillation has its own challenges, facilitators and barriers in various settings. This paper focuses on exploration of quality components related to practices, health system challenges and quality enablers from providers' perspectives with a focus on maternal health studied through a pilot research conducted in 2012–2013 in two states of India—Bihar and Jharkhand—with relatively poor indicators for maternal health.

Methods: Qualitative data through in-depth interviews of 49 health providers purposively selected from various cadres of public health system In two districts each from Bihar and Jharkhand states was thematically analysed using MAXQDA Version 10.

Results: Maternity management guidelines developed by the National Health Mission, India, were considered as a tool to learn instillation of quality in provision of health services in various selected health facilities. Infrastructure, human resources, equipments and materials, drugs, training capacity and health information systems were described as health system challenges by medical and paramedical health providers. On a positive note, the study findings simultaneously identified quality enablers such as appreciation of public-private partnerships, availability of clinical guidelines in the form of wall posters in health facilities, efforts to translate knowledge and evidence through practice and enthusiasm towards value of guidelines.

Conclusions: Against the backdrop of quality initiatives in the country to foster United Health Care (UHC), frontline health providers' perspectives about quality and safety need to be considered and utilized. The provision of adequate health infrastructure, strong health management information system, introduction of evidence-based education and training with supportive supervision must constitute parallel efforts.

Keyword: Healthcare quality, Maternal-child health services, Quality perspectives

Background

Globally, the maternal mortality ratio (MMR) has declined by 47 % over the past two decades with the highest reduction in Eastern Asia (69 %) and Southern Asia (64 %). In India, the National Rural Health Mission (NHM) launched by the Government of India is a leap forward in establishing effective integration and convergence of health services and affecting architectural correction in the healthcare delivery system in India [1]. It has developed a series of guidelines and has launched various programmes and initiatives such as the Janani Suraksha Yojana, the Janani Shishu Suraksha Karyakram and the Reproductive Maternal Neonatal Child and Adolescent Health (RMNCH+A) [2] for improving maternal health and quality of care. Additionally, it has set the Indian Public Health Standards (IPHS) for standardized service provision. However, the unfinished agenda of maternal and child mortality still exerts immense strain on the overstretched health systems in discrete locations.

Furthermore, the dichotomy in the health performance of various states of India draws attention towards

* Correspondence: frchpune@bsnl.in
Foundation for Research In Community Health, Pune, India

state-specific needs and priorities. The state of Kerala with an MMR as low as 61 [3] is striving to bring it further down, whereas vulnerable states such as Bihar [2] and Jharkhand [3] with MMR of 274 and 245, respectively, are struggling to reach the national MMR figure of 167 [3]. Besides, MMR percentage of home deliveries (Kerala—0.0, Bihar—42.1, Jharkhand—53.4) and unmet need of family planning (Kerala—19 [4], Bihar—31.5 and Jharkhand—22.3 [5]) highlight state disparity.

A systematic literature review showed that there is no universally accepted definition of quality of care which is widely accepted as multifaceted [6]. Outcomes of pregnancy and utilization of maternal healthcare services are studied to reflect lack of quality. Various studies [7–11] have highlighted health system challenges in terms of delay in obtaining obstetric care, service provisioning, access and cultural issues. Herein, fragmented and unregulated health-care delivery systems, poor availability of trained human resources for health and social determinants of health have been identified as some of the issues to be addressed for achieving universal health coverage by 2022 [12]. Most of the studies have addressed users' perspectives regarding health system challenges or are based on empirical evidence collected by researchers. Relatively less is known about the perspectives and practices of health providers at multiple levels even in international literature. Two studies present provider perspectives to understand health system challenges [13, 14]. Provider perspectives are important since they impinge on adherence to quality standards, professional team work, quality and training of medical education and interaction with the communities that are served by them.

Achieving quality maternal health care is the ultimate desired outcome at the national level; however, the strategies to achieve the outcome need to have state-specific contexts. This paper focuses on case studies of two vulnerable states—Bihar and Jharkhand—conducted in 2012–2013 based on exploration of quality components related to practices, services, systems and human resources from providers' perspectives with a focus on maternal health.

Methods

The pilot research was conducted in two selected states—Bihar and Jharkhand (two districts each)—during October 2012–May 2013. During the initial visits, a study team of two public health researchers interacted with local key organizations to understand maternal health situation in the state and to learn specific characters of districts. The state governments were approached for seeking formal approval to conduct the research. The district selection was governed by district statistics for maternal health, logistic feasibility for data collection

and suggestion from the state government. Attempts were made to include two contrasting districts from each district. Healthcare providers primarily from various health cadres in the public health sector formed the sample for this study.

Selected states and districts

Bihar has 38 districts with a total population of 103 million. The state has launched several initiatives, mostly in collaboration, such as the Family Friendly Hospital Initiative under the SWASTH programme [15] focusing on patient care, patient safety, patient stay and patient feedback and the Ananya programme with the Bill and Melinda Gates Foundation with an objective to ensure that mothers and babies survive and remain healthy during pregnancy, childbirth, and early childhood. Additionally, there are public-private partnership (PPP) schemes for service provisions. Bihar has implemented HIS strengthening project in collaboration with UNFPA since October 2009 [16].

Jharkhand state from eastern India was carved out of the southern part of Bihar in November 2000. The state has a population of 32 million residing in 24 districts. The state implements several collaborative initiatives such as the MCHIP programme of USAID for implementation of the RMNCH+A approach for reduction in mortality through focused maternal and child health interventions or UNICEF initiative focusing on child health and immunization, skilled birth attendance and basic emergency obstetric care (BEmOC). The state has initiated implementation of Electronic Health Management Information System (e-HMIS) in 2012 (Table 1).

Table 1 Key maternal health indicators for selected states of Bihar and Jharkhand

Health indicator	Bihar	Jharkhand
Total population (million) [3]	104	32.9
Decadal growth (%) [3]	25	22.34
Crude birth rate [5]	26.1	23
Natural growth rate [5]	19.3	18.1
Sex ratio [3]	918	947
Child sex ratio [3]	935	943
Infant mortality rate [5]	48	36
Maternal mortality ratio [5]	274	245
Total fertility rate [5]	3.5	2.7
Percentage of women with institutional delivery [5]	55.4	46.2
Percentage of women who had delivery at home [5]	42.1	53.4
Home delivery assisted by skilled persons [5]	30	27.4
Percentage of safe delivery [5]	64.5	56.2
Mothers who had three or more ANC [5]	36.7	60.2

Health facilities

All Indian states have a three-tiered rural healthcare system with the health sub-centre (HSC) as the most peripheral contact point generally serving a population of 5000. The primary health centre (PHC) is a referral unit for about six sub-centres with four to six beds generally serving a population of 30,000. The third tier—Community Health Centre (CHC)—is a 30-bedded referral hospital with four PHCs and having specialized services, generally serving a population of 120,000 [17]. In Bihar and Jharkhand, few health sub-centres were upgraded to serve as delivery points aiming to cater for maternity services. Personnel from health facilities at each of the three levels from the selected districts were included in the pilot research for understanding quality perspectives and health system challenges (Table 2).

The district health teams as well as local NGOs helped the research team for planning the field work.

Profile of the respondents

In all 49 health providers based at 32 selected health facilities from the two states were interviewed. They included doctors, nurses (staff nurses and auxiliary nurse midwives), private practitioners and academicians from formal public health sector, and informal health providers (quacks) involved in provision of maternal health services were also interviewed. The selection of health providers was purposive depending upon their involvement in provision of maternal health care in the selected district and availability at the time of interview (Fig. 1).

Study tool

The project focused on the following domains of maternal healthcare, viz. antenatal care, delivery practices, intra and post-natal care and family planning. Data was primarily derived from in-depth interviews of health providers in English and Hindi (for nurses). An interview guide was designed with the following themes: (a) clinical practices related to maternity management, (b) experience of provision of maternal health care including challenges, and (c) perceptions regarding guideline-based management and quality enablers.

Additionally, field observations made by the study team supported the primary data collected from the interview, for instance, number of beds in the health facility or the functionality of an intensive care unit.

Ethics considerations

The research proposal received ethics clearance from the Institutional Research and Ethics Committee of Foundation for Research in Community Health (IREC/2012/22/9). Written permission to conduct this research was obtained from the state health officials of the respective state. Each respondent was interviewed one-on-one at the health facility, subsequent to seeking written informed consent for conducting and audio-recording of the interview. Privacy during interview, anonymity and confidentiality of information shared were strictly maintained. At times, additional precaution had to be taken during the interviews of paramedical staff to avoid interference from their senior staff to influence their responses.

Data management and analysis

Qualitative data were transcribed and translated in English, wherever necessary. Thematic codes—inductive and deductive—were generated, viz. key clinical practices, perceptions of quality, health infrastructure challenges, community dynamics and attitude towards guidelines. The data were processed with the software MAXQDA Version 10.

Results

The results are presented under three categories—practices in maternity management, health system challenges and quality enablers.

Practices in maternity management

Maternity management guidelines developed by NHM were considered as a standard of quality for provision of health services in various selected health facilities. Respondents were asked about practices for provision of key components of maternity management including routine antenatal care investigations, the use of partograph for monitoring progress of labour and management

Table 2 Profile of health facilities (n = 32) visited during the study

Type of health facilities visited during the study	Bihar (n = 17)			Jharkhand (n = 15)		
	Public	Private	Informal	Public	Private	Informal
District hospitals	2	2	1	2	3	1
Sub-district/referral hospitals	2			0		
Block level hospitals	3			3		
Peripheral hospital-primary health centres/health sub-centres	6			6		
ANM training school	1					

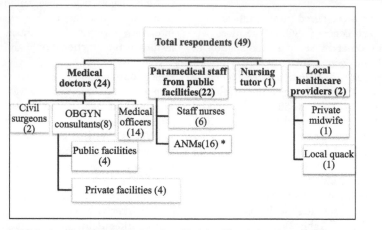

* ANMs- Auxiliary Nurse Midwives from block level hospitals, primary health centres and health sub-centres

Fig. 1 Profile of respondents based on their designation

of obstetric complications. The medical doctors and nurses reported several deviations from NHM guidelines in terms of non-compliance with the recommended investigations and examinations. Three key variations which emerged were as follows:

A) "Non"-use of partograph—partograph is a composite graphical record of key data (maternal and foetal) during labour entered against time on a single sheet of paper and provides progress of labour. One of the key messages regarding "Care during labour and delivery" in the "SBA Guidelines for Skilled Attendance at Birth" [17] states that "partograph will help the nurse recognize the need for action at the appropriate time and thus ensure timely referral".. Relevant measurements include cervical dilation, foetal heart rate, duration of labour and vital signs. The nurses mentioned about not using the partograph because of various reasons such as overload of women in labour or nurses perceived insignificance of partograph.

Partograph is not so useful because in most of the primi cases it suggests referral, but actually it is not so. We cannot refer them in real life situation due to delay and poor access and the woman delivers here. ANM, CHC, Jharkhand

B) Early augmentation of labour at the time of delivery—the training curriculum for skilled birth attendants does not recommend the use of drugs for augmentation of labour in case of normal labour [17]. However, the health providers frequently

mentioned about community dynamics as one of the major reasons for early augmentation of labour.

When the woman comes with labour pains, she is in a hurry. The attendant also feels like getting it over fast. Oxytocin dilates the cervix and is used for augmentation. Medical doctor, block PHC, Bihar

Subsequently, the NHM guideline about post-natal stay at health facility to be at least of 48 h was also compromised due to reasons such as insufficient beds or lack of warmers during the winter season.

C) No screening for HIV during pregnancy—facility for HIV testing as a desirable component of ANC investigation needs to be available at the CHC [17]. However, HIV testing was not routinely practiced either due to unavailability of laboratory equipments and/or trained human resources.

We have the necessary testing kits. Our lab technician is trained for HIV testing, but he has forgotten everything. We do not conduct any HIV testing here, but only prescribe the same. Medical officer, CHC, Jharkhand

Deviations in practices related to maternity management were the overall result of the lack of knowledge about the guideline recommendations, skill or attitude of a health provider, perceived community pressure or infrastructural challenges in implementation of the recommendations.

Health system challenges

Technical and non-technical components viewed as health system challenges by medical and paramedical health providers from the visited public health facilities are as follows:

Inadequacy of quality infrastructure

The reference point for gauging infrastructure was the IPHS promoted by the NHM [18]. Bihar and Jharkhand have poor distribution of health facilities, including First Referral Units (FRU). Some of the block PHCs have excessive population coverage and cater to a population of more than 0.2 millions. As per the policy, one block PHC caters to a population of 80,000 to 120,000 [19]. Health providers highlighted challenges in terms of inadequacy of health infrastructure including physical infrastructure, equipments, materials and poorly functioning transport. About 75 % of the health facilities, including the district hospitals, had shortage of beds, at times resulting in patients being required to lie on the floor. The supply of adequate electricity and running water was observed only in 50 % of the visited health facilities. Non-availability of ultrasound machines at the sub-district, referral and even district hospitals compromised early identification of high-risk pregnancies. This was in contravention to the *Operational guidelines for quality assurance in public health facilities* [20]

> If we cannot manage the eclampsia patients here, we refer them to Patna [neighbouring district]. If on assessment we know the woman has PROM [Premature Rupture of Membrane] or foetal distress then we will not open her here. We do not have the facilities here. If she developed some respiratory problem, there is no ventilator support here. Obstetrician, sub-district hospital, Bihar

Poor availability of treatment for eclampsia in public facilities forces women to seek eclampsia care mostly from the private sector and incurs heavy out of expenditure [21].

Forty percent of the visited health facilities did not have a regular supply of essential drugs such as folic acid tablets as was mentioned by the health providers and/or observed by the researchers in the study team. Shortage of contraceptives, IFA tablets and pregnancy testing kits [22] and drugs for treatment of eclampsia certainly affects preparedness of health providers to manage pregnancies or emergency obstetric care.

> The district societies are supported with funds for procurement of drugs; however it was noticed that the funds are underutilized. State level health official, Bihar

> Medicines are not available so we cannot provide the services. What is point in talking about protocols or guidelines? Medical officer, PHC, Bihar

Non-availability of drugs either deprived the women from availing the necessary drugs or increased their out-of-pocket expenditure since they were asked to procure the drugs from private drug stores.

Guideline implementation for referral of obstetric cases with high risks or complications can only be effected with functional transport arrangements. Both states have a toll-free facility of ambulance referred as "108" which works exclusively for transport of women in labour to hospital and to their homes, 48 h after delivery. However, an occasional breakdown of these vehicles and unduly extended repair was a problem in the peripheral health facilities.

> The ambulance had broken down for one month. Local leaders even got up to beating us. If we do something today and cannot offer it tomorrow, my complaint will go to the higher authority. Because of this fear, we cannot start anything. Medical officer, PHC, Bihar

Inadequate EmOC services in both the states especially Jharkhand further compromised quality of maternal health care. This was reflected both in shortage of trained staff at even as high as the district level hospital and lack of ultra sonography facilities as cited by the health providers and observed during the study visits. Subsequently, referral cases either had to visit private facilities or were managed by other informal health providers including local quacks. There were also incidents of involvement of local quacks for unnecessary augmentation of labour. The study team approached one such quack in Jharkhand. He was an agriculturist settled down in one of the study districts and provided medical aid upon demand from a community starved of formally trained providers.

> I inject drug Syntecinone to augment labour, on demand from the community. Local quack, Jharkhand

Shortage of trained workforce

About 90 % of the visited health facilities reported a problem of managing workload against the available trained manpower due to vacancies in the posts, e.g. one of the districts of Bihar had 27 medical doctors posted against the sanctioned number of 106 [23]. In general, there are significant vacancies for doctors, nurses and paramedical staff in Bihar [22].

A shortage of specialists was a problem even at the district hospital level.

> When a baby is premature and critical, we refer. We do have a pediatric ICU here, but there is no pediatrician which makes it difficult to monitor the baby 24 hrs. Obstetrician, district hospital, Jharkhand

In Jharkhand, only one out of ten auxiliary nurse mid-wife (ANM) training centres were functional. Hence, quality as well as quantity of trained human resource was a challenge for the health system. In recognition of the gaps in pre-service training, the government conducted in-service training for all their staff towards implementation of guidelines. Nevertheless, technical and non-technical (soft) skills were emphasized as gaps in such trainings in these two states.

> Necessary things [infrastructure and equipment] are here but we are not trained, for e.g. for laparoscopy, and hence we cannot do it. Also we need to train paramedical staff in order to have significant contribution from them as a team member. Obstetrician, district hospital, Bihar

> Nursing staff are trained for various issues such as breastfeeding. However training them for counselling is needed especially to understand community behaviour and to counsel relatives about women's stay the health facility for two days post-labour. Civil Surgeon, Bihar

Traditional birth attendants (TBA) locally referred as "Dais" and other informal healthcare providers played a crucial role because they were available in provision of accessible neighbourhood maternity management services. Adding value to their role by orientation and training towards safe delivery was considered as a needed approach for ensuring safe maternity management practices by both local NGOs and private practitioners.

> We can train Dais (TBAs) and community health workers in basic and routine health checkups. They can be taught and trained regards to risk factors, warning sign, etc and design tools around that. Private obstetrician, Jharkhand

Challenges in translating knowledge into practice

Translating knowledge or recent evidence into practice has multiple dimensions such as knowledge based on needs, field level challenges, perceived importance of experience-based learning over knowledge from books and value of guideline-based management. Ninety percent of the medical doctors and obstetricians interviewed in this study mentioned about following text books in their medical education. The obstetricians were aware about the availability of guidelines for management of obstetric complications, the need for evidence and their updating through attending conferences and personal readings.

> Guidelines are changed. RCOG guideline, for example, changes [gets updated regularly]. We follow the same here. Obstetrician, Bihar

The experience of providers was simultaneously mentioned as a crucial guiding factor.

> Earlier there used to be trained traditional birth attendants [dai]. These Dais would know about conducting deliveries. They used to tell us, teach us. Experience is the big thing, not only the knowledge from the book. We need to have experience. Medical officer, Bihar

> There is no fixed protocol in medical science. Patient is there with you and with your experience and knowledge, you have certain judgment. Patient should be safe as soon and as much as possible. Obstetrician, Bihar

Though there was awareness about recent evidence and guidelines among the obstetricians from both states, a clear preference for experience over evidence-based clinical management was perceived.

Perceived community dynamics

Managing community dynamics was equally challenging for healthcare providers while attempting to deliver quality services. The study highlighted community dynamics affecting delivery of quality services, as perceived by the health providers. The health providers mentioned poor awareness among community about the importance of post-natal care. As per the Indian guidelines [17], the duration of post-natal stay should be of 48 h. The doctors and nurses frequently mentioned about non-compliance with this recommended duration of post-natal stay at health facility because of the pressure from the family for early discharge of the woman from the health facility. The providers felt that the early exit of the new mother from the health facility was due to the prevalent unfriendly atmosphere and poor infra-structure. This was supported also by observations by the study researchers.

The language divide between the providers and users were barriers in the maintenance of a friendly atmosphere.

It further resulted in gaps in health education and counselling particularly towards preventive aspects of maternity management.

> We face some language problems so we are not able to have much communication with the women on issues such as their diet during pregnancy. Medical doctor, CHC, Jharkhand

At times, the reluctance of these communities towards the use of formal public health services proved to be a great challenge in provision of maternal health services. "The importance of efforts to take the services to their doorstep" was mentioned to be the key strategy to improve uptake of services by one of the district health officials from Jharkhand.

Lack of a robust HMIS

Both states claimed to have developed a robust HMIS; however, its implementation was observed to be rudimentary. The electronic HMIS was still in its infancy stage in both states.

> Data entry by ANMs is a challenge. There is only one data entry operator at a block level generally catering a population of about 200,000. Internet connectivity is poor. There is reluctance from medical doctors for any type of computerized monitoring. HMIS expert at the State level, Bihar

Additionally, there was a lack of analytical capacity for translation of uploaded information into action plans at the district as well as the state level. During the visit, the study team could not observe a functional electronic data upload in any of the peripheral health facilities including primary health centres of the two states. The information regarding referrals between health facilities could not be retrieved by the health officials at the district as well as sub-district level. There were instances of incomplete primary data at sub-centre level, e.g. a blank column of information regarding PROM for the past 1 year.

Quality enablers

The study findings simultaneously highlighted quality enabling features in the states.

Both states appreciated the need to partner with the private sector and generated several PPP initiatives. Most of the PPPs focused on provision of services. To illustrate, Bihar initiated formal partnerships with the private sector in the form of outsourcing of services such as pathology centres and hospital maintenance services. These services were provided free of cost to the patients in the public health system; however, there was

a need to ensure the availability and accessibility of these services at all the stipulated health facilities. There was state level monitoring of the PPPs through state data centres [24] but its benchmarks were unclear.

Both states initiated programmes and schemes for quality improvement in maternal health such as the creation of delivery points at health sub-centre level for the increase of outreach of obstetric services and focused efforts such as provision of comprehensive care in the areas of RMNCH+A in Jharkhand. As per the central mandate regarding implementation of adolescent reproductive and sexual health strategy, Adolescent Reproductive Sexual Health (ARSH) clinics have been established at the CHCs. Though such a centre was present in one of the CHCs visited during the study, implementation of key features to ensure quality of ARSH services, viz. creating conducive environment in the community, could not be confirmed.

Health facilities from both states displayed wall posters depicting certain treatment algorithms and were considered as an important check-list for the paramedical staff.

> Such posters [pointing at the poster on importance of breast feeding within ½ an hour after delivery] are helpful especially for the paramedicals. Medical officer, Block PHC, Bihar

However, it was mentioned that other than the protocols displayed in the form of wall posters, the health providers did not receive any quick reference document as "guidelines" from the public sector.

A section of the medical doctors from Bihar expressed the need for better dissemination of guidelines as even the doctors over and above the nurses were largely unaware about NHM guidelines. Obstetricians from the private sector in Jharkhand highlighted the need to have an apex body for generating guidelines and their local adaptations.

> There is no national body or uniform procedure for developing guidelines. Government guidelines are there, but not well circulated especially in the private sector. Further, there is no instruction for how to follow these guidelines, whether it is compulsory or not, what would be the legal aspects of (not) following various guidelines is not clear. Private obstetrician, Jharkhand

The emphasis on the need for well-developed guidelines and their accessibility is a highly positive indication for their acceptance and implementation.

The enthusiasm of health providers especially the young nurses drew special attention during the study. Enthusiasm to acquire knowledge regarding clinical practices and to seek inputs for improvisation in routine clinical skills was appreciable. The aspiration of a young ANM from one of the remote CHCs of Jharkhand about being "perfect in giving the episiotomy cut" was one striking example of expression of yearning for quality by primary healthcare providers.

Discussion

The utility value of the present study lies in the identification of the perspectives that challenge or facilitate the nesting of quality initiatives in India. These insights gathered from largely challenged settings are valuable since they are likely to be representative of several similar areas within India.

The development of guidelines in India since 2005 has itself been an imperfect exercise [25]. Indian guidelines in the field of maternity management are weak on documentation about the guideline development process, incorporation of patient views, weak emphasis on collection, collation and updating of evidence and formulating recommendations [26]. Additionally, the current study highlights the poor availability of guideline recommendations in the appropriate quick reference formats to the peripheral levels of health providers. No quick response guides are available, and the guidelines in poster formats which paramedical providers find useful may not have been strictly vetted for their quality-based content. Adherence to standard treatment protocols needs improvement across states because they are either not available or poorly followed with no mechanism of quality assurance [27] or quality benchmarks [28].

Good health outcomes require a downstream chain of events beginning with well-developed guidelines. The subsequent vital steps comprise of definition of quality benchmarks or standards that should percolate to providers at all levels and information systems and audits that measure and question health outcomes. In India, HMIS is used more for monitoring of tasks completed by peripheral workers rather than for programme management and designing [29]. Though large volumes of data are recorded, there is poor evidence about the use of this information in decision-making [22] and improvement of service. Facility level audits to analyse elements of causality similar to the set of clinical audits developed by NICE International [30] can also augment HMIS for local and regional improvements and should be adopted as a part of the quality fabric at all facilities. Investment in training for this at both pre and in-service stage is of paramount necessity.

Even if such evidence-based guidelines were made available and the standards defined, well-trained human resource and the lack of adequate infrastructure constitute an obvious potent block in the delivery of quality healthcare [31]. The percentage of shortfall of health

facilities in Jharkhand is 35, 66 and 22 at sub-centre, primary health centre and community health centre levels, respectively [27].

Bihar currently has 12 government medical colleges [32] and 18 government ANM training schools [33], whereas Jharkhand has three government medical colleges and ten government ANM training schools [27]. Despite the efforts to increase the number of seats for medical and paramedical courses, the availability of quality trained human resource in the public health sector especially the specialists, MBBS doctors, staff nurses and ANMs is a problem in the state [22]. While in-service training are provided by the states, e.g. Intra Uterine Contraceptive Device (IUCD) training for nurses and Integrated Management of Neonatal and Childhood Illnesses (IMNCI) training for doctors, gaps in clinical as well as communication and counselling skills are recorded particularly among primary care providers. These are crucial especially when providers are expected to deal with tribal and vulnerable population who may be overtly resistant to absorbing health messages and practices. Inbuilt mechanism for training and re-training, supportive supervision and, very importantly, opportunities for knowledge exchange and update are also desirable approaches for inclusion.

In a wider context, the situation on the ground advocates for a timely reform of medical education in India focusing on quality and evidence-based learning. Hopefully, the recent initiative of the Medical Council of India in introducing a competency-based education with learner-centric approaches, integration of ethics, attitudes and professionalism and skill development would address the need [34]. Imparting of communication and behavioural change skills to health providers may be an important incorporation during reforms in medical and paramedical education in both pre and in-service training.

A number of studies in infectious diseases highlight the gap between "know" and "do" with respect to the provider [35]. The inability of education to change provider behaviour may need to be supplemented through more efficient regulation. Clinical governance is the main vehicle for continuously improving quality of care [36] as was acknowledged in the late nineteenth century by the NHS in England. This will be important for adopting universal health coverage as a developmental imperative in India [37].

The current study highlights PPP as one of the potential quality enablers. However, the history of PPP in India with unclear definitions of roles, expectations and poor commitments [38, 39] does not give rise to optimism. It can be used only as a stop gap in a narrow window of time because private participation in public health depends heavily on external funding which drives incentivization inherent in PPP models [39]. The Kerala

Government's partnership with the Kerala Federation of Obstetricians and Gynaecologists for development and utilization of quality benchmarks with inputs from NICE International [28] is an example of well-planned PPP model. Since there has been a systematic commitment from the state for implementing quality, this PPP positively influences the health infrastructure, education and community mobilization for uptake of health services. The accountability for ensuring safe quality care should however ultimately rest with the public health sector.

Community dynamics was mentioned as negatively influencing guideline implementation or quality compliance. How does the doctor continue to exert good practices and good judgement against community demand which may be at variance with good practice? Despite the fact that Kerala has made a firm commitment for quality in healthcare, provider perspectives and community dynamics continue to affect guideline-based clinical practice, e.g. high rate of caesarean section [22]. Community education, provider perspective and quality of provider-patient interaction therefore assume vital importance.

With gaps at multiple levels, the need for strengthening and skill building of human resources for quality healthcare should be afforded the highest priority. Besides the advantages in providing better quality of care, this will also enable the optimal utilization of contemporary point of care technologies poised for health and disease control [40].

Conclusions

Against the backdrop of quality initiatives in the country to foster United Health Care (UHC), addressing frontline health providers' perspectives about quality and safety need to be acknowledged, addressed and valued. Provision of requisite services including health infrastructure, strong health management information system, introduction of evidence-based education and training with supportive supervision must be a parallel exercise. Furthermore, the health providers must respect health as a fundamental right and medical errors as immoral, illicit and illegal. If not, quality health care will continue to be a mirage in the absence of motivated human resources.

Competing interests
The authors declare that they have no competing interests.

Authors' contributions
SK carried out research, participated in the data collection, data management, data analysis and drafted the manuscript. DS coordinated all the datacollection and data management. SC participated in the data management and data analysis. SK and NM conceived of the study, and participated in its design and coordination and helped to draft the manuscript. All authors read and approved the final manuscript.

Acknowledgements
The authors acknowledge the funding support from Population Foundation of India and Tata Steel, India. They appreciate the positive support and help received from the government bodies of both the study states—Bihar and Jharkhand for permitting the pilot research. The support and help received from various NGOs from the two states are deeply acknowledged. The authors thank all the study participants for willingness to share their experiences.

References
1. Lakshminarayanan S. Role of government in public health: current scenario in India and future scope. J Family and Community Medicine. 2011;18(1):26.
2. National Health Mission, Govt of India, RMNCH + A. http://nrhm.gov.in/nrhm-components/rmnch-a.html. Accessed 27 Aug 2015.
3. Census of India. Sample registration system. (n.d.). http://www.censusindia.gov.in/2011-Common/Sample_Registration_System.html. Accessed 27 Aug 2011.
4. Ministry of Health and Family Welfare, HMIS Portal, District Level Household Survey-2012-13 DLHS IV. https://data.gov.in/catalog/district-level-household-and-facility-survey-dlhs-4. Accessed 1 Sept 2015.
5. Census of India. Annual health survey 2012—13 fact sheet. http://www.censusindia.gov.in/vital_statistics/AHSBulletins/AHS_Factsheets_2012_13.html. Accessed 27 Sept 2015.
6. Raven JH, Tolhurst RJ, Tang S, van den Broek N. What is quality in maternal and neonatal health care? Midwifery. 2012;28(5):e676–83.
7. Rao PSS, Richard J. Socioeconomic and demographic correlates of medical care and health practices (Abstract). J Biosocial Sci. 1984;16(3):343-355. http://journals.cambridge.org/action/displayAbstract?fromPage=online&aid=1632396&fulltextType=RA&fileId=S0021932000015169. Accessed 18 Feb 2016.
8. Sarita PT, Tuominen R. Use of health care services in two rural communities in Tanzania. Community Dent Oral Epidemiol. 1993;21:133–5.
9. Kumar R, Singh MM, Kaur M, Impact of health centre availability on utilization of maternity care and pregnancy outcome in a rural area of Haryana(Abstract). J Indian Med Assoc. 1997; 95(8):448-50. http://www.ncbi.nlm.nih.gov/pubmed/9492451. Accessed 18 Feb 2016
10. Rohde J, Viswanathan H. The rural private practitioner. New York: Oxford University Press; 1995.
11. Shelton JD, Davis SS. Some priorities in maximizing access to and quality of contraceptive services. Adv Contracept. 1996;12(3):233–7.
12. Singh Z. Universal health coverage for India by 2022: a utopia or reality? Indian J Community Med. 2013;38(2):70–3.
13. Afari H, Hirschhorn LR, Michaelis A, Barker P, Sodzi-Tettey S. Quality improvement in emergency obstetric referrals: qualitative study of provider perspectives in Assin North district, Ghana. BMJ Open. 2014;4(5):e005052.
14. Graner S, Mogren I, Duong LQ, Krantz G, Klingberg-Allvin M. Maternal health care professionals' perspectives on the provision and use of antenatal and delivery care: a qualitative descriptive study in rural Vietnam. BMC Public Health. 2010;10(1):608.
15. Bihar State Health Society, Family Friendly Hospital Initiative, An NRHM Initiative. http://164.100.130.11:8091/quality_assurance/FFHI_Bihar_booklet.pdf. Accessed 18 Feb 2016.
16. UNFPA India, Rapid assessment of HMIS strengthening project in Bihar, summary of findings and way forward. http://countryoffice.unfpa.org/india/drive/RapidassessmentofHMIS-UNFPA.pdf. Accessed 6 Aug 2015.
17. National Rural Health Mission, Government of India, Skilled birth attendance guidelines for skilled attendance at birth, guidelines—Government of India. http://nrhm.gov.in/nrhm-components/rmnch a/maternal-health/guidelines.html. Accessed 27 Aug 2015.
18. Indian public health standards—Government of India. http://nrhm.gov.in/nhm/nrhm/guidelines/indian-public-health-standards.html. Accessed 27 Aug 2015
19. Ministry of Health and Family Welfare, Rural health care system in India. http://www.mohfw.nic.in/WriteReadData/l892s/rural%20health%20care%20system%20in%20india.pdf. Accessed 15 May 2015.
20. Operational guidelines for quality assurance in public health facilities and checklists-3 books, guidelines—Government of India. http://nrhm.gov.in/nrhm-components/rmnch-a/maternal-health/guidelines.html. Accessed 27 Aug 2015.

21. Chaturvedi S, Randive B, Mistry N. Availability of treatment for eclampsia in public health institutions in Maharashtra, India. J Health Popul Nutr. 2013; 31(1):86–95.

22. 8th Common Review Mission, Report 2014. http://nrhm.gov.in/images/pdf/monitoring/crm/8th-crm/Report/8th_CRM_Main_Report.pdf. Accessed 19 Jan 2016.

23. Office of civil surgeon and chief medical officer, Kishanganj, District Status for Human Resource for District Kishanganj, January 2013 [Report]

24. Bihar State Health Society, Public-private partnership (PPP)-outsourcing of private services, (IX) monitoring and evaluation. http://164.100.130.11:8091/ppp.html. Accessed 6 Aug 2013.

25. Sharma S, Sethi G, Gupta U, Chaudhury RR, Barriers and facilitators to development of standard treatment guidelines in India, WHO South-East Asia Journal of Public Health. 2015; 4(1):86-91. http://www.searo.who.int/publications/journals/seajph/issues/barriersandfacilitatorsindevelopmentofstandardtreatment.pdf. Accessed 18 Feb 2016

26. Sonawane DB, Karvande SS, Cluzeau FA, Chavan SA, Mistry NF. Appraisal of maternity management and family planning guidelines using the AGREE II instrument in India. Indian J Public Health. 2015;59:264–71.

27. 7th Common Review Mission – Jharkhand report 2013-14. http://nrhm.gov.in/images/pdf/monitoring/crm/7th-crm/report/7th_CRM_Report_Jharkhand.pdf. Accessed 19 Jan 2016.

28. Health Partnership Schemes in India, NICE International. https://www.nice.org.uk/about/what-we-do/nice-international/nice-international-projects/health-partnerships-scheme. Accessed 28 Aug 2015.

29. Sundararaman T, Gupta P, Mishra A, Vasisht I, Kauser A, Mairembam DS. Designing an information technology system in public health: observations from India. BMC Proceedings. 2012;6 Suppl 5:O19. http://download.springer.com/static/pdf/721/art%253A10.1186%252F1753-6561-6-S5-O19.pdf?originUrl=http%3A%2F%2Fbmcproc.biomedcentral.com%2Farticle%2F10.1186%2F1753-6561-6-S5-O19&token2=exp=1453202341~acl=%2Fstatic%2Fpdf%2F721%2Fart%25253A10.1186%25252F1753-6561-6-S5-O19.pdf*~hmac=d48b48c3c748d65216e1026736018fb21b956ea7f62c8b169642188033c39aa. Accessed 19 Jan 2016.

30. National Institute for Healthcare and Excellence (NICE) International, Audit and service improvement. https://www.nice.org.uk/about/what-we-do/into-practice/audit-and-service-improvement. Accessed 21 Jan 2016.

31. Spangler SA. Assessing skilled birth attendants and emergency obstetric care in rural Tanzania: the inadequacy of using global standards and indicators to measure local realities. Reprod Health Matters. 2012;20(39):133–41.

32. National Health Portal, Medical colleges in Bihar. http://www.nhp.gov.in/medical-colleges-in-bihar_pg. Accessed 19 Jan 2016.

33. Indian Nursing Council, List of colleges of nursing for ANM course recognized and permitted to admit students for the academic year. http://www.indiannursingcouncil.org/pdf/anm-recognized-nursing-institution.pdf. Accessed 3 Feb 2016.

34. Medical Council of India, Vision 2015, March 2011. http://www.mciindia.org/tools/announcement/MCI_booklet.pdf. Accessed 20 Aug 2015.

35. Satyanarayana S, Subbaraman R. et al. Quality of tuberculosis care in India: a systematic review. Int J Tuberc Lung Dis. 2015;19(7):751–63.doi: 10.5588/ijtld.15.0186. http://www.ncbi.nlm.nih.gov/pmc/articles/PMC4462173/pdf/nihms684760.pdf. Accessed 18 Feb 2016.

36. Scally G, Donaldson LJ. Clinical governance and the drive for quality improvement in the new NHS in England. BMJ. 1998;317(7150):61.

37. Universal Health Coverage- India, Why UHC for India? And how can it be achieved? All about UHC in India Available from: http://uhc-india.org/. Accessed 27 Aug 2015.

38. Rangan SG, Juvekar SK, Rasalpurkar SB, Morankar SN, Joshi AN, Porter JDH. Tuberculosis control in rural India: lessons from public-private collaboration. Int J Tuberc Lung Dis. 2004;8(5):552–9. http://docstore.ingenta.com/cgibin/ds_deliver/1/u/d/ISIS/86083199.1/iuatld/ijtld/2004/00000008/00000005/art00008/D9BC3448212FB8A01455787629BD2BD5417C3E5AE6.pdf?link=http://www.ingentaconnect.com/error/delivery&format=pdf.

39. Murthy KJR, Frieden TR, Yazdani A, Hreshikesh P. Public-private partnership in tuberculosis control: experience in Hyderabad, India. Int J Tuberc Lung Dis. 2001;5(4):354–9.

40. Ortiz E, Clancy C. Use of information technology to improve quality of healthcare in the United States. Health Serv Res. 2003;38:2. http://www.ncbi.nlm.nih.gov/pmc/articles/PMC1360897/pdf/hesr_127.pdf. Accessed 2 Feb 2016.

21

Out-of-pocket expenditure on prenatal and natal care post Janani Suraksha Yojana: a case from Rajasthan, India

Dipti Govil[1*], Neetu Purohit[2], Shiv Dutt Gupta[2] and Sanjay Kumar Mohanty[3]

Abstract

Background: Though Janani Suraksha Yojana (JSY) under National Rural Health Mission (NRHM) is successful in increasing antenatal and natal care services, little is known on the cost coverage of out-of-pocket expenditure (OOPE) on maternal care services post-NRHM period.

Methods: Using data from a community-based study of 424 recently delivered women in Rajasthan, this paper examined the variation in OOPE in accessing maternal health services and the extent to which JSY incentives covered the burden of cost incurred. Descriptive statistics and logistic regression analyses are used to understand the differential and determinants of OOPE.

Results: The mean OOPE for antenatal care was US$26 at public health centres and US$64 at private health centres. The OOPE (antenatal and natal) per delivery was US$32 if delivery was conducted at home, US$78 at public facility and US$154 at private facility. The OOPE varied by the type of delivery, delivery with complications and place of ANC. The OOPE in public health centre was US$44 and US$145 for normal and complicated delivery, respectively. The share of JSY was 44 % of the total cost per delivery, 77 % in case of normal delivery and 23 % for complicated delivery. Results from the log linear model suggest that economic status, educational level and pregnancy complications are significant predictors of OOPE.

Conclusions: Our results suggest that JSY has increased the coverage of institutional delivery and reduced financial stress to household and families but not sufficient for complicated delivery. Provisioning of providing sonography/ other test and treating complicated cases in public health centres need to be strengthened.

Keywords: OOPE, Antenatal care, Delivery care, Cash assistance scheme, India

Background

Since the millennium declaration, the global, national and regional efforts to improve health-related millennium goals (reduction of maternal mortality and child mortality) in developing countries were intensified. Improving the maternal health services become the leading strategy to reduce maternal and child mortality. Several innovative programmes from many developing countries including the conditional cash transfer schemes in India (Janani Surakhya Yojana), Nepal (safe delivery incentive program) and Bangladesh (maternal health voucher schemes in Bangladesh) were introduced to increase the demand for maternal health services specifically among poor and marginalised. A large and growing literature from these countries suggests the functioning, utility and limitations of these programmes [1–18]. Though these programmes were context specific and differ by design and implementation strategy, they had the common goal to reduce the out-of-pocket expenditure on maternal care and increase the access to maternal services among the poor and marginalised. A number of evaluation studies reported the spectacular success of the various schemes in increasing access to maternal services [9, 11, 16, 17, 19]. Despite these programmes in place, the progress in health-related Millennium

* Correspondence: diptigovil@gmail.com
[1]Department of Population Policies and Programs, International Institute for Population Sciences, Govandi Station Road, Deonar, Mumbai 400088, Maharashtra, India
Full list of author information is available at the end of the article

Development Goals is slow and largely uneven across regions, income groups and by social attributes [20–23].

India accounts one fourth of child mortality and one fifth of maternal mortality worldwide [24, 25]. The inequalities in health outcome and health care utilisation are large across geography, economic status and education [26–29] and largely resulting from financial, cultural and social constraints. In India, in the year 2004–2005, about one fourth of the mothers who did not deliver at health centre reported cost as barrier for not availing the services [30]. Especially poor households consider spending a huge amount on child-bearing deterrent, leading to low health care utilisation among them. This is also corroborated by the fact that the out-of-pocket expenditure on health care accounts about two thirds of the total health expenditure [31] and health expenditure is often catastrophic [32, 33]. Though the maternal health services were free in public health centres, there were charges on medicine, bed, user fees and bribe [34–37].

Recognising that an increase in the level of utilisation of health care for child birth may lead to a reduction in the maternal mortality and neonatal mortality, the Ministry of Health and Family Welfare, Government of India, launched conditional cash transfer scheme, i.e., *Janani Suraksha Yojana (JSY)* (*Janani* denotes to *mother*, *Surakasha* for *protection/safety* and *Yojana* means *scheme*), to address the delays of decision-making, transportation and access to services. The JSY is a flagship intervention programme under National Rural Health Mission (NRHM), launched in April 2005. The JSY scheme covered transport cost, delivery cost and incentive to Accredited Social Health Activists (ASHAs) for motivating women to opt for institutional delivery. It also facilitated public-private partnerships by providing accreditation to private hospitals/nursing homes for delivery services. The cash incentive of INR 1400 (US$30) to recent mothers was given at the time of discharge from the hospital after verifying all the records.

Since the implementation of NRHM, the institutional deliveries in India had increased from 41 % in 2005–2006 to 81 % in 2013–2014 [30, 38] and the infant mortality declined from 58 infant deaths in 2005 [39] to 35 infant deaths per 1000 live births in 2013–2014 [38]. The maternal mortality ratio (MMR) had declined from 254 in 2004–2006 to 167 per 100,000 live births in 2011–2013 [40, 41]. A number of state specific studies were also undertaken to inform the functioning and progress of NRHM in general and JSY in particular [15, 42–45]. The gap (for institutional deliveries) between low and high performing states started reducing despite the fact that there was no differential change in the availability and access of any health facility [43]. This indicated that people were able to

avail skilled care at the time of delivery irrespective of the economic status.

Studies on OOPE consistently report higher expenditure for deliveries conducted in private health care centres and for complicated deliveries and caesarean deliveries [32, 46–54]. The OOPE for antenatal care in child-bearing process was also found much higher than delivery care alone [55]. The expenses incurred during child bearing also varied with the place of antenatal care (ANC), indicating that the contact with private facility at any stage of pregnancy will increase cost per delivery [52]. A normal delivery in a health care facility in Nepal was US$64 compared to US$129 per caesarean delivery while excluding opportunity cost [54]. Similarly, in the case of India before NRHM, the cost per delivery in a public and private health institution was US$25 and USD$104, respectively, whereas average cost at antenatal care was US$10 [32]. For Bangladesh, these costs were US$85 and US$181 [56]. The cost per complicated delivery was significantly higher in Tanzania, Africa, Kenya, Burkina Faso and Lao PDR [46, 50–52].

Though a number of studies have examined on the coverage of maternal care services, differentials in OOPE by type of health facility, there are not many studies on cost of antenatal care and the coverage of JSY incentives. The aim of this study is to examine the variation in out-of-pocket expenditure in accessing maternal health services (antenatal and delivery care) and the extent to which the JSY incentives covered the burden of cost incurred.

The paper has been conceptualised with the rationale. First, the cost was one of the major barriers in availing the antenatal and natal care among poor and marginalised. This has particular bearing in the state of Rajasthan that has higher infant and maternal mortality than national average and large variation in maternal care utilisation among different population sub-groups within the state. Second, because of poor quality of the services at public health care institutions, utilisation of maternal health services from private sector increased over a period of time, which had a significant burden on the economic condition of households across various socio-economic groups. Also, women switch the service provider from public to private and vice versa during pregnancy and child birth. No attempt has been made to capture this pattern of service utilisation. Third, it is important to document to what extent the large investment on maternal care under the NRHM helped in the reduction of cost for end users. This is generally of great interest to policy makers and planners for evidence-based policy-making.

Methods

This paper is based on a cross-sectional study conducted in Rajasthan during April to May 2011. The state of Rajasthan with a population of 69 million in 2011 [57] had the second highest maternal mortality ratio in the country (255 per 100,000 live births) [41] and at low level of socio-economic development. The study was conducted in the four districts of Rajasthan, namely, Udaipur and Banswara (tribal districts—with 49.7 and 76.4 % tribal population, respectively), and Sikar and Sawai Madhopur (nontribal districts). A multi-stage sampling was used to select the sample. From each selected district, two blocks were identified based on the highest and lowest proportion of institutional deliveries. Data on number of deliveries was obtained from Pregnancy and Child Tracking System of Government of Rajasthan (Management Information System—MIS). In this system, information from each village of Rajasthan is being recorded with the help of ground level health care workers. Government claims to maintain the data on all the pregnancies occurred in Rajasthan. From each of the blocks, two primary health centres (PHCs) were selected based on their performance on institutional deliveries (highest and lowest). From each PHC (in total 16), two villages were selected randomly. All the women who gave births (JSY beneficiaries and non-beneficiaries) 1 year prior to survey (during April 2010–March 2011) were interviewed from 32 villages of four districts. A list of women who gave birth during the period was obtained from ASHA (Accredited Social Health Activist) and ANM (Auxiliary Nurse Midwife) of the village. A total of 424 women were successfully interviewed under the study. A structure interview schedule was prepared for data collection and pre-tested in a village before final survey. Data was collected on multiple issues related to accessibility, availability and utilisation of services including cost incurred during pregnancy, delivery and post-delivery and money received under JSY.

The direct cost incurred during childbearing (pregnancy and delivery) was termed as out-of-pocket expenditure (OOPE). The OOPE includes (a) expenditure during antenatal care such as registration fees, doctor' fee, medicine, tests, sonography and transportation and (b) expenditure incurred during delivery—registration, transportation, doctor, medicine, tests, bed and food. The amount spend on bribe and gift was not included in the study. The cost incurred during postnatal care primarily included the cost on child health, therefore not included in the expenditure on maternal care. The OOPE in the paper is synonymous to the total expenditure incurred during a pregnancy/delivery irrespective of JSY amount. There were a few cases where the expenditure was very large. To reduce the variation, we have levelled the value at 95 % level; e.g., those 5 % women with higher than OOPE (antenatal care) of US$179 were kept at US$179, and similar

approach was followed for computing expenditure during natal care. The total OOPE was adjusted to average US$ in the year 2010–2011 (US$1 = 46.2 INR) [58]. The term normal delivery is defined as the delivery without any complication.

Descriptive statistics (mean, confidence interval, per cent distribution) was carried out to understand the differentials in OOPE on antenatal and natal care. A log linear regression model was used to understand the significant predictors of OOPE. Log of OOPE (continues variable) is the dependent variable. The independent variables are both continuous and categorical. The continuous variables are education, age, duration of stay in hospital and birth order. The categorical variables are BPL status of the family, complications during pregnancy and delivery, received JSY incentives and place of ANC.

Ethics

Ethical clearance for conducting the study was taken from the ethical board of Indian Institute of Health Management Research (IIHMR), Jaipur. Verbal informed consent was taken from women participating in study with the assurance that confidentiality will be maintained and information obtained for this study will not be used for any other purposes except for research.

Results

Table 1 presents the descriptive statistics of the study population. The mean age of the women was 25.7 years, and about half of them were illiterate. Half of the women belonged to schedule caste/tribe, and more than half were working for wages or kind. About one third of the women were living below poverty line (BPL). Most of the women had received at least three or more antenatal check-ups with a mean of 3.5. The distribution of women by source of antenatal care showed that 43 % women availed the antenatal check-up exclusively from public facilities, 21 % from private facilities and 36 % from both public and private facilities. However, the coverage of full antenatal care (3 check-up + 2 tetanus toxoid (TT) injections + received 90 iron folic acid (IFA) tablets) was only 24 %. On the other hand, the proportion of institutional deliveries was 83: 62 % delivered in public health facilities, 17 % at private health facilities and 3.5 % at accredited private health facilities. Of total, 66 % of the women received incentives under JSY. Almost all women who delivered at public health facilities received JSY incentives (96 % had already received and 4 % were about to receive at the time of survey). More than half of the respondents (57 %) had received any postnatal care (PNC).

Table 1 Sample profile of the women covered under the study in Rajasthan, 2011 (N = 424)

Background characteristics	Percentage	n
Literacy rate	44.8	190
Caste		
Schedule caste	13.0	55
Schedule tribe	37.7	160
Other backward saste	34.7	147
Others	14.6	62
Working	52.8	224
Households possessing BPL card	33.3	141
Mothers received 3 or more ANC	76.9	326
Full antenatal care (3 ANC + 2 TT + received 90 IFA)	24.3	103
Place of antenatal care		
No ANC	1.2	5
Public facility	42.9	182
Private facility	20.5	87
At both public and private facility	35.4	150
Place of delivery		
Public facility	62.3	264
Accredited private facility	3.5	15
Private facility	17.2	73
Home	17.0	72
Mothers received incentives under JSY	65.8	279
Mothers received postnatal care	57.0	241

Figure 1 presents the out-of-pocket expenditure (OOPE) on antenatal care by place of antenatal care. It may be mentioned that the OOPE on antenatal services includes costs incurred on registration, fee to the doctor, medicines, blood and urine tests, sonography and transportation.

The mean OOPE on antenatal care was US$41 (95 % CI 37–45), US$26 in public health facilities and US$64 for those availed services at private health facilities. Women, who availed antenatal care services exclusively from private facility, spend nearly two and a half times higher than women who availed services exclusively from public health facility. Women who availed at both public and private health facilities spent UD$49.

Though all women reported the total cost on antenatal care, only 23 % could provide the expenditure incurred on various services during antenatal care. The share of medicine in OOPE was 59 % followed by sonography (18 %), blood tests (8 %), transporation (8 %) and doctor consultation (7 %). It varied almost in the similar proportion among women who received antenatal care exclusively from public facility, private facility or from both public and private facilities. If women received ANC from public sector, they spent 53 % on medicine, 19 % on sonography, 9 % on tests, 12 % on transportation and 7 % on doctor's fee of total OOPE. And, this proportion was 60, 17, 7, 9 and 7 %, respectively, if they went to private sector for antenatal care.

OOPE on delivery care

The OOPE on delivery care and antenatal and delivery care (together) by place delivery is presented in Table 2. The OOPE on delivery was US$44, US$51 for institutional deliveries and US$10 for home deliveries. The OOPE at public health centre was estimated at US$39 compared to US$88 in private health facilities and US$72 for accredited private health facilities. By considering the expenditure on antenatal and delivery care, the total OOPE expenditure was estimated at US$85. The OOPE expenditure on antenatal and delivery care in public health centre was significantly lower (US$78 per

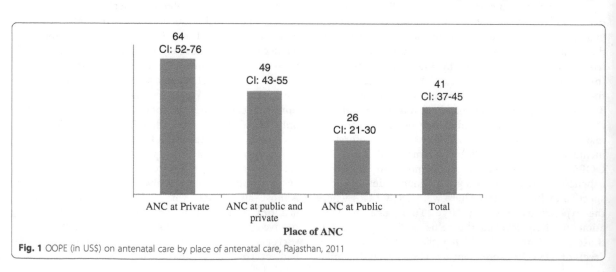

Fig. 1 OOPE (in US$) on antenatal care by place of antenatal care, Rajasthan, 2011

Table 2 OOPE[*] (in US$) on delivery care and antenatal and delivery care by place of delivery in Rajasthan, 2011

| Place of Delivery | Expenditure (in US$) during | | | | N |
| | Delivery care | | Antenatal and delivery care | | |
	Mean	95 % CI	Mean	95 % CI	
Institution[a]	51	46–56	96	87–105	352
Public facility	39	34–45	78	69–87	264
Accredited private facility	72	44–101	133	91–176	15
Private facility	88	75–102	154	131–176	73
Home	10	7–12	32	25–40	72
Total	44	39–49	85	78–93	424

[*]JSY incentive has not been deducted from OOPE
[a]Institutional includes private, public and accredited private health facilities

delivery) compared to US$154 in private health centre and US$133 at accredited private health centre.

A pregnant woman may avail antenatal care services from private health care facility and deliver at a public health facility or vice versa. This behaviour would affect the OOPE occurred during the child-bearing process. Percent distribution of women by place of antenatal care and delivery is shown in Table 3. Among women who delivered at public health centre, half of them obtained antenatal care services from public facility and nearly one third of them availed antenatal care services both from public and private facility. It is interesting to note that among women who delivered at private facility, 48 % of them received antenatal care services from both public and private health facility. Further analysis of OOPE revealed that the expenses incurred varied significantly with the place of antenatal care and delivery. When all antenatal check-ups were availed from public health facility, and the delivery too was conducted at public health facility, the average OOPE was US$59. However, when the place of delivery was private facility, the average expenditure increased to US$97 and exceeds spending of US$38 over the amount spent on delivery at public health facility (Table 3).

When a woman availed antenatal services at private health facility but chose to deliver at public facility, the OOPE was US$107. As expected, the respondents who received ANC services at private and delivered at private health facility spend US$183. OOPE among women who availed ANC services both from public and private

health facility or delivered at private revealed that the contact with private health facility at any stage of child-bearing process increased the OOPE.

Complications and OOPE

Table 4 describes the OOPE on antenatal and delivery care by complications. In general, the OOPE increases with complications both during pregnancy and delivery. For example, a normal delivery without any complication at home costs an average of US$14, US$44 at public facility and US$92 at private facility. Complications during pregnancy alone had contributed to increase in expenditure. Respondents who suffered from complications during pregnancy and delivered at public health facility had spent US$72. Women who suffered from complications both during pregnancy and delivery spent an average of US$145 in public facility delivery and US$197 for private health facility delivery.

Share of JSY incentives on cost of antenatal and delivery care

Figure 2 provides OOPE and JSY incentives provided by government per delivery. As stated elsewhere, the OOPE in public facility was US$78. Further, it was US$44 and 145 for normal and complicated delivery, respectively. Since the government was reimbursing US$34 directly to the beneficiary as JSY incentive, it was deducted from OOPE to get the actual expenditure made by the beneficiary per delivery. After deducting JSY incentives, OOPE per delivery was estimated at US$44. The government

Table 3 Place of delivery by place of ANC (%) and OOPE[*] by place of delivery and antenatal care (in US$) in Rajasthan, 2011

| Place of antenatal care | Place of delivery | | | | | |
| | Percentage | | | OOPE (in US$) | | |
	Public facility	Private facility	Home	Public facility	Private facility	Home
Public facility	52.7	14.8	44.9	59 (CI 50–69)	97 (CI 39–154)	21 (CI 12–30)
Private facility	13.4	37.5	27.5	107 (CI 75–140)	183 (CI 149–217)	32 (CI 17–48)
Both public and private facility	34.0	47.7	27.5	97 (CI 82–111)	141 (CI 115–167)	55 (CI 39–72)

[*]JSY incentive has not been deducted from OOPE

Table 4 OOPE[*] (in US$) on antenatal and delivery care by pregnancy and delivery complications[#] and place of delivery in Rajasthan, 2011

Complications		Place of delivery			
		Institutional	Public	Private	Home
Normal deliveries	Mean	52	44	92	14
	95 % CI	41–62	33–55	61–124	8–20
	N	83	70	13	29
Complications during pregnancy but not during delivery	Mean	90	72	141	44
	95 % CI	80–100	63–81	118–164	33–56
	N	189	140	49	36
Complications during pregnancy and delivery	Mean	163	145	197	48
	95 % CI	139–187	124–173	152–243	13–84
	N	76	50	26	7
Complications during pregnancy or delivery	Mean	110	90	160	45
	95 % CI	99–120	80–101	138–183	34–55
	N	269	194	75	43

[*]JSY incentive has not been deducted from OOPE
[#]the number of cases was less (four each in public and private facility delivery) in the case of no complication during pregnancy but complications during delivery, therefore, dropped from analysis

share accounts 44 % of OOPE per delivery, 77 % for normal delivery, 38 % for delivery that had complications during pregnancy or delivery and 23 % for those deliveries who had complications both during delivery and pregnancy.

Socio-economic differentials in OOPE

Table 5 provides the socio-economic differentials in institutional delivery and OOPE. Comparatively larger proportion of younger women opted for institutional deliveries than older women. After deducting JSY incentives the mean OOPE of younger women (below 25 years) was US$57 compared to US$48 among women aged 25 years and above (US$57 vs. US$48). Similarly, women with general caste spend almost double than other caste women even after deducting JSY incentives. Nearly two-third women from BPL and 59 % from APL

delivered at public health centre. Among these, a BPL family spends US$56 on antenatal and delivery care compared to US$91 among APL families. JSY incentives were received by both the sections. JSY incentives reduced the total cost by 47 % among BPL families and 32 % among APL families. Almost the same proportion of literate and illiterate women delivered in public facilities; their expenditure on antenatal and delivery care varied significantly (for illiterate US$68; for literate US$91). Results were similar by husband's literacy status; in the case of literate husband, the spending on antenatal and natal care was almost double than when husband was illiterate. JSY incentives shared the expenditure to a greater extend in the family where husband was illiterate, even more than where a woman was illiterate. As the birth order increased, the proportion who delivered at institution and the expenditure on

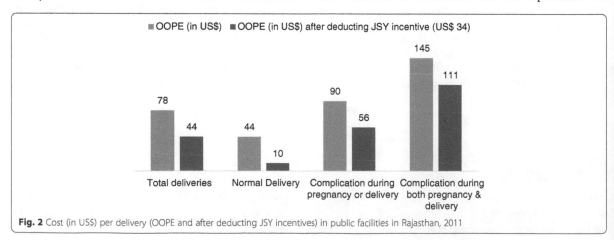

Fig. 2 Cost (in US$) per delivery (OOPE and after deducting JSY incentives) in public facilities in Rajasthan, 2011

Table 5 Place of delivery and expenditure by background characteristics. Percentage distribution of women by place of delivery, mean OOPE (in US$) and JSY incentive as percentage of total cost per delivery by background characteristics in Rajasthan, 2011

Background characteristics	N	Percentage of women delivered at public facilities	Percentage of women delivered at private facilities	Expenditure during antenatal and natal care by place of delivery				
				Public facility			OOPE in private facility	OOPE in home delivery
				Total cost	Actual OOPE less of JSY incentives	Incentives as % of total cost		
Age								
Less than 25	206	65.0	20.9	84	57	31.7	168	44
25 and above	218	59.6	20.6	72	48	33.6	134	24
Caste								
General	62	54.8	35.5	116	82	28.8	177	32
Others	362	63.5	18.2	72	45	37.9	141	32
Economic status								
BPL cardholder	141	69.5	12.8	56	30	46.4	101	22
APL	283	58.7	24.7	91	61	32.4	163	38
Type of family								
Nuclear	111	55.8	15.3	92	63	31.5	162	24
Joint/extended family	313	64.6	22.7	74	46	38.0	147	39
Literacy								
Illiterate	234	64.9	12.4	68	42	38.6	134	26
Literate	190	59.0	31.1	91	60	33.8	158	35
Work status								
Not working	200	72.0	20.5	73	45	38.3	142	43
Working	224	53.6	21.0	71	55	22.8	157	23
Husband's literacy								
Illiterate	84	60.7	14.3	48	23	51.3	117	24
Literate	340	62.6	22.3	85	56	34.1	155	36
Birth order								
One	140	66.5	22.9	92	61	33.2	165	50
Two	124	58.2	27.5	82	54	34.0	149	29
Three and above	160	61.9	13.8	62	36	42.2	149	27
Place of ANC[a]								
Public facility	182	75.9	7.1	59	34	42.4	97	21
Private facilities	87	40.3	38.0	107	76	29.7	183	32
Both public and private facilities	150	59.3	28.0	97	65	33.0	141	55
Duration of stay in hospital after delivery[b]								
Less than 48 h	145	65.5	34.5	59	34	43.3	115	NA
More than 48 h	207	81.6	18.4	88	59	33.5	197	NA
N	424	279	145	264	264	264	88	72

[a]Includes home deliveries
[b]Only institutional deliveries

antenatal and delivery care reduced. Women, who delivered for the first time, spend US$90 as compared to women who delivered their second, third and more order births (US$82 and 62, respectively). Therefore, the reduction in the OOPE due to JSY was greater in the higher-order birth than in the lower-order birth. Nearly 60 % of the women who delivered their children in the hospital stayed for more than 48 h. Women who stayed for more than 48 h, 82 % of them delivered in public facilities. Increase stay in hospital also increased the expenditure on child birth. Those who stayed in public hospital for 48 h paid US$29 additional as compared to woman who stayed less than 48 h (US$59 vs. 88). This gap widened (US$82), when the delivery was conducted at private facility. The reduction in OOPE due to JSY was less among women staying for longer duration.

Determinant of OOPE

To understand the determinants of OOPE, a log linear regression model is used for all nonzero cases. Further log linear regression model is suitable for OOPE as the OOPE is skewed in nature. All variables except age and place of ANC (private) are significant in the model (Table 6). Educational attainment, duration of stay and complications are positively associated with OOPE. For example, with increase in educational attainment by 1 year, the OOPE is likely to increase by 2 %. The APL households are likely to incur 35 % more OOPE than BPL households. Those women experienced pregnancy complications are likely to spend 61 % more than normal deliveries. These results are in agreement with bivariate analyses and in expected direction. Those who received JSY were likely to spend 46 % less than those not under JSY categories. Similarly, those who had ANC at public hospital were less likely to spend more compared to others. The R^2 value was .408 indicating that 41 % variation in the model is being explained. The F statistics (25.7) was significant, indicating the overall significance of the model.

Table 6 Determinant of out-of-pocket expenditure (OOPE): dependent variable—log of out-of-pocket expenditure

Independent variables	Unstandardized beta coefficients	Sig.	95.0 % CI	
			Lower limit	Upper limit
Age (in completed years)	−.010	.477	−.037	.018
Education (in completed years)	.020	.047	.000	.041
Birth order	−.084	.214	−.217	.049
Duration of stay in the hospital (in hr.)	.005	.000	.003	.006
Economic status of family (BPL®)				
APL	.353	.001	.149	.557
Complications during pregnancy/delivery (No®)				
Yes	.612	.000	.392	.832
Received JSY incentives (No®)				
Yes	−.458	.000	−.691	−.225
Place of ANC—public (No®)				
Yes	−.544	.000	−.753	−.334
Place of ANC—private (No®)				
Yes	.095	.468	−.160	.351
(Constant)	7.833	.000	7.127	8.538

Discussion

In India, enormous efforts were made by the government, nongovernmental organisations and bilateral and multi-lateral donors to increase the level of skilled birth attendance while launching or supporting dedicated policies and programmes since 1990s. In this series, National Rural Health Mission emerged as a milestone. About two third of national health budget is being spent on NRHM, and the NRHM is said to bring considerable changes in whole health care delivery system in India especially in reducing infant and maternal mortality. However, the national average conceals large disparities across the states and socio-economic group in the country. Numerous studies have shown the socio-economic inequality in the utilisation of health care services, and the increased services do not necessarily benefit the poor and marginalised. Prior to the launch of NRHM, empirical evidences and research studies suggest that the cost of the health care services was one of the major barriers for poor households to avail the services [30, 32, 59–62] especially for child bearing. After one decade of the implementation of NRHM, especially *Janani Suraksha Yojana* (JSY), the largest conditional cash transfer programme in the world [9], a phenomenal increase was observed in institutional deliveries across Indian states [38]. This study attempts to understand the OOPE by pattern of antenatal care and delivery care in post-NRHM period in the state of Rajasthan.

The following are the salient findings of this study. First, we found about three-fourth mothers received three and more antenatal care and nine out of ten women delivered in a health centre. This is significantly higher compared to 41 % coverage of three or more antenatal care and 32 % institutional delivery in Rajasthan in 2005–2006 [30]. It may be mentioned that majority of women in our sample were from scheduled caste and scheduled tribe. Hence, this is indicative that the NRHM may have resulted in positive effect on antenatal care and institutional delivery in the state of Rajasthan particularly among the poor and marginalised. The finding is in line with studies on the impact of JSY [44, 63, 64]. Second, we found varying OOPE on antenatal care by the type of provider. The mean OOPE of antenatal care among those availed from public health centre was US$26, US$64 from private health centres and US$49 for those who availed from both private and public health centres. This was higher than the cost of antenatal care in the state during pre-NRHM period [32] possibly due to increasing contact and awareness on institutionalised maternal care and the price effect. Third, half of the OOPE on antenatal care and delivery care was on medicines followed by sonography/test and transportation irrespective of type of service provider. Fourth, the JSY covered 77 % of the cost for normal delivery and 23 % of the cost of complicated delivery with an average of 44 %.

This result of our study was higher than the study conducted by Gopalan et.al., where they mentioned that JSY covered 26 % of the maternal healthcare cost in rural areas [65]. The women, who suffered from complications during pregnancy and delivery, spent about three and a half times higher than those who had a normal delivery. The cost per complicated delivery was also significantly higher in African countries [46, 50].

The overall findings of the study suggest that JSY has been successful in reducing the OOPE of the beneficiaries opting for delivery at public health facility. Since the incentive was the highlight of the scheme, the increase in institutional deliveries could be attributed to the satisfaction with the incentives attached to the scheme [66]. Evidences support that incentives provided under JSY were able to meet the cost incurred by the family for the delivery to some extent. Therefore, the incentives worked in favour of institutional delivery addressing the financial barriers and enhancing utilisation of maternal care services in Rajasthan. Also, the NRHM strengthened the public health care system while addressing the other barriers for poor health care utilisation [67]. NRHM focused on the facilitating environment for safe motherhood, i.e., utmost care and attention provided to pregnant women and newborns by strong health care delivery system, i.e., availability of skilled health personnel, adequate health care facilities, equipment, medicines and emergency care along with the community mobilisation [67].

Conclusions

Based on the extent of antenatal and natal care coverage in our study, it is evident that most of the women were availing the services. Therefore, it can be said that the government's intention to encourage mothers to deliver at a health facility by providing incentives along with improvement in health care system is reducing disparity and bringing women to the health care centre. Hence, the cash incentive should continue and extend to sonography/test during pregnancy period and complicated deliveries. Since complicated deliveries are largely carried out at private health centres, provisioning of financial incentive to complicated deliveries irrespective of the type of provider should be considered. The incentives have been able to substantially reduce the financial burden faced by the women who delivers at an institution. Last, the population based survey should not only collect the cost of delivery care but also cost of antenatal care.

Limitation of the study

The study followed a cross-sectional design due to limited resource and time. The study could not segregate the post-delivery care cost from child care cost, therefore addressed the expenditure related to prenatal and natal care.

Acknowledgements

We express our heartfelt thanks to express our gratitude to UNFPA, Bangkok, for funding the study; the officials at the Department of Health and Family Welfare, Rajasthan, for their support and co-operation in granting the permission to conduct the study in the State and providing relevant information. We are extremely grateful to our research staff Dr. Vrinda Mehra, Mr. Lalit Mohan Nayak and Dr. Sonia Luna for their assistant in collecting the data for the study.

Authors' contributions

DG conceived and implemented (data collection) the study and drafted and finalised the manuscript. NP coordinated the research and helped in carrying out the data collection, analysis, and drafting of the manuscript. SDG participated in the design of the study, guided the whole process and edited the manuscript. SKM participated in the statistical analysis, sequence alignment and editing. All authors read and approved the final manuscript.

Competing interests

The authors declare that they have no competing interests.

Author details

[1]Department of Population Policies and Programs, International Institute for Population Sciences, Govandi Station Road, Deonar, Mumbai 400088, Maharashtra, India. [2]The IIHMR University, 1, Prabhu Dayal Marg, Near Sanganer Airport, Jaipur 302029, Rajasthan, India. [3]Department of Fertility Studies, International Institute for Population Sciences, Govandi Station Road, Deonar, Mumbai 400088, Maharashtra, India.

References

1. Xu L, Liu X, Sun X, Fang L, Hindle D. Maternal and infant health prepayment schemes in Shandong, China: a survey of demand and supply. Aust Health Rev. 2002;25(3):15–25.
2. Ensor T, Clapham S, Prasad D. What drives health policy formulation: insights from the Nepal maternity incentive scheme? Health Policy. 2009;90: 247–53. doi:10.1016/J.healthpol.2008.06.009.
3. Urquieta J, Angeles G, Mroz T, Lamadrid-Figueroa H, Hernández B. Impact of oportunidades on skilled attendance at delivery in rural areas. Econ Dev Cult Change. 2009;57:539–58.
4. Anastasia M. Bolivia tackles maternal and child deaths. Lancet. 2009;374:442. dx.doi.org/10.1016/S0140-6736(09)61438-0.
5. Bhat R, Mavalanker DV, Singh PV, Singh N. Maternal healthcare financing: Gujarat's Chiranjeevi scheme and its beneficiaries. J Health Popul Nutr. 2009; 27(2):249–58.
6. Morris SS. Conditional cash transfer programs and health. In: Adato M, Hoddinott J, editors. Conditional cash transfer in Latin America. Baltimore: The John Hopkins University Press; 2010. p. 212–30.
7. Schmidt JO, Ensor T, Hossain A, Khan S. Vouchers as demand side financing instruments for health care: a review of the Bangladesh maternal voucher scheme. Health Policy. 2010;96(2):98–107. doi:10.1016/J. healthpol.2010.01.008.
8. Ir P, Horemans D, Souk N, Damme WV. Using targeted vouchers and health equity funds to improve access to skilled birth attendants for poor women: a case study in three rural districts in Cambodia. BMC Pregnancy Childbirth. 2010;10(1):1–11. doi:10.1186/1471-2393-10-1.
9. Lim SS, Dandona L, Hoisington JA, James SL, Hogan MC, Gakidou E. India's Janani Suraksha Yojana, a conditional cash transfer programme to increase births in health facilities: an impact evaluation. Lancet. 2010; 375(9730):2009–23.
10. de Brauw A, Peterman A. Can conditional cash transfers improve maternal health and birth outcomes? Evidence from El Salvador's Comunidades Solidarias Rurales. IFPRI discussion paper no. 01080, International Food Policy Research Institute, Washington DC, 2011. p.12-17.
11. Ahmed S, Khan MM. A maternal health voucher scheme: what have we learned from the demand side financing scheme in Bangladesh? Health Policy Plan. 2011;26(1):25–32.
12. Sosa-Rubí SG, Walker D, Serván E, Bautista-Arredondo S. Learning effect of a conditional cash transfer programme on poor rural women's selection of delivery care in Mexico. Health Policy Plan. 2011;26:496–507.

13. Agha S. Impact of a maternal health voucher scheme on institutional delivery among low income women in Pakistan. Reprod Health. 2011;8:10. doi:10.1186/1742-4755-8-10.

14. Abuya T, Njuki R, Warren CE, Okal J, Obare F, Kanya L, et al. A policy analysis of the implementation of a reproductive health vouchers program in Kenya. BMC Public Health. 2012;12:540. doi:10.1186/1471-2458-12-540.

15. Randive B, Diwan V, De Costa A. India's conditional cash transfer programme (the JSY) to promote institutional birth: is there an association between institutional birth proportion and maternal mortality? PLoS. 2013; 8(6):e67452. doi:10.1371/journal.pone.0067452.

16. Nguyen HTH, Hatt L, Islam M, Sloan NL, Chowdhury J, Schmidt J, et al. Encouraging maternal health service utilization: an evaluation of the Bangladesh voucher program. Soc Sci Med. 2014;74:989–96.

17. Poel EV, Flores G, Ir P, O'Donnell O, Doorslaer EV. Can vouchers deliver? An evaluation of subsidies for maternal health care in Cambodia. Bull World Health Organ. 2014;92(5):331–9. doi:10.2471/BLT.13.129122.

18. Arur A, Gitonga N, O'Hanlon B, Kundu F, Senkaali M, Ssemujju R. Insights from innovations: lessons from designing and implementing family planning/reproductive health voucher programs in Kenya and Uganda. Bethesda: Private Sector Partnerships-One project, Abt Associates Inc; 2009. p. 23–38.

19. Grainger C. Lessons from sexual and reproductive health voucher program design and function: a comprehensive review. Int J Equity Health. 2014;13: 33. doi:10.1186/1475-9276-13-33.

20. Lawn JE, Costello A, Mwansambo C, Osrin D. Countdown to 2015: will the Millennium Development Goal for child survival be met? Arch Dis Child. 2007;92:551–6. doi:10.1136/adc.2006.099291.

21. Houweling TAJ, Ronsmans C, Campbell OMR, Kunst AE. Huge poor-rich inequalities in maternity and child care in developing countries. Bull World Health Organ. 2007;85(10):745–54.

22. Barros AJD, Ronsmans C, Axelson H, Loaiza E, Bertoldi AD, França GVA, et al. Equity in maternal, newborn, and child health interventions equity in maternal, newborn, and child health interventions in Countdown to 2015: a retrospective review of survey data from 54 countries. Lancet. 2012;379: 1225–33.

23. United Nations. The millennium development goals report. New York: United Nations; 2014. p. 4–5.

24. UNICEF. The situation of children in India: a profile. New Delhi: United Nations Children's Fund (UNICEF); 2011. p. 3.

25. WHO, UNICEF, UNFPA, WB, UNDP. Trends in maternal mortality: 1990 to 2013. Geneva: World Health Organization; 2014. p. 21.

26. Say L, Raine R. A systematic review of inequalities in the use of maternal health care in developing countries: examining the scale of the problem and the importance of context. Bull World Health Organ. 2007;85(10):812–9.

27. Hatt L, Stanton C, Makowiecka K, Adisasmita A, Achadic E, Ronsmans C. Did the strategy of skilled attendance at birth reach the poor in Indonesia? Bull World Health Organ. 2007;85(10):774–83. doi:10.2471/BLT.06.033472.

28. Mohanty SK, Pathak PK. Rich-poor gap in utilization of reproductive and child health care services in India, 1992-2005. J Biosoc Sci. 2009;41(3): 381–98.

29. Balarajan Y, Selvaraj S, Subramanian SV. Health care and equity in India. Lancet. 2011;377(9764):505–15. doi:10.1016/S0140-6736(10)61894-6.

30. International Institute for Population Sciences and Macro International. National Family and Health Survey (NFHS 3) 2005-06—India, vol. I. Mumbai: IIPS; 2007. p. 210.

31. Government of India, National Health Accounts Cell. National Health Accounts, India, 2004–05. New Delhi: Ministry of Health and Family Welfare, Government of India; 2009. p. 30.

32. Bonu S, Bhushan I, Rani M, Anderson I. Incidence and correlates of 'catastrophic' maternal health care expenditure in India. Health Plann Policy. 2009;24:445–56.

33. Skordis-Worrall J, Pace N, Bapat U, Das S, More NS, Joshi W, Pulkki-Brannstrom A, Osrin D. Maternal and neonatal health expenditure in Mumbai slum (India): a cross sectional study. BMC Public Health. 2011;11: 150. doi:10.1186/1471-2458-11-150.

34. Sengupta A, Nundy S. The private health sector in India is burgeoning, but at the cost of public health care. Br Med J. 2005;331:1157–8.

35. Chatterjee P. How free healthcare became mired in corruption and murder in a key Indian state. Br Med J. 2012;344:e453. doi:10.1136/bmj.e453.

36. Chattopadhyay S. Corruption in healthcare and medicine: why should physicians and bioethicists care and what should they do? Indian J Med Ethics. 2013;10(3):153–9.

37. Bajpai V. The challenges confronting public hospitals in India, their origins, and possible solutions. Advances in Public Health 2014; Article ID 898502. http://dx.doi.org/10.1155/2014/898502. Accessed 9 May 2016.

38. National Health Mission. Annual Report 2013-2014. Department of Health & Family Welfare, Ministry of Health & Family Welfare, Government of India. 2014; p.371. http://nrhm.gov.in/images/pdf/media/publication/Annual_Report-Mohfw.pdf. Accessed 10 May 2016.

39. Registrar General of India. SRS Bulletin. New Delhi, Vital Statistical Division; 2006; 41(1):1-6. ISSN 0971-3549. http://www.censusindia.gov.in/vital_statistics/SRS_Bulletins/SRS_Bulletins_links/SRS_Bulletin-October-2006.pdf. Accessed 10 May 2016.

40. Registrar General of India. Special bulletin on maternal mortality in India 2004-06. New Delhi: Vital Statistical Division; 2009. p. 3.

41. Registrar General of India. Maternal mortality ratio bulletin. Sample Registration System. New Delhi: Vital Statistical Division; 2014. http://www.censusindia.gov.in/vital_statistics/mmr_bulletin_2011-13.pdf. Accessed 10 May 2016.

42. Khan ME, Hazra A, Bhatnagar I. Impact of Janani Suraksha Yojana on selected family health behaviour in rural Uttar Pradesh. J Fam Welf. 2010; 56(Special Issue):9–22.

43. Dongre A. Effect of monetary incentives on institutional deliveries: evidence from the Janani Suraksha Yojana in India. Munich Personal RePEc Archive (MPRA), 2010; Paper No. 26339. https://mpra.ub.uni-muenchen.de/id/eprint/26339. Accessed on 10 May 2016.

44. United National Population Fund. Concurrent assessment of Janani Suraksha Yojana (JSY) in selected states Bihar, Madhya Pradesh, Orissa, Rajasthan, Uttar Pradesh. New Delhi: UNFPA; 2009.

45. Modugu HR, Kumar M, Kumar A, Millett C. State and socio-demographic group variation in out-of-pocket expenditure, borrowings and Janani Suraksha Yojana (JSY) programme use for birth deliveries in India. BMC Public Health. 2012;12:1048.

46. Kowalewski M, Mujinja P, Jahn A. Can mother afford maternal health care costs? User costs of maternity services in rural Tanzania. Afr J Reprod Health. 2001;6(1):65–73.

47. Borghi J, Hanson K, Acquah CA, Ekanmian G, Filippi V, Ronsmans C, et al. Costs of near-miss obstetric complications for women and their families in Benin and Ghana. Health Policy Plan. 2003;18(4):383–90.

48. Mukherjee S, Singh A, Chandra R. Maternity or catastrophe: a study of household expenditure on maternal health care in India. Health. 2013;5(1): 109–18. http://dx.doi.org/10.4236/health.2013.51015.

49. Mohanty SK, Srivastava A. Cost and utilization of hospital based delivery care in Empowered Action Group (EAG) States of India. Matern Child Health J. 2013;17(8):1441–51. doi:10.1007/s109995-012-1151-3.

50. Perkins M, Brazier E, Themmen E, Bassane B, DjenebaDiallo D, Mutunga A, Mwakajonga T, Ngobola O. Out-of-pocket costs for facility-based maternity care in three African Countries. Health Policy Plan. 2009;24(4):289–300.

51. Douangvichit D, Liabsuetrakul T, McNeil E. Health care expenditure for hospital-based delivery care in Lao PDR. BMC Res Notes. 2012;5:30. doi:10.1186/1756-0500-5-30.

52. Levin A, Dymatraczenko TT, McEuen M, Ssengooba F, Mangani R, Van Dyck G. Costs of maternal health care services in three Anglophone African Countries. Int J Health Plann Manag. 2003;18:3–22.

53. Borghi J, Sabina N, Blum LS, Hoque ME, Ronsmans C. Household costs of healthcare during pregnancy, delivery and the postpartum period: a case study from Matlab, Bangladesh. J Health Popul Nutr. 2006;24:446–55.

54. Borghi J, Ensor T, Neupane BD, Tiwari S. Financial implications of skilled attendance at delivery in Nepal. Trop Med Int Health. 2006;11:228–37.

55. Tripathi N, Saini SK, Prinja S. Impact of Janani Shishu Suraksha Karyakram on out-of-pocket expenditure among urban slum dwellers in Northern India. Indian Pediatr. 2014;51:475–7.

56. Khan SH. Free does not mean affordable: maternity patient expenditures in a public hospital in Bangladesh. Cost Eff Resour Alloc. 2005;3:1. doi:10.1186/1478-7547-3-1.

57. Registrar General and Census Commissioner of India. Census of India, 2011, Provision Population Totals, Paper 1 of 2011, 1. India: Government of India; 2011.

58. Reserve Bank of India. Handbook of statistics on Indian economy, 2011-12. Mumbai: Reserve Bank of India, Central Office Building; 2012. p. 236.

59. Kouyarw B, Flessa S. Catastrophic household expenditure for health care in low-income society: a study from Nouna District, Burkin Faso. Bull World Health Organ. 2006;84:21–7.

60. Agarwal S, Satyavada A, Kaushik S, Kumar R. Urbanization, urban poverty and health of the urban poor: status, challenges and the way forward. Demography India. 2007;36(1):121–34.

61. Simkhada B, Van Teijlingen ER, Porter M, Simkhada P. Factors affecting the utilization of antenatal care in developing countries: systematic review of the literature. J Adv Nurs. 2008;61(3):244–60. doi:10.1111/j.1365-2648.2007. 04532.x.

62. International Institute for Population Sciences. District level household and facility survey (DLHS-3), 2007-08. India: International Institute for Population Sciences, Ministry of Health and Family Welfare Government of India; 2010. p. 74–5.

63. Powell-Jacksona T, Mazumdar S, Mills A. Financial incentives in health: new evidence from India's Janani Suraksha Yojana. J Health Econ. 2015;43: 154–69. http://dx.doi.org/10.1016/j.jhealeco.2015.07.001.

64. Gupta SK, Pal DK, Tiwari R, Garg R, Shrivastava AK, Sarawagi R, Patil R, Agarwal L, Gupta P, Lahariya C. Impact of Janani Suraksha Yojana on institutional delivery rate and maternal morbidity and mortality: an observational study in India. J Health Popul Nutr. 2012;30(4):464–71.

65. Gopalan SS, Varatharajan D. Addressing maternal healthcare through demand side financial incentives: experience of Janani Suraksha Yojana program in India. BMC Health Serv Res. 2012;12:319. doi:10.1186/1472-6963-12-319.

66. Mohanty SK, Srivastava A. Out-of-pocket (OOP) expenditure on institutional delivery in India. Health Policy and Plan. 2012;28(3):247–62. doi:10.1093/heapol/czs057.

67. Government of India. Report of the working group on National Rural Health Mission (NRHM) for the twelfth five year plan (2012-2017), WG1: progress and performance of National Rural Health Mission (NRHM) and suggestions 2011; No. 2(6)2010-H&FW, Planning Commission, GoI. http://planningcommission.nic.in/aboutus/committee/wrkgrp12/health/WG_1NRHM.pdf

22

Are there changes in the nutritional status of children of *Oportunidades* families in rural Chiapas, Mexico? A cohort prospective study

Esmeralda García-Parra[1], Héctor Ochoa-Díaz-López[1*], Rosario García-Miranda[1], Laura Moreno-Altamirano[2], Roberto Solís-Hernández[1] and Raúl Molina-Salazar[3]

Abstract

Background: In Mexico, despite that the fact that several social programs have been implemented, chronic undernutrition is still a public health problem affecting 1.5 million children of <5 years. Chiapas ranks first in underweight and stunting at national level with a stunting prevalence of 31.4 % whereas for its rural population is 44.2 %. The purpose of this paper is to determine if the nutritional status of a cohort of children living in poor rural communities under *Oportunidades* has changed. We were interested in assessing the nutrition evolution of the children who were initially diagnosed as stunted and of those who were diagnosed as normal. Oportunidades is an anti-poverty program of the Mexican government consisting mainly in monetary transfers to the families living in alimentary poverty.

Methods: A 9-year cohort prospective study was conducted with nutritional evaluations of 222 children. Anthropometric indices were constructed from measurements of weight, height, and age of the children whose nutritional status was classified following WHO standards.

Results: The results showed that although these children were Oportunidades beneficiaries for 9 years and their families improved their living conditions, children still had a high prevalence of stunting (40.1 %) and 69.6 % had not recovered yet. Children who were initially diagnosed with normal nutritional status and became stunted 2 years later had a higher risk (relative risk (RR) 5.69, 2.95–10.96) of continuing stunted at school age and adolescence.

Conclusions: Oportunidades has not impacted, as expected, the nutritional status of the study population. These findings pose the question: Why has not the nutritional status of children improved, although the living conditions of their families have significantly improved? This might be the result of an adaptation process achieved through a decrease of growth velocity. It is important to make efforts to watch the growth of the children during their first 3 years of age, to focus on improving the diet of women at fertile age and pay special attention to environmental conditions to break the vicious cycle of malnutrition.

Keywords: Child malnutrition, Stunting, Social programs, Poverty, *Oportunidades / Prospera*, Chiapas, Mexico

* Correspondence: hochoa@ecosur.mx
[1]Health Department, El Colegio de la Frontera Sur, Carretera Panamericana y Periférico Sur s/n C.P. 29290, Barrio de María Auxiliadora, San Cristóbal de las Casas, Chiapas, Mexico
Full list of author information is available at the end of the article

Background

In the world, there are two billion people who have some deficiency of micronutrients and 1400 million are overweight, out of which 500 million are obese [1]. In spite of this, the malnutrition problems for short height (stunting) affect almost 200 million children under 5 years old in the world. In Latin American and Caribbean countries, the incidence data registers differences of up to 14 % points between the rural and the urban areas [2]. In Mexico, stunting affects 1.5 million children under 5 years of age [3]. Nowadays, Mexico faces the problem of malnutrition, which is expressed, on the one hand, with a great proportion of overweight and obese children, and on the other hand, infantile stunting and anemia [4]. Almost half of the children under five (27.5 %) who live in rural areas are stunted [5]. Between 2008 and 2010, the population living in poverty increased from 48.8 million to 52 million people (from 44.5 to 46.2 %), and ten million children (approximately 25 %) were unable to afford reasonable access to food, the so-called food poverty [2, 6].

The last National Health and Nutrition Survey (ENSA-NUT 2012) reported that the preschool and school populations of the southern region of Mexico still have a high prevalence of stunting (19.2 %) [5]. The most affected areas are the rural localities with a prevalence of 27.5 % compared with the national average of 13.6 %. Chiapas, Guerrero, and Oaxaca are among the less developed Mexican states, with the highest indexes of poverty, the poorest nutrition indicators, and the highest stunting prevalence [7]. Chiapas, where this study was conducted, comes first at national level in underweight and stunting prevalence, e.g., the prevalence of stunting among children under 5 years of age is 31.4 % at state level and for children living in rural area is 44.2 % [7].

Different social programs to combat poverty and undernutrition in Mexico have been implemented in the last four decades [8]. In 1997, Mexico launched a new incentive-based poverty reduction program, initially known as *Progresa*, in 2006 changed to *Oportunidades*, and since 2014 renamed as *Prospera*. Oportunidades focuses on enhancing the human capital of those living in extreme poverty [9]. According to the World Bank (2010), it is the principal anti-poverty program of the Mexican federal government and its aim is to break the intergenerational cycle of poverty by using cash transfers, targeted to the poorest families and conditioned to regular school attendance and family health clinic visits. In addition, households with young children are provided with a fortified food supplement (*Nutrisano*), and pregnant and breastfeeding mothers receive a fortified food (*Nutrivida*) [10].

The objective of this study was to identify the changes in the nutritional status of a prospective cohort, initiated in 2002, of children under 5 years from families affiliated to Oportunidades who live in poor rural communities of Chiapas. We were interested in assessing the nutrition evolution of the children who were initially diagnosed as stunted and of those who were diagnosed as normal.

Methods

Study area

Chiapas is a Mexican state, located in the south-eastern area of the country. According to the 2010 National Population Census, Chiapas has a population of 4,796,580 inhabitants out of which 51 % live in the rural area [11]. Chiapas is divided into 15 socioeconomic and geographic regions [12]. The results of the present research are based on the VII region called *De los Bosques*.

Study population

This research was developed in four rural communities: *La Competencia*, *Ramos Cubilete*, *Rivera Domínguez*, and *El Jardín*. These municipalities were selected by a purposive sampling technique according to their level of marginalization [12], for being an indigenous area and a priority area for the Chiapas State Ministry of Health (SSA). The four communities were selected according to the following criteria: geographical access (two of difficult access and two near the head of the municipality), proportion of indigenous population, and health system that attends them, and the other two communities being served by the SSA and two under the health system of the federal government for the uninsured population operated by the Mexican Social Security Institute (IMSS), both institutions are the ones that operate the health component of Oportunidades.

The cohort study started with a first evaluation (baseline) conducted in 2002–2003 through a census of children under 5 years of age living in the four communities, registering a total of 407 children. Three hundred seventy-nine children out of the total were children from Oportunidades families, and the other 28 were non-Oportunidades children. For the second evaluation (2004–2005), to accomplish the study objectives, only the children under 5 years who still were receiving the benefits of Oportunidades, such as supplementary foods (*Nutrisano*), were included in the follow-up. Thus a total of 237 children met these criteria and were measured during the second evaluation; the other 142 children measured in the first evaluation did not fulfill the selection criteria for the second one. During the third evaluation (2010–2011), 15 children out of these 237 were lost (6.3 %), obtaining a total final sample of 222 children who participated in the three evaluations.

Data source and study design

The data for the three evaluations were collected by household interview surveys under a prospective cohort design. During the baseline evaluation, three groups were defined according to the nutritional status of the children: stunted, normal, and high height. These three groups were followed up and evaluated twice more (2004–2005 and 2010–2011). The questionnaire used was designed and validated by the research team. The questionnaire included demographic (age of the mothers, gender, kinship, local language spoken) and socioeconomic (schooling, occupation, benefits from Oportunidades, access to social security, household conditions, and assets) information and nutritional status data. The fieldwork was done with the help of community health workers, local language speakers, who were not members of the communities under study.

Anthropometric measures

Anthropometric measurements included weight and height data of all children living in the household included in the sample.

The anthropometric measurements were conducted by students (undergraduates in nutrition) and nutritionists who were trained according to the techniques described and recommended by the World Health Organization [13] with the help of community health workers for translating and interviewing. The fieldwork staff was trained and standardized according to conventional procedures [14, 15]. To measure the weight of children under five, in the first two evaluations, we used standardized spring loaded Salter scale. For children weighing more than 20 kg, we used standardized scale class III with a capacity for 150 kg. To measure the length of the under 2-year-olds, we used an acrylic infantometer of 85 cm, with a precision up to ±0.5 cm. To measure the height of those children older than 24 months of age, we used wall estadiometer (DAY designs BREU) of acrylic material with capacity of 2 m. During the third evaluation, we used the same scale and estadiometer as in the first and second evaluation. The calibration of the equipment was done by the nutritionist responsible of the fieldwork team. To calibrate the balances weights of 5, 10 and 20 kg were used. To calibrate the estadiometers, rods of 0.5, 1.0, and 1.5 m were used [16, 17].

The cutoff points used for classifying the nutritional status of the children were defined as follows: stunting (height-for-age): <-2 standard deviations (SD) from the reference median [18].

Ethical approvals

According to Mexican health regulations, this study was considered as exempt from IRB review due to the non-invasive methods used. Informed consent was obtained verbally from all participants.

Table 1 Changes in the living conditions of the participant's families during follow-up period

Year of evaluation	2002–2003	2004–2005	2010–2011	p^a
Number of people	1093	1106	1060	
Mean age in years of the children's mothers (SD)	27.31 (6.77)	29.43 (8.05)	36.83 (7.95)	$p = 0.000$
Children under 5 years old, global and by sex[b]				
Total	26.2 %	23 %	10.6 %	$p = 0.000$
Men	11.7 %	11.2 %	4.8 %	$p = 0.000$
Women	14.5 %	11.8 %	5.8 %	$p = 0.000$
Illiterate population over 15 years old	35.2 %	30.7 %	22.4 %	$p = 0.000$
No-schooling population over 15 years old	31.7 %	27.3 %	22.5 %	$p = 0.000$
Number of homes visited	159	157	157	
Homes with dirty floor	93.7 %	84.3 %	15.1 %	$p = 0.000$
Houses with electricity	93.1 %	97.5 %	100.0 %	$p = 0.001$
Homes with refrigerator	9.4 %	14.5 %	40.3 %	$p = 0.000$
Houses with TV	32.7 %	50.9 %	66.7 %	$p = 0.000$
Households with piped water	78.6 %	81.8 %	97.5 %	$p = 0.000$
Overcrowded housings	91.2 %	92.5 %	72.3 %	$p = 0.000$
Families who eat red meat once a month	23.3 %	30.8 %	40.3 %	$p = 0.005$
Average income from *Progresa-Oportunidades* per person (USD)	$6.91	$8.91	$29.38	$p = 0.000$

[a]On a chi-square test for proportions and F test for averages
[b]In the first, second, and third evaluation, all children were under 5 years of age. In the second evaluation, only cohort children still under 5 years of age were included; the other children were their brothers and sisters who fulfill the criteria of being under 5 years of age. In the third evaluation, any children from the cohort were included for being older than 5 years of age

During the induction of the study in the study area, permissions for conducting fieldwork activities were obtained from the health community authorities at each locality. Before the administration of the questionnaires, a verbal informed consent explaining the purpose of the interview and giving assurances of the confidential use of the information was obtained from the head of each of the households visited. Those cases of children with nutritional problems were immediately referred to the nearest health center for their medical attention.

Statistical analyses

In the data entry phase, the information was processed in SPSS version 15.0.1, while for the anthropometry data, according to the age of the children; we used WHO AnthroV.3.1.0 [19] for children of 0–60 months; and WHO AnthroPlus V.1.0.2 [20] for children between 5 to 13 years of age based on WHO tables of reference [18]. These tables were used to obtain Z values for the height/age index. For the analysis of differences between proportions, chi-square test and F test were used. We calculated crude and stratified (age and sex) relative risk (RR) with a 95 % confidence interval to assess the risk of continuing stunted (cases) in the third evaluation among the children under study by comparing stunted children

(exposed group) *vs* normal and high height (non-exposed group) in the second evaluation. For this analysis, we used Stata/SE 10.0 for Windows, (2008).

Results
Living conditions of the study population

Table 1 describes the living conditions of the children's families under study. We focused on analyzing changes in demographic and socioeconomic characteristics after 9 years from the first evaluation. In general, all the living conditions indicators have improved significantly. The educational level improved as the number of illiterates diminished 12.8 percentage points (from 35.2 to 22.4 %), the number of people without schooling decreased (from 31.7 to 22.5 %), while the mean years of schooling among people over 15 years old increased 1.45 years. Housing conditions also improved during the study period. For example, the number of households with dirty floors decreased significantly and the number of household with piped water has increased. Consumption of meats, utilized as income indicator, increased significantly during the 9-year period, as it is shown in Table 1.

The age distribution of the cohort of children was as follows: 114 females of whom 56 were 0–23 months of

Table 2 Evolution of the movement of the prospective cohort of children in the different categories of nutritional status

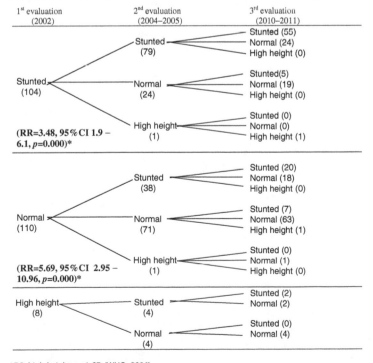

Stunted: <−2SD, normal: −2 to +1DS, high height: >+1 SD (WHO, 2006)
*To calculate the RRs of stunted children of each cohort, stunted children in the 2nd evaluation (2004–2005) were used as exposed group and normal + high height as non-exposed group. Stunted children in the 3rd evaluation (2010–2011) were defined as cases and normal children + high height as non-cases

age, 58 were 24–60 months; 108 males of whom 56 were 0–23 months of age and 52 were 24–60 months of age.

Cohort analysis of the nutritional status of the children

During the first evaluation, children were classified in three categories according the height/age index. These categories were as follows: stunting children, normal children, and children with high height for their age. Children in each category were followed up and their nutritional status was assessed to ascertain how many of them recovered and how many got worse.

Table 2 describes the movement between the nutritional status categories of the prospective cohort of the children during the follow-up period. It also shows that after 9 years of the first evaluation, the stunting problem still persists. Within the initial group of children diagnosed as stunted (104), 76 % of these children were still stunted in the second evaluation and 69.6 % children were still in the same nutritional category in the third evaluation. Likewise, 110 children who were diagnosed as normal in the first evaluation in the second

evaluation, 34.5 % of these children were identified as stunted and in the third evaluation 52.6 % children (out of 38) were still in this same condition. From the group of children diagnosed as normal the second evaluation (71), only 88.7 kept being diagnosed as normal during the third evaluation.

As far as the risk analysis is concerned, we observed that children who were stunted and did not recover for the second evaluation had 3.4 times higher risk of being stunted in the third evaluation, than children who were firstly diagnosed as stunted but they recovered in the second evaluation, whereas children, who started with a normal nutritional status and in the second evaluation were diagnosed as stunted, had a higher risk of 5.7 times of being stunted in the third evaluation than children who remained with a normal nutritional status in the second evaluation. Following this analysis, the RR was stratified for sex and age (Tables 3 and 4), finding that the statistical significance of the pattern of risk shown in Table 4 did not disappear.

Table 3 Risk analysis of the children of the cohort according to the height for age index by sex

1st. evaluation 2002 (n=222)	2nd. evaluation 2004–2005 (n=222)	3rd. evaluation 2010-2011 (n=222)	RR (95%CI) p value
Stunted male (56)	Stunted 76.8%	Stunted 74.4% / Normal 25.6%	4.8 (2.1–10.9) p=0.000
	Normal 23.2%	Stunted 15.4% / Normal 84.6%	
Stunted female (48)	Stunted 75%	Stunted 63.9% / Normal 36.1%	2.5 (1.2–5.7) p=0.042
	Normal 25%	Stunted 25% / Normal 75%	
Normal male (52)	Stunted 38.5%	Stunted 60% / Normal 40%	4.1 (2.1–7.8) p=0.000
	Normal 61.5%	Stunted 6.3% / Normal 93.8%	
Normal female (66)	Stunted 33.3%	Stunted 45.5% / Normal 11.4%	4.0 (1.7–9.6) p=0.003
	Normal 66.7%	Stunted 54.5% / Normal 88.6%	

Stunted: <–2SD, normal: –2 to +1SD and >+1 SD (WHO, 2006). To calculate RR, stunted children were used as exposed group and normal children as non-exposed group (2nd evaluation 2004–2005). Stunted children were defined as cases and normal children as non-cases (3rd evaluation 2010–2011)

Table 4 Risk analysis of the children of the cohort according to the height for age index by age

1st. evaluation 2002 (n=222)	2nd. evaluation 2004–2005 (n=222)	3rd. evaluation 2010–2011 (n=222)	RR (95%CI) p value
Stunted 0–23months of age (35)	Stunted 65.7%	Stunted 69.6% / Normal 30.4%	4.1 (1.6–10.9) p=0.030
	Normal 34.3%	Stunted 16.7% / Normal 83.3%	
Stunted 24–60months of age (69)	Stunted 81.1%	Stunted 69.6% / Normal 30.4%	3.0 (1.5–6.1) p=0.001
	Normal 18.9%	Stunted 23.1% / Normal 76.9%	
Normal 0–23months of age (77)	Stunted 38.9%	Stunted 53.3% / Normal 46.7%	5.0 (2.3–10.9) p=0.000
	Normal 61.1%	Stunted 10.6% / Normal 89.4%	
Normal 24–60months of age (41)	Stunted 29.3%	Stunted 50% / Normal 50%	7.2 (2.1–25.1) p=0.001
	Normal 70.7%	Stunted 6.9% / Normal 93.1%	

Stunted: <−2SD, normal:−2 to +1SD and >+1 SD (WHO, 2006). To calculate RR, stunted children were used as exposed group and normal children as non-exposed group (2nd evaluation 2004–2005). Stunted children were defined as cases and normal children as non-cases (3rd evaluation 2010–2011).

Discussion

The purpose of this study was to identify the changes in the nutritional status of a cohort of children of rural communities of Chiapas beneficiaries of Oportunidades on a 9-year follow-up period. Specifically, we were interested in determining the risk for children to continue with their nutritional status diagnosed at the baseline. The main finding of this study was that children who did not recover nutritionally before 3 years of age have a higher risk of continuing with the problem of stunting regardless their gender. While children who were diagnosed at the baseline evaluation as normal, but identified as stunted between 3 and 5 years of age, were at greater risk of continuing with this nutritional condition at school age and adolescence, compared with those who remained normal in the second evaluation or were stunted at the baseline evaluation but recovered in the second evaluation. In spite of the benefits of the Oportunidades program, the population is still at risk of continuing with the vicious circle of the malnutrition. The studied children who in the first evaluation were diagnosed with stunting problems (69.6 %) continued

with this health problem after almost 10 years from the first evaluation.

These findings leave us the question, why has not the nutritional status of children improved? A possible answer might be the low effectiveness of Oportunidades in improving the quality of the diet [21] together with the lack of high-quality nutritional surveillance and orientation. As shown in another component of our research, yet unpublished, where we assessed the children's diet and their families' diet habits, children are consuming a hypercaloric diet (mainly carbohydrate) with an increase of the industrialized food consumption and a decrease of fruits and vegetables consumption during the follow-up period.

Nevertheless, we recognize the limitation of not having a group of children without the benefits of Oportunidades, due to all families in these communities being included in the Oportunidades program.

Stunting during the first 3 years of life is a negative promoter for a good economic situation in the adulthood; by contrast, an adequate nutrition in the first 2 years of life is essential for the formation of human capital [22, 23]. Chronic malnutrition that occurs in the first years of life causes a shorter size, which explains the smaller size of individuals in developing countries [1, 2]. Several longitudinal studies have shown that the nutritional status of children under 3 years of age determine their adult nutritional status [24–27]. Families of the children in this research have lived in highly marginalized conditions for a long time. Therefore, the short stature of children might be associated to an intergenerational nutritional factor [28]. The intergenerational cycle of growth failure has been described in many developing countries, that is, girls who were stunted in early childhood became stunted women and are more likely to give birth to low birth-weight children [29]. Muzzo suggests that the height of the mother is strongly associated with the height of their children, rather than the height of the father is. There might have a genetic factor that influences growth; however, the extent of the genetic potential might be affected by the socioeconomic and environmental conditions of the children [30].

Our results suggest that the study children might be under the so-called "the double burden of malnutrition transition" [31–33], which implies the coexistence of malnourished children and adults with overweight and obesity within the same families due to the presence of stunting. This situation has been observed in Mexican rural communities of the south of the country [34–36]. During the period of this research, significant changes were observed in the living conditions of the families; it is remarkable to note the increase in the literacy levels and the higher number of assets and better housing conditions of these families. For instance, these families increased their income in $22.94 USD per person in average during the last evaluation (from $6.9 in 2002–2003 to $29.38 USD in 2010–2011). Although their living conditions have significantly improved, these improvements are not reflected in a better nutritional status of their children. This might be the result of an adaptation process achieved through a decrease of growth velocity. The more severe and the longer the malnutrition is, the greater the negative effects on all body measurements are [37, 38]. The results of this research agree with the ones presented in the cited study.

Conclusions

From the findings of this study, we can conclude that despite the studied population has being exposed to the benefits of Oportunidades during a long time, the problem of stunting persists and affects mostly children who are between 3 and 7 years of age. Therefore, it might be expected that a great proportion of these children will be overweight or obese in their adulthood due to their halted growth and a short stature, which in its turn determines that their weight becomes greater than their size. Thus, it is important to make efforts to watch the growth of the children during their first 3 years of age, to focus on improving the diet of women at fertile age and pay special attention to environmental conditions to break the vicious cycle of malnutrition.

Competing interests
The authors declare that they have no competing interests.

Authors' contributions
All authors contributed to the research design, interpretation and analysis of the results, and writing of the manuscript. RSH built the data base and performed the statistical analysis. All authors read and approved the final manuscript.

Acknowledgements
The authors would like to thank Alain Basail-Rodríguez, Erin I. J. Estrada-Lugo, and Helda E. Morales for their comments on the preliminary analysis, and we are indebted to all the children's families who have participated in this research. This project would have not been possible without the enthusiasm of all research team.
We also thank BA Deborah Colvin for her patience in the revision and correction of the manuscript.

Funding
This project was funded by the Alliance for Health Services Research and Health Policies, WHO, State of Chiapas Fund for Research (2004–2006), and El Colegio de la Frontera Sur, Chiapas, México.

Author details
[1]Health Department, El Colegio de la Frontera Sur, Carretera Panamericana y Periférico Sur s/n C.P. 29290, Barrio de María Auxiliadora, San Cristóbal de las Casas, Chiapas, Mexico. [2]Public Health Department, Faculty of Medicine, Universidad Nacional Autónoma de México, Circuito Interior, Ciudad Universitaria, Av. Universidad 3000, CP 04510 Mexico City, Mexico. [3]Department of Economics, Universidad Autónoma Metropolitana—Iztapalapa, Av. San Rafael Atlixco 186, Col. Vicentina C.P. 09340 Delegación Iztapalapa, Mexico City, Mexico.

References|
1.   Food and Agriculture Organization of the United Nations. The state of food and agriculture, 2013. Food Systems for Better Nutrition. Online. Retrieved from http://www.fao.org/docrep/018/i3300e/i3300e00.htm. On 15th August 2013.
2.   Fondo de la Naciones Unidas para la Infancia . Informe Annual 2010. Online. Retrieved from: http://www.unicef.org/mexico/spanish/informeUNICEF2010_final_baja.pdf. On 10th September 2013.
3.   Rivera J, Cuevas L, González T, Shamah T, García R. Stunting in Mexico in the last quarter century: analysis of four national surveys. Salud Publica Mex. 2013;55 suppl 2:S161–9.
4.   Ávila A, Shamah T, Galindo C, Rodríguez G, Barragán LM. La desnutrición infantil en el medio rural mexicano. Salud Publica Mex. 1998;40:150–60.
5.   Instituto Nacional de Salud Pública. Encuesta Nacional de Salud y Nutrición 2012. Cuernavaca, Morelos, México:INS,2012;147–154.
6.   Consejo Nacional de Evaluación de la Política de Desarrollo Social. Informe de Evaluación de la Política de Desarrollo Social en México, México D.F: CONEVAL 2012; 28–47.
7.   Instituto Nacional de Salud Pública. Encuesta Nacional de Salud y Nutrición 2012. Resultados por entidad federativa. Chiapas. Cuernavaca, Morelos, México: INS; 2012. p. 63–88.
8.   Chávez A, De Chávez M, Roldán A, Bermejo S, Avila A, Madrigal H. The food and nutrition situation in Mexico: a food consumption, nutritional status and applied programs tendencies report from 1960 to 1990. México, D.F: Editorial Pax México; 1996.

9. Levy S. Progress against poverty: sustaining Mexico's *Progresa-Oportunidades Program*. Washington D.C.: Brookings Institution press; 2006. p. 21–30.

10. World Bank. Shanghai poverty conference: case study summary. Retrieved from: Julio 2014 http://web.worldbank.org/archive/website00819C/WEB/PDF/CASE_-62.PDF.

11. Instituto Nacional de Estadística y Geografía. Panorama Sociodemográfico de Chiapas, México. INEGI 2012.

12. Consejo Nacional de Población. Chiapas, región norte. Grado de marginación por municipio, 2010. Retrieved from: Julio 2014 http://cuentame.inegi.org.mx/monografias/informacion/chis/default.aspx?tema=me&e=07

13. World Health Organization. Physical status: the use and interpretation of anthropometry. Report of a WHO Expert Committee. Geneva: WHO Technical Report Series; 1995. No. 854.

14. Lohman T, Roche A, Martorell R. Standardization reference manual. Champlaign, IL: Human Kinetics; 1988.

15. Habitch. Standardization of anthropometric methods in the field. PHAO Bull. 1974;76:375–84.

16. Sguassero Y, Moyano C, Aronna LA, Fain H, Orellano A, Carroli B. Validación clínica de los nuevos estándares de crecimiento de la OMS: análisis de los resultados antropométricos en niños de 0 a 5 años de la ciudad de Rosario, Argentina. Arch argent pediatr [online]. 2008;106:198–204. ISSN 1668-3501.

17. Peláez ML, Torre P, Ysunza A. Elementos prácticos para el diagnóstico de la desnutrición. Centro de capacitación integral para promotores comunitarios. México, D.F: Instituto Nacional de la Nutrición Salvador Zubiran; 1993.

18. World Health Organization, World Health Organization. Multicentre Growth Reference Study Group. WHO child growth standards: length/height-for-age, weight-for-age, weight-for-length, weight-for-height and body mass index-for-age: methods and development. Geneva: WHO; 2006.

19. World Health Organization. Anthro for personal computers, version 3.1: software for assessing growth and development of the world's children. Geneva: WHO; 2010. http://www.who.int/childgrowth/software/en/.

20. World Health Organization AnthroPlus for personal computers, version 1.0.2: Software for assessing growth of the world's children and adolescents. Geneva: WHO; 2009. http://www.who.int/growthref/tools/en/.

21. Ramírez-Silva I, Rivera JA, Leroy JL, Neufeld LM. The Oportunidades programs fortified food supplement, but not improvements in the home diet, increased the intake of key micronutrients in rural Mexican children aged 12–59 months. J Nutr. 2013;143:656–63.

22. Martorell R, Melgar P, Maluccio J, Ayreh D, Rivera J. The nutrition intervention improved adult human capital and economic productivity. J Nutr. 2010;140:411–4.

23. Victora C, Adair L, Fall C, Hallal P, Martorell R, Richter L, et al. Maternal and child undernutrition: consequences for adult health and human capital. Lancet. 2008;371:340–57.

24. Victora C, de Onis M, Hallal P, Blossner M, Shrimpton R. Worldwide timing of growth faltering: revisiting implications for interventions. Pediatrics. 2010;125:473–80.

25. Prader A, Largo R, Molinari L, Issler C. Physical growth of Swiss children from birth to 20 years of age. First Zurich longitudinal study of growth and development. Helvetica Paediatrica Acta. 1995;Supplementum 52:1–125.

26. Roche A, Wainer H, Thissen D. Predicting adult stature for individuals. Monographs in paediatrics. 3rd ed. Basel: Karger; 1975.

27. Tanner J, Goldstein H, Whitehouse R. Standards for children's height at ages 2–9 years allowing for height of parents. Arch Dis Child. 1970;45:755–62.

28. Emanuel I, Kimpo C, Moceri V. The association of grandmaternal and maternal factors with maternal adult stature. Int J Epidemiol. 2004;33:1243–8.

29. UNICEF. Estado Mundial de la Infancia. Ginebra: UNICEF; 1998. p. 98–101.

30. Muzzo B. Crecimiento normal y patológico del niño y del adolescente. Rev Chil Nutr. 2003;30:92–100.

31. Leroy JL, Habicht JP, González de Cossío T, Ruel MT. Maternal education mitigates the negative effects of higher income on the double burden of child stunting and maternal overweight in rural Mexico. J Nutr. 2014;144:765–70.

32. Ihab AN, Rohana AJ, Manan WMW, Suriati WNW, Zalilah MS, Rusli AM. The coexistence of dual form of malnutrition in a sample of rural Malaysia. Int J Prev Med. 2013;4:690–4.

33. Doak C, Adair L, Bentley M, Monteiro C, Popkin B. The dual burden household and the nutrition transition paradox. Int J Obes. 2005;29:129–36.

34. Gurri FD. La doble carga de la transición nutrimental en zonas rurales de la Península de Yucatán, ¿consecuencia de la alteración de los sistemas agrícolas de subsistencia tradicionales en la segunda mitad del siglo XX? En: Muñoz Cano JM. Obesidad: Problema Multifactorial. (Coord), septiembre 2011:65–84.

35. Arroyo P, Fernandez V, Loria A, Pardio J, Laviaga H, Vargas-Ancona L, et al. Obesity, body morphology, and blood pressure in urban and rural population groups of Yucatan. Salud Publica de Mex. 2007;49:274–85.

36. Malina R, Peña M, Tan S, Buschang P, Little B. Overweight and obesity in rural Amerindian population in Oaxaca, southern Mexico, 1968–2000. Am J Hum Biol. 2007;19:711–21.

37. Restrepo BN, Restrepo MT, Beltrán JC, Rodríguez M, Ramírez RE. Estado nutricional de niños y niñas indígenas de hasta seis años de edad en el resguardo Embera-Katío, Tierralta, Córdoba, Colombia. Biomédica [revista en la Internet]. 2006;26(4):517–27. Disponible en: http://www.scielo.org.co/scielo.php?script=sci_arttext&pid=S0120-41572006000400006&lng=es.

38. Svedberg P. Poverty and undernutrition: theory, measurement and policy. New York: United Nations Universuty (UNU/WIDER) Oxford University Press; 2000.

Bacteriological quality of bottled drinking water versus municipal tap water in Dharan municipality, Nepal

Narayan Dutt Pant[1*], Nimesh Poudyal[2] and Shyamal Kumar Bhattacharya[2]

Abstract

Background: Water-related diseases are of great concern in developing countries like Nepal. Every year, there are countless morbidity and mortality due to the consumption of unsafe drinking water. Recently, there have been increased uses of bottled drinking water in an assumption that the bottled water is safer than the tap water and its use will help to protect from water-related diseases. So, the main objective of this study was to analyze the bacteriological quality of bottled drinking water and that of municipal tap water.

Methods: A total of 100 samples (76 tap water and 24 bottled water) were analyzed for bacteriological quality and pH. The methods used were spread plate method for total plate count (TPC) and membrane filter method for total coliform count (TCC), fecal coliform count (FCC), and fecal streptococcal count (FSC). pH meter was used for measuring pH.

Results: One hundred percent of the tap water samples and 87.5 % of the bottled water samples were found to be contaminated with heterotrophic bacteria. Of the tap water samples, 55.3 % were positive for total coliforms, compared with 25 % of the bottled water. No bottled water samples were positive for fecal coliforms and fecal streptococci, in contrast to 21.1 % and 14.5 % of the tap water samples being contaminated with fecal coliforms and fecal streptococci, respectively. One hundred percent of the tap water samples and 54.2 % of the bottled water samples had pH in the acceptable range.

Conclusions: All of the municipal tap water samples and most of the bottled drinking water samples distributed in Dharan municipality were found to be contaminated with one or more than one type of indicator organisms. On the basis of our findings, we may conclude that comparatively, the bottled drinking water may have been safer (than tap water) to drink.

Keywords: Bacteriological quality, Fecal coliform count, Fecal streptococcal count, Total plate count, Total coliform count

Background

The quality of drinking water is of great concern to mankind, but drinking water supplies have a long history of being contaminated by a wide spectrum of microbes including the fecal coliforms [1]. Contaminated water can cause a spectrum of diseases ranging from self-limiting gastrointestinal disturbances to severe life-threatening infections [2]. According to World Health Organization (WHO), 80 % of the diseases in developing countries are either water or sanitation related [3].

Recently, there has been a considerable worldwide increase in the consumption of bottled water due to consumer's awareness regarding bottled water as a healthy alternative to tap water. However, bottled water is not necessarily safer than tap water. Many studies have reported the presence of heterotrophic bacteria along with coliforms in bottled water in counts, exceeding national and international standards [4].

World Health Organization (WHO) has reported that about 30,000 people and children die everyday from water-related diseases, more critically, in developing or least developing countries. According to the data published by public health department, Nepal government,

* Correspondence: ndpant1987@gmail.com
[1]Department of Microbiology, Grande International Hospital, Dhapasi, Kathmandu, Nepal
Full list of author information is available at the end of the article

every year, about 3500 children die due to water-related illnesses [5].

So, it has become imperative to assess the quality of drinking water to ensure that if it is acceptable for human consumption. We tested the bacteriological quality and pH of the municipal tap water and bottled drinking water and compared their quality.

Methods
Study design
The present study was a community-based cross-sectional study conducted in the Department of Microbiology, B. P. Koirala Institute of Health Sciences (BPKIHS) from July 2011 to June 2012. Twenty-four bottled water samples and 76 tap water samples collected from Dharan municipality were tested for bacterial contamination, pH, and temperature.

Sample size calculation
In most of the studies conducted in developing countries including Nepal, the prevalence of bacterial contamination (due to heterotrophic bacteria) for tap water was around 95 % and that for bottled water was around 99 %. So, by using the following formula, the sample sizes for both tap water and bottled water were calculated.

$$\text{Sample size} = Z^2 P(1-P)/C^2$$

where
$Z = Z$ value (1.96 for 95 % confidence level)
P = prevalence
C = confidence interval (0.05)

The sample size for tap water was calculated to be 73 and that for bottled water was calculated to be 15. But, we took comparatively larger sample size.

Water sample collection
Since this study was conducted in a low-income country with limited resources, we chose the sample size according to the availability of the resources. For the collection of tap water, the Dharan municipality was divided into 19 approximately equal parts. Within each area, a main street was identified and the samples were collected from each fifth tap on alternating sides of the street until four samples were collected, for a total of 76 samples. For tap water, two sterile bottles, each of 200-ml capacity containing sodium thiosulfate (to neutralize any chlorine if present) were used. The mouth of the tap was cleaned by using clean cloth to remove any dirt if present. Then, the sterilization of the mouth of the tap was done with the help of flame. The tap was turned on and allowed the water to run for 1–2 min at a medium flow. Sterilized bottle was opened and filled with water

by leaving a small air space to make shaking before analysis easier. Finally, a stopper was placed on the bottle and a brown paper protective cover was fixed with the string. For the collection of the bottled drinking water, the numbers of registered bottled drinking water distributors in the Dharan municipality were identified. There were 8 bottled drinking water distributors distributing 8 different brands of bottled drinking water. A total of 24 bottled drinking water samples (3 samples from each brand) were collected. The basic assumptions for the sampling strategy we have followed were; almost every area of the Dharan was included and no bottled water brand present in the market of Dharan at the time was left. And the main purpose of choosing the particular sampling strategy was to include different water samples with different bacteriological qualities; as the tap water from different areas might have a very different quality due to different factors like leakage in distribution system, difference in quality of water supplied from sources or reservoir tanks, etc.

Transport and analysis of samples
pH was measured by using pH meter and temperature was measured by using thermometer. The pH and temperature were measured at the sites of sample collection. The water samples were transported to the water bacteriology laboratory of BPKIHS in ice box within 2 hrs of collection. Analysis of the water sample was done within 6 hrs of collection. Detection of bacterial contamination in water samples was done in terms of total plate count (TPC) (by spread plate method); and total coliform count (TCC), fecal coliform count (FCC) and fecal streptococcal count (FSC) (by membrane filter method) [6–8].

Identification of the bacterial isolates
All the bacteria grown on bile esculin agar (BEA), eosine methylene blue agar (EMB), m-endo agar les (MEA), and plate count agar (PCA) were subjected to identification. The *Pseudomonas* spp., *Acinetobacter* spp., and *Staphylococcus* spp. were detected in plate count agar. *Citrobacter* spp., *Enterobacter* spp., *Klebsiella* spp., *Serratia marcescens*, and *Chromobacterium violaceum* were detected in m-endo agar les (MEA). After filtering the water through the membrane filter, it was kept on m-endo agar les (MEA), which showed the growth of different types of colonies after 48 hrs of aerobic incubation at 37 °C, and on identification, these colonies were found to be of *Citrobacter* spp., *Enterobacter* spp., *Klebsiella* spp., *S. marcescens*, and *C. violaceum*. Similarly, *Enterococcus* spp. was detected by membrane filter technique by using BEA. The bacterial isolates were identified with the help of colony morphology, Gram's staining, and biochemical properties. The biochemical tests used were catalase test, oxidase test, citrate utilization test, urease test, sulfide

indole motility test, triple sugar iron test, methyl-red Voges Proskauer test, lysine decarboxylase test, slide coagulase test, tube coagulase test, growth on bile esculin agar at 44.5 °C, etc. In case of some bacteria like fecal coliforms, total coliforms, and fecal streptococci, their colony morphology in selective media like eosin methylene blue agar, m-endo agar les, and bile esculin agar, respectively, further helped in identification.

Data analysis
The data obtained were entered into Microsoft (MS) excel and analyzed using Statistical Package for Social Sciences (SPSS) version 11.0. Mean and standard deviation were calculated, and according to the nature of the data, P value was determined by applying T test, Mann-Whitney U test, chi-square test, and Fisher's exact test. P value <0.05 was taken as significant.

Results
Different characteristics of water samples
The temperatures of the tap water and bottled water were found to be 16.01 ± 3.62 °C and 17.75 ± 0.44 °C, respectively. Similarly, the pH of the tap water was found to be 7.63 ± 0.50 and that of the bottled water was 6.5 ± 0.57. The TPC/0.1 ml, TCC/100 ml, FCC/100 ml, and FSC/100 ml of the tap water were found to be 18.58 ± 17.70, 10.61 ± 22.49, 2.95 ± 9.26, and 3.33 ± 9.68 respectively, while TPC/0.1 ml and TCC/100 ml of the bottled water were 120.88 ± 85.82 and 19.33 ± 48.52, respectively. But, no bottled water were found to be contaminated with fecal coliforms and fecal streptococci. There were significant differences between the temperature, pH, TPC, and FCC of the tap water and those of the bottled water ($P < 0.05$) (Table 1).

Water samples unacceptable on the basis of different criteria
According to the WHO criteria for drinking water, on the basis of pH, no tap water samples were found to be unacceptable for drinking while 45.8 % of the bottled water samples were unacceptable and the difference was significant ($P < 0.05$). Similarly, on the basis of

TPC, all the tap water samples and 87.5 % of the bottled water samples were unacceptable according to WHO criteria for drinking water ($P < 0.05$). On the basis of TCC, 55.3 % of the tap water samples and 25 % of the bottled water samples were found to be unacceptable and was statistically significant ($P < 0.05$). Similarly, on the basis of FCC and FSC, 21.1 % and 14.5 % of the tap water samples respectively were found to be unacceptable while no bottled water samples were unacceptable for drinking (Table 2).

Percentage of water samples found to be contaminated with different bacteria
The most prevalent bacteria in tap water samples were gram-positive rods (100 %) followed by *Pseudomonas* spp. (76.3 %). Other bacteria isolated from tap water samples were *Citrobacter* spp. (36.8 %), *Acinetobacter* spp. (30.3 %), *Enterobacter* spp. (23.7 %), *Escherichia coli* (21.1 %), *Klebsiella* spp. (17.1 %), *Enterococcus* spp. (14.5 %), *Proteus* spp. (3.9 %), *Serratia* spp. (2.4 %), and *Staphylococcus* spp. (2.4 %). Similarly, the most prevalent bacteria in bottled water samples were *Pseudomonas* spp. and *Acinetobacter* spp. (87.5 %). Other bacteria isolated from bottled water samples were *Citrobacter* spp. (25 %), *C. violaceum* (12.5 %), and gram-positive rods (12.5 %) (Table 3).

Discussion
In our study, the bacteriological quality of bottled water was found to be better than that of tap water which was in agreement with the findings of Yasin et al. in Rawalpindi and Islamabad-Pakistan [9], Islam et al. in Dhaka [10], and Kassenga et al. in Tanzania [11]. The worse condition of the bacteriological quality of the tap water might be due to the ineffectiveness of the disinfection processes used for the treatment of water before distribution or distributing from contaminated sources without prior disinfection. But unlike our study, no significant difference was found in the bacteriological quality of tap water and bottled water by Mythri et al. in Karnataka India [12] and Ahmad and Bajahlan in Yanbu, Saudi Arabia [13]. The wrong practice of filling

Table 1 Different characteristics of water samples

Characteristics	Type of water		P value
	Tap water (mean ± SD)	Bottled water (mean ± SD)	
Temperature (°C)	16.01 ± 3.62	17.75 ± 0.44	<0.05
pH	7.63 ± 0.50	6.5 ± 0.57	<0.05
TPC/0.1 ml	18.58 ± 17.70	120.88 ± 85.82	<0.05
TCC/100 ml	10.61 ± 22.49	19.33 ± 48.52	0.102
FCC/100 ml	2.95 ± 9.26	0	<0.05
FSC/100 ml	3.33 ± 9.68	0	0.050

Table 2 Water samples unacceptable on the basis of different criteria

Characteristics	Type of water		P value
	Tap water %	Bottle water %	
pH	0	45.8	<0.05
TPC	100	87.5	<0.05
TCC	55.3	25	<0.05
FCC	21.1	0	<0.05
FSC	14.5	0	0.062

Table 3 Percentage of water samples found to be contaminated with different bacteria

Bacteria	Tap water %	Bottle water %	P value
Pseudomonas spp.	76.3	87.5	0.241
Acinetobacter spp.	30.3	87.5	<0.05
Gram-positive rods (GPR)	100	12.5	<0.05
Enterobacter spp.	23.7	0	<0.05
Citrobacter spp.	36.8	25	0.286
Klebsiella spp.	17.1	0	<0.05
Escherichia coli	21.1	0	<0.05
Enterococcus spp.	14.5	0	0.062
Chromobacterium violaceum	0	12.5	<0.05
Serratia marcescens	2.6	0	1
Proteus spp.	3.9	0	1
Staphylococcus spp.	2.6	0	1

the bottle directly from tap water and sealing it without any prior treatment which is generally done by the bottled water manufacturers for financial benefit might be one of the reasons behind the same bacteriological quality of tap water and bottled water found in some countries. Further, in contrast to our findings, tap water was found to be superior by Abed and Alwakeel in Riyadh, Saudi Arabia [14], and Silva et al. in Brazil [15]. Due to storage of the already contaminated bottled water for a long time, its bacteriological quality may have further deteriorated to worse condition. And further, the government body responsible for monitoring the quality of bottled water might not be strict in the places where the bottled water was found to be more contaminated.

In our study, 87.5 % of the bottled water samples were contaminated with heterotrophic bacteria which was comparable with the findings by Kassenga [11] and El-Salam et al. [16]. One hundred percent of the bottled water samples were contaminated with heterotrophic bacteria in the study done by Majumder et al. in Bangladesh [17] and Khaniki et al. in Tehran [18]. Comparatively, lower rates of contamination were detected by Islam et al. (50 %) in Dhaka city [10] and Yasin et al. (30 %) in Rawalpindi and Islamabad-Pakistan [9]. Bhandari et al. found only 28 % of the bottled water samples not meeting the Nepal standards [5]. Similar concentrations of heterotrophic bacterial contamination in bottled water as in our study were also reported by Majumder et al. (1 to >500 cfu/ml) [17], Yarsin et al. (80 to 3000 cfu/ml) [9], and Lalumandier and Ayer (0.01 to 4900 cfu/ml) [19]. Much higher concentration (10^4 to 10^6 cfu/ml) was reported by Karem and Hassan [20]. The bacterial concentration in bottled water generally depends on the disinfection processes used by the factory [15]. And in bottled drinking water, bacteria may be indigenous from the natural source of water or may be introduced during

processing or handling [11, 21]. Although the microbial concentration in processed water is initially low, it can develop into high level during storage [22]. The reasons for this may be due to the high level of oxygen provided to the water during processing, larger surface area provided by the container, higher temperature, and the nutrients arising in the container [23, 24]. Higher concentration of the bacteria may also occur through carriers like introduced flakes of human skin, particularly in non-ozonated and non-carbonated water [25]. Though 25 % of the bottled water samples we had tested were contaminated with total coliforms, fecal coliforms were not detected in any of the samples. Similar type of result was also found by El-Salam et al. [16]. But in contradiction, Kassenga et al. (1.3 %) [11], Yarsin et al. (10 %) [9], and Abayasekara et al. (15 %) [26] detected fecal coliforms from bottled water. In our study, 45.8 % of the bottled water had pH below the minimum level of 6.5 recommended by WHO. The higher percentage of bottled water with unacceptable pH may be due to the higher numbers of heterotrophic bacteria per milliliter we found in most of the bottled water samples. The temperature of the bottled water ranged from 17 to 18 °C, and it depends upon the temperature of the environment in which it has been stored. The bacteria isolated from bottled water in our study were *Pseudomonas* spp. (87.5 %), *Acinetobacter* spp. (87.5 %), *Citrobacter* spp. (25 %), gram-positive rods (12.5 %), and *C. violaceum* (12.5 %). The presence of different species of bacteria in supposedly bacteria-free bottled water is of high concern. Whether the species of bacteria present in the water samples are pathogenic or not, the fact that these are present, the hazards of contamination, and health risks to consumers should not be taken for granted [14]. Neither epidemiological studies nor correlation with occurrence of waterborne pathogens has provided the evidence of heterotrophic plate count (HPC) values alone being directly related to health risk [27]. However, some strains of bacterial species which are the part of heterotrophic bacteria can cause infections in immune-compromised persons [27].

The use of bottled water is only based on the assumption of purity and this can be misleading [14]. In our study, the method of purification of bottled water was found to be mentioned on labeling of bottled water as UV treatment, ozonation, reverse osmosis, and microfiltration. Although, bottled water should have a shelf life of 30 days unopened [16], most bottled water companies label showed that the water is valid for 6 to 9 months. In our study, one hundred percent of tap water samples were found to be contaminated with heterotrophic bacteria. Similar rates of contamination were also found by Islam et al. in Dhaka city [10] and Chaidez et al. in Mexico [28]. But, slightly low rates of contamination were found by Anwar (91.3 %) in Punjab [29] and Nguendo-Yongsi et al. (95 %) in Yaounde [30]. Most of the natural water sources are highly contaminated [31], and in a study done by Pant et al., most of the sources and reservoirs supplying drinking water to Dharan municipality were found to be heavily contaminated [32]. Further, bacteria may enter and colonize the distribution systems through the failure to disinfect water or maintain a proper disinfection residual, excessive network leakages and improper along with inadequate disposal of sewage [33]. In our study, 55.3 % of the tap water samples were contaminated by total coliforms which was similar to the percentage detected by Kassenga et al. (49.2 %) [11] and Chaidez et al. (46 %) [28]. But, higher percentages were detected by Rai et al. (85.7 %) in Nepal [34] and Yarsin et al. (64 %) in Pakistan [9]. Fecal coliforms were isolated from 21.1 % of the tap water samples which was in agreement with the results of Kassenga et al. (26.2 %) [11] and Chaidez et al. (28 %) [28]. Quite high percentage was found by Rai et al. (67.4 %) [34]. The concentration of heterotrophic bacteria in tap water in our study ranged from 10 to1200 cfu/ml which were higher in the study done by Yasin et al. (80–3000 cfu/ml) [9] and Chaidez et al. (1–5320 cfu/ml) [28], but less numbers were detected by Lalumandier and Ayer (0.2–2.7 cfu/ml) [19]. The difference in these results obtained from different studies might be due to the different maintenance conditions of the water distribution systems, different bacteriological quality of water of sources and reservoirs supplying drinking water, and the difference in effectiveness of the disinfection processes used.

The microorganisms isolated in our study from tap water were *Pseudomonas* spp. (76.3 %), *Acinetobacter* spp. (30.3 %), Gram-positive rod (100 %), *Citrobacter* spp. (36.8 %), *Enterobacter* spp. (23.7 %), *Klebsiella* spp. (17.1 %), *E. coli* (21.1 %), *Enterococcus* spp. (14.5 %), *Serratia* spp. (2.6%), *staphylococcus* spp. (2.6 %), and *proteus* spp. (3.9 %). Similarly, in a study done by Islam et al., *E. coli* (60 %), *Klebsiella* spp. (40 %), *Enterobacter* spp. (20 %), *Pseudomonas* spp. (70 %), *Proteus* spp. (10 %), *Staphylococcus* spp. (40 %) were found [10].

In our study, all the tap water samples had acceptable pH. Similar types of results were also found by Chaidez et al. [28] and Abed and Alwakeel [14]. The average temperature was between 28.7 °C and 29.38 °C in the study by Chaidez et al. [28], which was between 11 °C and 26 °C in our study. The temperature of water is influenced by the temperature of the environment.

Finally, from the literatures we have reviewed, it can be concluded that bacteriological contamination of drinking water is a significant problem not only in Nepal but also in other south Asian countries and other parts of the world like Sudan [35], Makkah al-Mokaarama [36], Egypt [37], Canada [38], and Mexico [28].

Limitations of the study

Since this study was conducted in a low-income country, with limited resources, we could not process large numbers of the samples. Further, we could not use molecular technology for the identification of the bacteria isolated. The use of large numbers of the samples in the study would have generated more significant results. And the molecular methods are the best methods for the proper identification of the organisms. We could not include the detection of pathogens like pathogenic bacteria (*Salmonella* spp., *Vibrio cholerae*, etc.), viruses, fungi, and parasites (protozoa and helminths) in our study. These microorganisms may be present in the water and may be responsible for large numbers of infections, but for their detection, more effort and additional resources are needed. In different seasons, the microbial flora presenting in the water may differ due to different environmental conditions of the surrounding. But in this study, we could not study the seasonal variation of the microorganisms present in the water, as for this more samples needed to be processed and for which we did not have sufficient resources.

Conclusions

One hundred percent of the municipal tap water samples and most of the bottled drinking water samples distributed in Dharan were found to be contaminated with indicator organisms in counts exceeding WHO standards. The findings of our study suggest that comparatively, the bottled drinking water may be safer (than tap water) to drink.

Abbreviations
BEA, bile esculin agar; BPKIHS, B. P. Koirala Institute of Health Sciences; EMB, eosine methylene blue agar; FCC, fecal coliform count; FSC, fecal streptococcal count; GPR, gram-positive rods; HPC, heterotrophic plate count; MEA, m-endo agar les; ml, milliliter; MS, Microsoft; PCA, plate count agar; SD, standard deviation; SPSS, statistical package for social sciences; TCC, total coliform count; TPC, total plate count; WHO, World Health Organization

Acknowledgements
The authors would like to thank the staffs of Nepal Drinking Water Corporation, Dharan, for their kind support to provide the necessary information. We would like to appreciate the opportunity provided by B. P. Koirala Institute of Health Sciences to conduct this research.

Authors' contributions
NDP was involved in designing of the study, collection and processing of the water samples, collection and analysis of data, and preparation of the manuscript. NP and SKB were involved in designing and monitoring of the study. All authors read and approved the final manuscript.

Competing interests
The authors declare that they have no any competing interests.

Author details

[1]Department of Microbiology, Grande International Hospital, Dhapasi, Kathmandu, Nepal. [2]Department of Microbiology, B. P. Koirala Institute of Health Sciences, Dharan, Nepal.

References

1. Sadeghi GH, Mohammadian M, Nourani M, Peyda M, Eslami A. Microbiological quality assessment of rural drinking water supplies in Iran. J Agri Soc Sci. 2007;3:31–3.
2. Akoto O, Adiyiah J. Chemical analysis of drinking water from some communities in the Brong Ahafo region. Int J Environ Sci Tech. 2007;4(2):211–4.
3. Prasanna RB, Reddy MS. Bacteriological examination of drinking water with reference to coliforms in Jeedimetla, Hyderabad, India. Afr J Biotechnol. 2009;8(20):5495–6.
4. Semerjian LA. Quality assessment of various bottled waters marketed in Lebanon. Environ Monit Asses. 2011;172(1-4):274–85.
5. Bhandari MR, Gautam DN, Joshi S, Bhattarai UK. Quality assessment of drinking water commercially available in Kathmandu valley Nepal. Food Res Bulletin. 2009;2:5–13.
6. World Health Organisation. Guidelines for drinking water quality, Surveillance and control of community supplies, vol. Volume 3. 2nd ed. Geneva: WHO; 1997.
7. World Health Organisation. Guidelines for drinking-water quality. 4th ed. Geneva: WHO; 2011.
8. Senior BW. Examination of water, milk, food and air. In: Collee JG, Fraser AG, Marmion BP, Simmons A, editors. Mackie and McCartney practical medical microbiology. 14th ed. India: Elsevier India Private Limited; 2007. p. 883–921.
9. Yasin N, Shah N, Khan J, Saba N, Islam Z. Bacteriological status of drinking water in the peri-urban areas of Rawalpindi and Islamabad-Pakistan. Afr J Microbiol Res. 2012;6(1):169–75.
10. Islam S, Begum HA, Nill NY. Bacteriological safety assessment of municipal tap water and quality of bottle water In Dhaka city: health hazard analysis. Bangladesh J Med Microbiol. 2010;4(1):9–13.
11. Kassenga GR. The health-related microbiological quality of bottled drinking water sold in Dar es Salaam, Tanzania. J Water Health. 2007;5(1):179–85.
12. Mythri H, Chandu G, Prashant G, Subba RW. Fluoride and bacterial content of bottled drinking water versus municipal tap water. Indian J Dent Res. 2010;21(4):515–7.
13. Ahmad M, Bajahlan AS. Quality comparison of tap water vs bottled water in the industrial city of Yanbu, Saudi Arabia. Environ Monit Assess. 2009; 159(1-4):1–14.
14. Abed KF, Alwakeel SS. Mineral and microbial contents of bottled and tap water in Riyadh, Saudi Arabia. Middle-East J Sci Res. 2007;2(3-4):151–6.
15. Zamberlan da Silva ME, Santana RG, Guilhermetti M, Filho IC, Endo EH, Ueda-Nakamura T, et al. Comparison of the bacteriological quality of tap water and bottled mineral water. Int J Environ Health. 2008;211(5-6):504–9.
16. El-Salam MMMA, El-Ghitany EMA, Kassem MMM. Quality of bottled water brands in Egypt part II: biological water examination. J Egypt Public Health Assoc. 2008;83:467–86.
17. Majumder AK, Islam KN, Nite RN, Noor R. Evaluation of microbiological quality of commercially available bottled water in the city of Dhaka, Bangladesh. Stamford J Microbiol. 2011;1(1):24–30.
18. Khaniki GRJ, Zarei A, Kamkar A, Fazlzadehdavil M, Ghaderpoori M, Zarei A. Bacteriological evaluation of bottled water from domestic brands in Tehran market, Iran. World Appl Sci J. 2010;8(3):274–8.
19. Lalumandier JA, Ayers LW. Fluoride and bacterial content of bottled water vs tap water. Arch Fam Med. 2000;9(3):246–50.
20. Karem HA, Hassan AA. Quality assessment of Egyptian drinking water supplies and disinfecting using ultraviolet radiation. Pak J Biol Sci. 2000;3:772–6.
21. Warburton DW, Dodds KL, Burke R, Johnston MA, Laffey PJ. A review of microbiological quality of bottled water sold in Canada between 1981 and 1989. Can J Microbiol. 1992;38(1):12–9.
22. Stickler DJ. The microbiology of bottled natural mineral waters. J R Soc Health. 1989;109(4):118–24.
23. Warburton DW, Bowen B, Konkle A. The survival and recovery of Pseudomonas aeruginosa and its effect upon salmonellae in water: methodology to test bottled water in Canada. Can J Microbiol. 1992;40(12):987–92.
24. Warburton DW. The microbiological safety of bottled waters. In: Farber JM, Ewen ED T, editors. Safe handling of foods. New York: Marcel Dekker; 2000.
25. Kassenga GR, Mbuligwe SE. Comparative assessment of physico-chemical quality of bottled and tap water in Dar es Salaam, Tanzania. Int J Biol Chem Sci. 2009;3(2):209–17.
26. Abayasekara CL, Herath WHMAT, Adikaram NKB, Chandrajith R, Illapperuma SC, Sirisena AD, et al. Microbiological quality of bottled water in Sri Lanka: a preliminary survey. In: Proceedings of the Peradeniya university research sessions; Sri Lanka. 2007;12:30.
27. Bartram J, Cotruvo J, Exner M, Fricker C, Glasmacher A. Heterotrophic plate counts and drinking-water safety: the significance of HPCs for water quality and human health. London: IWA Publishing; 2003.
28. Chaidez C, Soto M, Martinez C, Keswick B. Drinking water microbiological survey of the Northwestern State of Sinaloa, Mexico. J Water Health. 2008; 6(1):125–9.
29. Anwar MS, Chaudhry NA, Tayyab M. Bacteriological quality of drinking water in Punjab: evaluation of H2S strip test. J Pak Med Assoc. 1999;49(10):237–41.
30. Nguendo-Yongsi HB. Microbiological evaluation of drinking water in a sub-Saharan urban community (Yaounde). Am j biochem and mol bio. 2011;1(1): 68-81.
31. Stukel A, Greenberg ER, Dain BJ, Reed FC, Jacobs NJ. A longitudinal study of rainfall and coliform contamination in small community drinking water supplies. Environ Sci Technol. 1990;24:571–5.
32. Pant ND, Poudyal N, Bhattacharya S. Bacteriological quality of drinking water sources and reservoirs supplying Dharan municipality of Nepal. Ann Clin Chem Lab Med. 2016;2(1):19–23.
33. Lee EJ, Schwab KJ. Deficiencies in drinking water distribution systems in developing countries. J Water Health. 2005;3(2):109–27.
34. Rai SK, Ono K, Yanagida JI, Kurokawa M, Rai CK. Status of drinking water contamination in Mountain Region, Nepal. Nepal Med Coll J. 2009;11(4):281–3.
35. Abdelrahman AA, Eltahir YM. Bacteriological quality of drinking water in Nyala, South Darfur, Sudan. Environ Monit Assess. 2011;175(1-4):37–43.
36. Mihdhdir AA. Evaluation of bacteriological and sanitary quality of drinking water stations and water tankers in Makkah Al-Mokarama. Pak J Biol Sci. 2009;12(4):401–5.
37. Ennayat MD, Mekhael KG, El-Hossany MM, Abd-El K, Arafa R. Coliform organisms in drinking water in Kalama village. Bull Nutr Inst Arab Republic of Egypt. 1988;8:66–81.
38. Levesque B, Simard P, Gauvin D, Gingras S, Dewailly E, Letarte R. Comparison of the microbiological quality of water coolers and that of municipal water systems. Appl Environ Microbiol. 1994;60(4):1174–8.

Permissions

The contributors of this book come from diverse backgrounds, making this book a truly international effort. This book will bring forth new frontiers with its revolutionizing research information and detailed analysis of the nascent developments around the world.

We would like to thank all the contributing authors for lending their expertise to make the book truly unique. They have played a crucial role in the development of this book. Without their invaluable contributions this book wouldn't have been possible. They have made vital efforts to compile up to date information on the varied aspects of this subject to make this book a valuable addition to the collection of many professionals and students.

This book was conceptualized with the vision of imparting up-to-date information and advanced data in this field. To ensure the same, a matchless editorial board was set up. Every individual on the board went through rigorous rounds of assessment to prove their worth. After which they invested a large part of their time researching and compiling the most relevant data for our readers.

The editorial board has been involved in producing this book since its inception. They have spent rigorous hours researching and exploring the diverse topics which have resulted in the successful publishing of this book. They have passed on their knowledge of decades through this book. To expedite this challenging task, the publisher supported the team at every step. A small team of assistant editors was also appointed to further simplify the editing procedure and attain best results for the readers.

Apart from the editorial board, the designing team has also invested a significant amount of their time in understanding the subject and creating the most relevant covers. They scrutinized every image to scout for the most suitable representation of the subject and create an appropriate cover for the book.

The publishing team has been an ardent support to the editorial, designing and production team. Their endless efforts to recruit the best for this project, has resulted in the accomplishment of this book. They are a veteran in the field of academics and their pool of knowledge is as vast as their experience in printing. Their expertise and guidance has proved useful at every step. Their uncompromising quality standards have made this book an exceptional effort. Their encouragement from time to time has been an inspiration for everyone.

The publisher and the editorial board hope that this book will prove to be a valuable piece of knowledge for researchers, students, practitioners and scholars across the globe.

List of Contributors

Elma Z. Ferdousy and Mohammad A. Matin
Department of Statistics, Jahangirnagar University, Savar, Dhaka

G. Tubatsi, M. C. Bonyongo and M. Gondwe
Okavango Research Institute, University of Botswana, Private Bag 285, Maun, Botswana

Sophia R. Stroud, Tania Ruiz Maya and Christopher R. Plaman
School of Medicine, MSC09 5040, University of New Mexico, Albuquerque, NM 87131, USA

Angelo Tomedi
School of Medicine, MSC09 5040, 1 University of New Mexico, Albuquerque, NM 87131, USA
Department of Family and Community Medicine, School of Medicine, Albuquerque, NM, USA

Mutuku A. Mwanthi
School of Public Health, University of Nairobi, Nairobi, Kenya

Donna Espeut and Stan Becker
Department of Population, Family and Reproductive Health, Johns Hopkins University, Baltimore, USA

Michael P. Murrays
Department of Economics, Bates College, Lewiston, ME 04240, USA

Raisa Sharmin
University of Waterloo, Waterloo, Canada

Li Tang Colin W. Binns and Andy H. Lee
School of Public Health, Curtin University, GPO Box U 1987, Perth, WA 6845, Australia

Fenglian Xu
National Drug and Alcohol Research Centre, University of New South Wales, Sydney, NSW, Australia

Taotao Zhang
School of Medicine, Shihezi University, Shihezi, Xinjiang, China

Jun Lei
Xinjiang Tumour Hospital, Urumqi, Xinjiang, China

Leo Pruimboom
Natura Foundation, Edisonstraat 66, 3281 NC Numansdorp, Netherlands
Department of Laboratory Medicine, University Medical Center Groningen (UMCG), University of Groningen, P.O. Box 30.001, 9700 RB Groningen, Netherlands

Karin de Punder
Natura Foundation, Edisonstraat 66, 3281 NC Numansdorp, Netherlands
Institute of Medical Psychology, Charité University Medicine Berlin, Hufelandweg 14, 10117 Berlin, Germany

Jane O. Ebot
Service Delivery Improvement Division, Office of Population and Reproductive Health, Bureau for Global Health, United States Agency for International Development (USAID), 2100 Crystal Drive, Arlington, VA 22202, USA

Nkechi G. Onyeneho, Ngozi Idemili-Aronu and Ijeoma Igwe
Department of Sociology/Anthropology, University of Nigeria Nsukka, Nsukka 410001, Nigeria

Felicia U. Iremeka
Humanities Unit, School of General Studies, University of Nigeria, Enugu Campus, Enugu, Nigeria

Kranti Suresh Vora
Indian Institute of Public Health Gandhinagar, Drive-in-Road, Ahmedabad, Gujarat 380054, India

Sally A. Koblinsky
University of Maryland, College Park,, Prince George's

Marge A. Koblinsky
USAID, Washington D.C, USA

Mitravinda S. Savanur and Padmini S. Ghugre
Department of Food Science and Nutrition, Sir Vithaldas Vihar, S.N.D.T. Women's University, Juhu Road, Mumbai 400049, Maharashtra, India

Neda Dolatkhah
Department of Nutrition Sciences, Shahid Beheshti University of Medical Sciences (SBUMS), International Branch, tehran, iran

Majid Hajifaraji
Nutrition Society, National Nutrition and Food Technology Research Institute, Faculty of Nutrition and Food Technology, Beheshti University of Medical Sciences, Baran 3, West Arghavan, Farahzadi Blvd., Shahrak Qods, 19395-4741, Istanbul 1981619573, turkey

Fatemeh Abbasalizadeh
Department of Obstetrics & Gynecology, Tabriz University of Medical Sciences, tabriz, iran

Naser Aghamohammadzadeh
Section of Endocrinology & Metabolism, Department of Internal Medicine, Tabriz University of Medical Sciences, Tabriz, Iran

Yadollah Mehrabi
Department of Biostatistics & Epidemiology, Shahid Beheshti University of Medical Sciences, Tehran, Iran

Mehran Mesgari Abbasi
Drug Applied Research Center, Tabriz University of Medical Sciences, Tabriz, Iran

Johanna Maria Axelsson
Department of Medicine, Copenhagen University Hospital Glostrup, Glostrup, Denmark

Sofie Hallager
Department of Infectious Diseases, Hvidovre University Hospital, Hvidovre, Denmark

Toke S. Barfod
Department of Medicine, Roskilde University Hospital, Roskilde, Denmark

Mostafizur Rahman
University of Rajshahi, Rajshahi, Bangladesh

Asma Ahmad Shariff and Rohayatimah Md. Tahir
Centre for Foundation Studies in Science, University of Malaya, Kuala Lumpur, Malaysia

Aziz Shafie
Department of Geography, Faculty of Arts and Social Sciences, University of Malaya, Kuala Lumpur, Malaysia

Rahmah Saaid
Department of Obstetrics and Gynaecology, Faculty of Medicine, University of Malaya, Kuala Lumpur, Malaysia

I. Naidoo and B. Cassim
Department of Geriatrics, University of KwaZulu-Natal, Durban, South Africa

Karen E. Charlton
School of Medicine, Faculty of Science, Medicine and Health, University of Wollongong, Wollongong, Australia

TM Esterhuizen
Centre for Evidence Based Health Care, Department of Interdisciplinary Health Sciences, Faculty of Medicine and Health Sciences, Stellenbosch University, Stellenbosch, South Africa

Helen Harris-Fry, Leila Younes, Anthony Costello and Edward Fottrell
UCL Institute for Global Health, 30 Guilford Street, London, WC1N 1EH, UK

Kishwar Azad, Abdul Kuddus, Sanjit Shaha, Badrun Nahar and Munir Hossen
Perinatal Care Project, Diabetic Association of Bangladesh, 122 Kazi Nazrul Islam Avenue, Dhaka 1000, Bangladesh

Taranum Ruba Siddiqui, Safia Bibi and Sobiya Mohiuddin Ayaz
Gastroenterology and Hepatology unit, Pakistan Medical Research Council, Research Center, Jinnah Postgraduate Medical Center, Refiquee Shaheed Road, Karachi 75510, Pakistan

Muhammad Ayaz Mustufa
Pakistan Medical Research Council, Research Center, National Institute of Child Health, Karachi, Pakistan

Adnan Khan
Microbiology Department, University of Karachi, Karachi, Pakistan

Dickson A. Amugsi, Elizabeth Kimani and Blessing U. Mberu
African Population and Health Research Centre, APHRC Campus, P.O. Box 10787-00100, Nairobi, Kenya

Anna Lartey
Nutrition Division, Economic and Social Department, Food and Agriculture Organization, Rome, Italy

Tahera Akter, Fatema Tuz Jhohura, Fahmida Akter, Tridib Roy Chowdhury, Sabuj Kanti Mistry, and Mahfuzar Rahman
BRAC Research and Evaluation Division, BRAC Centre, 75 Mohakhali, Dhaka 1212, Bangladesh

Digbijoy Dey and Milan Kanti Barua
BRAC Water, Sanitation and Hygiene Programme, BRAC Centre, 75 Mohakhali, Dhaka 1212, Bangladesh

Md Akramul Islam
BRAC Tuberculosis Programme, BRAC Centre, 75 Mohakhali, Dhaka 1212, Bangladesh BRAC Water, Sanitation and Hygiene Programme, BRAC Centre, 75 Mohakhali, Dhaka 1212, Bangladesh

Shilpa Karvande, Devendra Sonawane, Sandeep Chavan and Nerges Mistry
Foundation for Research in Community Health, Pune, India

Dipti Govild
Department of Population Policies and Programs, International Institute for Population Sciences, Govandi Station Road, Deonar, Mumbai 400088, Maharashtra, India

Neetu Purohit and Shiv Dutt Gupta
The IIHMR University, 1, Prabhu Dayal Marg, Near Sanganer Airport, Jaipur 302029, Rajasthan, India

Sanjay Kumar Mohanty
Department of Fertility Studies, International Institute for Population Sciences, Govandi Station Road, Deonar, Mumbai 400088, Maharashtra, India

Esmeralda García-Parra, Héctor Ochoa-Díaz-López, Rosario García-Miranda and Roberto Solís-Hernández
Health Department, El Colegio de la Frontera Sur, Carretera Panamericana y Periférico Sur s/n C.P. 29290, Barrio de María Auxiliadora, San Cristóbal de las Casas, Chiapas, Mexico

Laura Moreno-Altamirano
Public Health Department, Faculty of Medicine, Universidad Nacional Autónoma de México, Circuito Interior, Ciudad Universitaria, Av. Universidad 3000, CP 04510 Mexico City, Mexico

Raúl Molina-Salazar
Department of Economics, Universidad Autónoma Metropolitana—Iztapalapa, Av. San Rafael Atlixco 186, Col. Vicentina C.P. 09340 Delegación Iztapalapa, Mexico City, Mexico

Narayan Dutt Pant
Department of Microbiology, Grande International Hospital, Dhapasi, Kathmandu, Nepal

Nimesh Poudyal and Shyamal Kumar Bhattacharya
Department of Microbiology, B. P. Koirala Institute of Health Sciences, Dharan, Nepal

Index

A

Akaike Information Criterion (aic), 113
Antiretroviral Therapy (art), 104
Asian Esophageal Cancer Belt, 48

B

Bacteriological Quality, 202-205, 207

C

Caesarean Delivery (c-section), 113
Carrier Rate, 144, 149-150
Case-control Study, 19, 48-49, 172
Cash Transfer Schemes, 80, 183
Chemical Parameters, 161-162, 167-169, 171-172
Child Malnutrition, 7, 160, 194
Child Morbidity, 1, 3, 5-7
Child Survival Safe Motherhood (cssm), 81
Childhood Morbidity, 1
Community Health Workers (chws), 28
Composite Index of Anthropometric Failure (ciaf), 89, 95
Confidence Interval (ci), 49

D

Demographic Health Surveys (dhs), 62
Depressive Symptoms, 124-125, 127, 129, 131
Dietary Diversity, 132-133, 135, 137, 139-143, 153-160

E

Education Attainment, 38-45, 47

F

Fasting Blood Sugar (fbs), 96, 98
Fecal Coliform Count, 202, 206
Fecal Streptococcal Count, 202-203, 206
Fertility Estimation, 27
Food Availability Determinants, 139, 141

G

Gestational Diabetes Mellitus, 96-101, 103

Gluten-containing Cereals, 53
Groundwater Arsenic, 38-41, 43-47

H

Hazard Ratios, 115-116
Healthcare Quality, 173
Height-for-age (haz), 89
High Risk of Malnutrition, 124-125, 127, 129, 131
Higher Dietary Diversity, 142, 153-155, 157, 159
Honest Significant Difference (hsd) Test, 11
Household Autonomy and Health, 61
Household Decision-making, 63-64, 153, 155-159
Household Food Security, 132-135, 137, 139-143
Households' Diarrheal Encounters, 8-9, 11, 13-19
Human Immunodeficiency Virus (hiv), 104

I

Immunization, 61-69, 174
Insecticide Treated Bednets, 70-71, 75, 77, 79
Intermittent Presumptive Treatment, 70-72, 77-79
Intimate Partner Violence, 1, 3, 5-7, 62, 69

J

Janani Suraksha Yojana
(jsy), 80-81, 87, 183-184

L

Logistic Regression, 1, 3, 30, 33, 48-49, 51, 64, 66, 80, 82, 113, 115, 118, 120-122, 124, 126-127, 134, 138, 153, 155, 157-158, 183
Logistic Regression Models, 1, 51, 127, 153

M

Magnitude of Undernutrition, 89-91, 93, 95
Malaria-in-pregnancy, 70
Maternal Health Services, 80-87, 179, 183-184
Maternal Mortality Ratio (mmr), 173, 184
Maternal-child Health Services, 173
Mid-upper Arm Circumference (muac), 125
Mini Nutritional Assessment, 124, 130
Mortality Estimation, 27-28

N

National Hydrochemical Survey (nhs), 38-39
National Rural Health Mission (nrhm), 81, 183, 193
Nephelometric Turbidity Units (ntu), 9
Non-adherence, 104, 110-111
Nutrition Assessment, 132
Nutrition Screening, 124, 130

O

Odds Ratio (or), 49
Oportunidades Families, 194-195, 197, 199, 201

P

Poor Rural Women, 80, 191
Pregnancy Histories, 27-37
Prenatal Care (pnc), 20 Probiotic Supplements, 96-97, 99, 101-103

Q

Quality Perspectives, 173, 175

R

Randomized Clinical Trial, 96-97, 99, 101, 103
Regional Typhoid Endemicity, 144
Relative Risk Ratio (rrr), 132
Risk Factors, 8, 18-19, 49, 52, 113-123, 130, 148-149, 151-152, 160, 178

S

Salinity (nacl) Levels, 166

Salmonella Enterica Serovars, 144-145, 147, 149, 151
Skilled Birth Attendants (sba), 20
Sustainable Development Goals (sdgs), 161

T

Total Coliform Count, 202-203
Total Plate Count, 202-203, 206
Traditional Birth Attendant (tba), 20
Typhoid Fever, 144, 148-152

U

Undernutrition, 7, 89-95, 132-133, 139, 141-142, 159, 194, 201

W

Water Quality, 8-9, 11, 13-19, 161-165, 167, 169, 171-172, 205, 207
Water Quality Index, 161-163, 165, 167, 169, 171-172
Water Quality Index (wqi), 161-162, 165, 167, 171
Water Storage, 8-9, 19
Water Treatment, 8-9, 11-12, 18
Water Use Practices, 8-9, 11, 13, 15, 17-19
Waterborne Diseases, 8, 12, 19
Weight-for-height (whz), 89
White Rice Consumption, 48-52
Women's Dietary Diversity Score, 132, 141

Printed in the USA
CPSIA information can be obtained
at www.ICGtesting.com
JSHW051326221024
72173JS00006B/1297